Buy "TRANCE AS A Coping MECHANISM"
by FRANKEL

"THE DISSOCIATION OF A PERSONALITY"
by MORTON PRINCE 1906

Diagnosis and Treatment of
MULTIPLE PERSONALITY DISORDER

FOUNDATIONS OF MODERN PSYCHIATRY
David J. Kupfer and Richard Jed Wyatt, Editors

DIAGNOSIS AND TREATMENT OF
MULTIPLE PERSONALITY DISORDER
Frank W. Putnam

MOVEMENT DISORDERS:
A NEUROPSYCHIATRIC APPROACH
James B. Lohr and Alexander A. Wisniewski

UNDERSTANDING AND TREATING
TARDIVE DYSKINESIA
Dilip V. Jeste and Richard Jed Wyatt

Diagnosis and Treatment of
MULTIPLE PERSONALITY DISORDER

FRANK W. PUTNAM, MD

THE GUILFORD PRESS
New York   London

© 1989 Frank W. Putnam
Published by The Guilford Press
A Division of Guilford Publications, Inc.
72 Spring Street, New York, NY 10012

Printed in the United States of America

Last digit is print number: 9 8 7 6 5

Library of Congress Cataloging-in-Publication Data

Putnam, Frank W., 1947–
    Diagnosis and treatment of multiple personality disorder / Frank
W. Putnam.
        p.   cm. — (Foundations of modern psychiatry)
    Bibliography: p.
    Includes index.
    ISBN 0-89862-177-1
    1. Multiple personality.   I. Title.   II. Series.
    [DNLM: 1. Multiple-Personality Disorder—diagnosis.   2. Multiple-
Personality Disorder—therapy.   WM 173.6 P989d]
    RC569.5.M8P87 1989
    616.85′236—dc 19
    DNLM/DLC
    for Library of Congress   88-11217
                                                                    CIP

To my loving wife, Karen

Preface

The impetus to write this book came from the daily phone calls I received from therapists seeking help with newly diagnosed multiple personality disorder (MPD) patients. I found myself hearing the same questions and concerns and repeating the same information over and over again, typically three to four times a week and often three to four times a day. Over the years, I attempted to supplement the phone consultations by mailing out reference lists and selected articles that addressed questions and concerns commonly raised by therapists. This was time-consuming at best since I do my own copying and mailing. I kept wishing for a book that could serve as an introduction for therapists new to the disorder. Eventually it became clear that if I wanted such a book I would have to write it.

Diagnosis and Treatment of Multiple Personality Disorder is intended to be a book for therapists unfamiliar with dissociative disorders. It is a synthesis of ideas, techniques, and treatment philosophies gleaned from experienced therapists and work with many patients. It is designed to integrate and convey to clinicians in the mental health field the mainstream thinking and experience of the MPD therapist community. The book is extensively referenced and cross-referenced to serve both as a primer and as a reference work. Above all, I have sought to make it pragmatic.

I have tried to present a balanced view of the issues and to credit those who made significant contributions to our knowledge. In many cases it is difficult to know who should receive primary credit for some ideas or interventions as their origin is lost in the oral history and clinical lore that forms the bedrock of our knowledge. One of the compelling observations made by those who witnessed the course of the recent explosion of interest in MPD is the frequency with which therapists independently make the same observations and discover the utility of specific interventions and techniques. Not surprisingly there are many claims of credit for common discoveries.

One of my goals is to demystify MPD and to place it within its rightful historical context as a pivotal disorder that has contributed substantially to the development of dynamic psychiatry and the science of psychology. I believe that MPD has much to offer in the future and will reclaim its former role as the centerpiece for models of human consciousness. MPD is an experiment of nature that provides us insight into the range of possibilities for the human condition and a window into the psychobiological linkages between state of mind and body. The treatment of MPD is a natural extension of the art of psychotherapy and has much to teach us about how the "talking therapies" heal. We need to take advantage of the lessons MPD offers rather than engage in meaningless debates about whether it is "real."

I would like to thank Julie Guroff for the help and support she provided during the development of this book and Evan DeRenzo for her editing skills. I greatly appreciate the advice and encouragement offered over the years by Richard Loewenstein, Robert Post, David Rubinow, and Richard Wyatt. I would especially like to thank my patients and friends with MPD who shared their thoughts, feelings, and lives to help me learn about multiple personality disorder.

Contents

Diagnosis and Treatment of
MULTIPLE PERSONALITY DISORDER

CHAPTER ONE

Dissociation

There is a renewed interest in the psychopathological role of dissociation in a variety of psychiatric disorders. A number of specific dissociative disorders have been identified and diagnostic criteria established (American Psychiatric Association, 1980a, 1987). In addition, the contribution of the dissociative process to other disorders (e.g., posttraumatic stress disorder, anxiety disorders, somatoform disorders, impulse disorders, gender and sexual disorders, and some Axis II personality disorders such as borderline personality disorder) is being actively investigated (Bernstein & Putnam, 1986). Traditionally, dissociative disorders have been thought of as acute, time-limited reactions that closely follow a traumatic precipitant. The existence of chronic dissociative pathology, either as a primary disorder (such as multiple personality) or as a major pathophysiological process contributing to other disorders (such as posttraumatic stress disorder), is only now being recognized. The dissociative process is also receiving attention as a research window into the psychophysiological mechanisms of psychosomatic phenomena and as a model for understanding the impact of trauma on such crucial developmental tasks as the consolidation of a sense of self.

THE HISTORY OF DISSOCIATION

Janet's Work

Most scholars discussing the history of dissociation begin with the work of Pierre Janet (1859–1947) (Hart, 1926; White & Shevach, 1942; Kirshner, 1973; Hilgard, 1977). Janet, however, after rediscovering the work of the "magnetizers" such as Puységur and Bertrand, always scrupulously acknowledged his debt to these earlier pioneers (Ellenberger, 1970). The contributions of the "magnetizers" and the roots of dynamic psychiatry have been identified in Ellenberger's (1970) impressive history of dynamic psychiatry. Jean-Martin Charcot, who taught that in hysteria the stream of consciousness breaks up into diverse elements, also influenced Janet's concept of and metaphors for dissociation (West, 1967). Janet, however, stands first among all clinicians and researchers who have inquired into the nature of dissociation.

Janet, born in 1859 to an upper-middle-class French family, was a brilliant student who won many national competitions and qualified for a position at the elite French academy, École Normale Supérieure. Although first trained as a philosopher, he closely followed the ideas of Jean-Martin Charcot, who was at that time re-establishing hypnosis as a legitimate focus of scientific inquiry. In 1883, Janet took a position as a professor in philosophy at the Lyceum in Le Havre, beginning upon arrival to search for patients for his doctoral thesis. A local physician, Dr. Gibert, introduced Janet to his patient, Léonie, who displayed the capacity to be hypnotized from a distance. Janet began a series of experiments with Léonie that were described in a paper read by his brother, Jules, at a scientific meeting in Paris in the fall of 1885. These initial experiments excited the interest of Charcot, Frederick Myers, Charles Richet, and other notable investigators and clinicians, many of whom visited Janet in Le Havre to examine Léonie personally. Janet's results with Léonie were confirmed, and this success, together with additional publications, soon established his reputation in philosophical and psychological circles.

Janet returned to Paris and in 1889 began his medical studies. He was allowed to waive certain requirements and thus was able to devote extensive time to examining Charcot's patients at the Salpêtrière. During this period he worked wtih Madame D, Marcelle, Isabelle, and Achille, who, together with Léonie, provided much of the material for his subsequent theories. Janet's studies with patients suffering from amnesias, fugues, "successive existences" (his description of alter personalities), and conversion symptoms led him to postulate that these symptoms were attributable to the existence of split-off parts of the personality (which he conceptualized as "subconscious fixed ideas") capable of independent life and development. He demonstrated that the dissociated elements that gave rise to the patient's symptoms or behavior had their origin in past traumatic experiences and could be treated by bringing into consciousness the split-off memories and affects, which were then transformed by further therapy (Ellenberger, 1970).

Janet never sought to expand his theories on dissociation into a larger model of the mind. He is widely acknowledged to have been a modest, thoughtful man who carefully recorded his observations and made conservative interpretations of the results (Ellenberger, 1970). He limited his explanations to the phenomena of hysteria and hypnosis, and did not seek to account for other forms of psychopathology or the nature of personality (Hart, 1926; Crabtree, 1986).

Janet's Contemporaries

On this side of the Atlantic, two prominent American writers, Boris Sidis and Morton Prince, further amplified Janet's concept of dissociation (Hilgard, 1977; Crabtree, 1986). Sidis, a student of the great psychologist William James, pursued the question of "suggestibility" in both normal and abnormal subjects. He concluded that there is within every person two streams of consciousness that constitute two separate selves, the "waking self" and the "subwaking self" (Crabtree, 1986). Sidis believed that the subwaking self was devoid of morality, willing to carry out any act, very susceptible to the emotional forces aroused by crowds and mobs, and without will or goals of its own.

Morton Prince, founder of the *Journal of Abnormal Psychology* and informal leader of a Boston salon of psychopathologists, also readily embraced Janet's ideas as the foundation for his own further speculations on dissociation. Prince suggested replacing Janet's term "subconscious" with "coconscious," which he felt more clearly expressed the simultaneous nature of the coactivity of the second consciousness (Crabtree, 1986). Prince also sought to de-emphasize the importance of amnesia, making the simultaneous activity of two or more systems within one individual the crucial factor in his model of dissociation. He is best known for his work with the multiple personality patient "Miss Beauchamp," described extensively in *Dissociation of a Personality* (M. Prince, 1906).

William James was clearly captured by Janet's ideas and discussed his work extensively in the 1896 Lowell Lectures (Taylor, 1982). James summarized his first lecture with the statement that "the mind seems to embrace a confederation of psychic entities" (quoted in Taylor, 1982, p. 35). James also drew heavily on the work of the Englishman Frederick Myers, whose investigations of dissociative phenomena led him to postulate the existence of a second self, which he termed the "subliminal self." In contrast to Sidis's "brutal self," Myers's second self was the individual's true self or greater self; the conscious self, or "supraliminal self," was merely a subordinate stream of consciousness required to exercise those activities necessary for existence in the world (Crabtree, 1986). James synthesized these two formulations of dissociation into a model that accounted for hypnotism, automatisms, hysteria, multiple personality, demonic possession, witchcraft, and genius (Taylor, 1982).

The Decline of Interest in Dissociation

Although Janet, Prince, and other contemporaries took an experimental approach toward the phenomena of dissociation, most of their experiments were carried out with single subjects exhibiting unusual dissociative capacities (a number of whom would probably meet *Diagnostic and Statistical Manual of Mental Disorders*, third edition [DSM-III] criteria for multiple personality) and lacked control groups. Typical experiments of the time focused on the ability of these dissociative virtuosos to simultaneously perform two or more complex tasks, such as adding sums and copying poetry. Prince's primary experimental interest was in establishing that simultaneous "coconscious" processes were in fact conscious and not merely purely automatic physiological processes. Prince recognized, however, that the activities of one coconscious process might affect the functioning of the other: "Certainly in many cases there is a halting flow of thought of the principal intelligence, indicating that the activities of the secondary intelligence tends to inhibit the untrammeled flow of the former" (M. Prince, 1929, p. 411).

Janet's successors, however, took the principle of "noninterference" between two simultaneously performed tasks as the *sine qua non* of dissociation. The careful experiments of Ramona Messerschmidt, under the tutelage of Clark Hull, convincingly demonstrated the existence of a significant degree of interference between simultaneous conscious and subconscious tasks (Messerschmidt, 1927–1928). Messerschmidt used two pairs of combined tasks: oral reading (conscious) with serial addition (subconscious), and oral serial addition (conscious) with serial addition by automatic writing (subconscious). Both sets of tasks produced massive interference, compared to the same tasks performed singly in a conscious manner. Although Messerschmidt's design has been criticized as failing to produce the optimal dissociative barriers between tasks (Erickson & Erickson, 1941; White & Shevach, 1942), her results nonetheless effectively ended experimental inquiry into this question until the much later work of Hilgard and others on automatic writing (Hilgard, 1977).

During the 1930s, dissociation ceased to be a subject for legitimate scientific investigation and clinically was demoted to the role of an obscure, minor phenomenon. Messerschmidt's studies were responsible in part, but other powerful developments in psychiatry were sweeping aside dissociative models of psychopathology and reinterpreting the same symptoms from the psychoanalytic perspective of repression. The conflict between the dissociative and psychoanalytic models had been foreshadowed in the early exchanges between Janet and Freud concerning credit for recognizing the mechanisms of hysteria. Janet, in his review of *Studies on Hysteria*, wrote: "I am happy to see that the results of my already old findings have been recently confirmed by two German authors, Breuer and Freud" (quoted in Taylor, 1982, p. 63). The psychoanalysts, in turn, were protesting that they were not finding the cases of dual or multiple personality reported by clinicians using hypnosis, and that these alter personalities were artifacts hypnotically induced, unwittingly or deliberately, by their therapists.

Dissociative psychopathology continued to be identified during the 1930s, and clinical research such as Abeles and Schilder's (1935) studies of psychogenic loss of identity and Kanzer's (1939) collection of amnesia victims remain landmark clinical investigations. Repression, however, with its putative active unconscious defensive function, was considered responsible for the banishment of unacceptable ideas, affects, memories, and impulses from conscious awareness and voluntary recall. This mechanism was central to Freud's idea of a dynamic unconscious. Amnesias and hysterical symptoms were thought to be the result of the active repressive process that was protecting the person from intolerable affects or drives. Many of the formulations of dissociative symptoms came to be based on Freudian dynamic concepts (Nemiah, 1981).

The Renewal of Interest in Dissociation

The rebirth of interest in dissociation is the result of several converging trends. Clinically, dissociative psychopathology, primarily multiple personality disorder (MPD), is being increasingly diagnosed. The current interest in posttraumatic stress syndromes has also called attention to the role of dissociative symptoms in other disorders. Public awareness of child abuse, one of the major causes of chronic dissociative pathology, has increased dramatically within the last few years and provides a backdrop for a greater acceptance of the traumatically induced dissociative disorders. Experimentally, research into the physiology of MPD (Putnam, 1984a, 1986a), and the work of Hilgard (1977, 1984) and others on the hidden-observer phenomenon, have stimulated a return to laboratory investigation of dissociation. Hypnosis is also receiving renewed interest, both as a therapeutic tool and as a trait associated with certain forms of traumatically induced psychopathology (Frankel & Orne, 1976; John *et al.*, 1983; Pettinati *et al.*, 1985).

DEFINITIONS AND DESCRIPTIONS OF DISSOCIATION

Most authorities recognize that dissociation occurs in both minor non-pathological and major or pathological forms (Spiegel, 1963; West, 1967; Hilgard, 1977; Nemiah, 1981; Ludwig, 1983). Many authors conceptualize these different forms of dissociation as lying on a continuum from the minor dissociations of everyday life, such as daydreaming, to the major pathological forms, such as multiple personality (Bernstein & Putnam, 1986). Thus most definitions of dissociation are primarily concerned with distinguishing when a person's consciousness, sense of identity, or behavior is sufficiently dissociated to represent an abnormal and/or pathological process.

Over the years, different authorities have emphasized different aspects of the dissociative process as the key elements in determining whether or not a particular example of dissociation is pathological. In modern times, disruption of normal integrative functions has been the critical issue in definitions of dissociation. West (1967) defined dissociation as a "psychophysiological process whereby information—incoming, stored, or outgoing—is actively deflected from integration with its usual or expected associations" (p. 890). Although acknowledging that not all such experiences are pathological, West defined a dissociation reaction as a "state of experience or behavior wherein dissociation produces a discernable alteration in a person's thoughts, feelings, or actions, so that for a period of time certain information is not associated or integrated with other information as it normally or logically would be" (p. 890).

Principles of Dissociative Psychopathology

John Nemiah (1981) has identified two principles that can be used to characterize most forms of pathological dissociation. The first is that the individual undergoing a dissociative reaction experiences an alteration in his or her sense of identity. This disturbance of personal identity may take a variety of forms—for example, complete amnesia for self-referential information such as name and age, as occurs in psychogenic amnesia or fugue states, or the existence of a series of alternating identities that claim independence from one another, as in MPD. The second principle is that there will be a disturbance in the individual's memory for events occurring during a period of dissociation. This disturbance of memory may range from complete amnesia to forms of detached or dreamlike recall of events. These two principles can be used to characterize dissociative disorders as defined in DSM-III and its revision (DSM-III-R) and are most useful clinically in examining behavior suspected of having dissociative elements.

A third principle that has emerged from the study of dissociative reactions is that the vast majority of dissociative disorders are traumatically induced (Putnam, 1985a). The wartime amnesic syndromes provide the best documentation of the connections between trauma and dissociative reactions. Dissociative phenomena such as amnesia, profound detachment, or depersonalized feelings during moments of extreme stress; out-of-body experiences; and dream-like recall of events are commonly reported by combat veterans when one systematically inquires about such experiences. In my experience of treating over 70 combat veterans, I have repeatedly heard them describe having experiences of extreme detachment and depersonalization during moments when they thought that they were about to die or when they killed others. A substantial percentage of veterans have partial or complete amnesia for their combat experiences (Henderson & Moore, 1944; Archibald & Tuddenham, 1965). Persistent feelings of detachment and estrangement, as well as more active dissociative phenomena such as flashbacks and abreactions, are often part of war-induced posttraumatic stress reactions (Ewalt & Crawford, 1981).

Estimates of the incidence of wartime dissociative syndromes, generally psychogenic amnesia or psychogenic fugue reactions, range from 5% to 14% of all psychiatric combat casualties (Henderson & Moore, 1944; Sargant & Slater, 1941; Torrie, 1944; Grinker & Spiegel, 1943; Fisher, 1945). In contrast, Kirshner (1973) has reported the overall rate of dissociative reactions at 1.3% among military psychiatric patients in peacetime. A direct relationship between the degree of combat-related stress and the frequency of dissociative reactions has been reported by some authors (Sargant & Slater, 1941; Henderson & Moore, 1944).

In peacetime, a similar relationship between traumatic events (usually psychological trauma) and dissociative reactions has been observed (Abeles & Schilder, 1935; Kanzer, 1939). Abeles and Schilder (1935), in their classic study of psychogenic amnesia patients presenting at Bellevue Hospital, observed that "Some unpleasant conflict, either financial or familial, was significant in the immediate cause of the amnesia" (p. 603). Reviewers of the psychogenic fugue syndrome have identified three general categories of traumatic precipitants. The first is a situation in which the person can neither fight nor flee danger (Berrington *et al.*, 1956; Fisher, 1947; Luparello, 1970; Herold, 1941). The second commonly identified precipitant is the loss or threatened loss of an important object (Geleerd *et al.*, 1945; Geleerd, 1956). The third frequently identified precipitant is the experience of an overwhelming, panic-inspiring impulse, such as a powerful suicidal or homicidal urge (Fisher, 1947; Stengel, 1941, 1943).

There is strong evidence that depersonalization syndromes frequently occur in persons who have experienced severe trauma. For example, there is a high incidence of depersonalization syndromes in survivors of sustained life-threatening experiences, such as internment in a concentration camp (Bluhm, 1949; Frankenthal, 1969; Krystal, 1969; Jacobson, 1977; Dor-Shav, 1978; Bettelheim, 1979). A second line of evidence linking depersonalization syndromes to traumatic experiences is based on the work of Noyes and his colleagues (Noyes & Kletti, 1977; Noyes *et al.*, 1977; Noyes & Slymen, 1978–1979) on acute psychological responses to life-threatening danger. They have identified the existence of a "transient depersonalization syndrome" that occurred in approximately one-third of their subjects who experienced life-threatening danger. Fullerton *et al.* (1981) identified a similar transient depersonalization syndrome in trauma patients with severe spinal cord injuries; there was a higher incidence of this in patients with more severe injuries. Noyes and colleagues compared the experience of depersonalization associated with life-threatening experiences with that reported by hospitalized psychiatric patients and concluded that the two experiences were essentially similar, although the accident victims tended to respond with an increased alertness, whereas the psychiatric patients reported a clouding of mental processes during depersonalization experiences.

As we shall see in Chapter Three, there is strong evidence linking the development of MPD to severe, recurrent traumatic experiences usually occurring during childhood or early adolescence. Childhood trauma has also been identified as a contributing factor in the genesis of hypnoid states. These abnormal states of consciousness were described by Breuer and Freud in *Studies on Hysteria* (1895/1957) as the *sine qua non* of hysteria. A number of psychoanalytically oriented authors have suggested a relationship between hypnoid states observed in their patients and early childhood trauma, including sexual abuse (Loewald, 1955; Dickes, 1965; Silber, 1979).

FUNCTIONS OF DISSOCIATION

The hypothesis that dissociation is a normal process that is initially used defensively by an individual to handle traumatic experiences and evolves over time into a maladaptive or pathological process has been expressed in a variety of forms over the years. Ludwig (1983) states, "The widespread prevalence of dissociative reactions and their many forms and guises argues for their serving important functions for man and their possessing great survival value" (p. 95). This concept of the adaptive value of dissociation is invoked by many of the descriptive models of MPD (Braun & Sachs, 1985; Kluft, 1984d; Spiegel, 1984).

The Dissociative Continuum

Central to the concept of the adaptive function(s) of dissociation is the idea that dissociative phenomena exist on a continuum and become maladaptive only when they exceed certain limits in intensity or frequency, or occur in inappropriate contexts. Although Janet, in his descriptions of dissociative phenomena, emphasized an "unusual separation" of the dissociated subsystem from the controlling influence of the conscious self (White & Shevach, 1942), his contemporaries conceptualized dissociation as a normative process that became pathological only in certain circumstances. Morton Prince (1909b/1975), for example, characterized dissociation as "a general principle governing the normal psycho-nervous mechanism and therefore in a highly marked form only is pathological" (p. 123). Taylor and Martin (1944), in their extensive review of multiple personality, express the idea that there is a continuum running from normal experiences (e.g., daydreaming) to multiple personality. Similar formulations were subsequently expressed by others (Murphy, 1947; Spiegel, 1963; Rendon, 1977; McKellar, 1977; Greaves, 1980; Beahrs, 1983; Braun & Sachs, 1985; Saltman & Solomon, 1982). Hilgard (1977), with his "neodissociative" theory of the mind, has probably been the most instrumental modern figure advocating the concept of a continuum of dissociation from the normal to the pathological. He has observed that "daily life is full of many small dissociations if we look for them" (Hilgard, 1973, p. 406).

Evidence to support the idea of a dissociative continuum comes from two sources. The first line of evidence is the research on the distribution of hypnotic susceptibility (also commonly referred to as hypnotizability; Weitzenhoffer, 1980) in the normal population. Hypnotic susceptibility has been closely linked to dissociative potential (Spiegel & Spiegel, 1978; Spiegel, 1984; Bliss, 1983, 1984a; Braun & Sachs, 1985). A number of studies demonstrate that there is a characteristic curve describing the distribution of hypnotizability within a sample population. The shape of this curve varies according to the type of scale used to measure hypnotic susceptibility and is influenced by the testing setting, with laboratory settings yielding different results than clinical settings (Frankel, 1979). All studies of the distribution of hypnotizability have demonstrated that in a normal population this capacity exists along a continuum.

A second line of evidence supporting the concept of a continuum of dissociative experiences—ranging from the simple dissociations of everyday life, such as daydreaming, "tuning out" of conversations, and "highway hypnosis," to major dissociative phenomena, such as amnesia and fugue episodes—comes from surveys using the Dissociative Experiences Scale (DES; Bernstein & Putnam, 1986). The DES is a short, self-administered questionnaire that asks the respondent to indicate, by marking on a 100-mm-line visual analogue scale, the frequency with which certain specific dissociative or depersonalization experiences occur. The instrument has high test–retest reliability, excellent split-half reliability, and good criterion-referenced validity (Bernstein & Putnam, 1986).

Figure 1-1 shows the continuum of dissociative phenomena based on total DES scores of a series of group samples, ranging from normal adults and adolescents to multiple personality patients. All of the psychiatric patients met DSM-III criteria for their respective diagnoses. The solid bar shows the median DES score for each diagnostic group, and the dots represent individual subject scores. The stepwise increasing median scores of the different groups demonstrate the overlapping continuum of dissociative experiences across different diagnostic groups. The highest DES scores were found in patients with MPD, a chronic dissociative disorder incorporating most of the dissociative symptoms found in the other DSM-III/DSM-III-R dissociative disorders (Putnam *et al.*, 1986).

The relatively high median total DES score for the normal adolescent group is in agreement with several studies, using other questionnaires, on the incidence of feelings of depersonalization in adolescents (Roberts, 1960; Sedman, 1966; Harper, 1969; Myers & Grant, 1970). Adolescents tend to report frequent experiences of "tuning out" to external or internal stimuli and to report contextual shifts in their sense of self-identity—a finding that should come as no surprise to parents of teenagers.

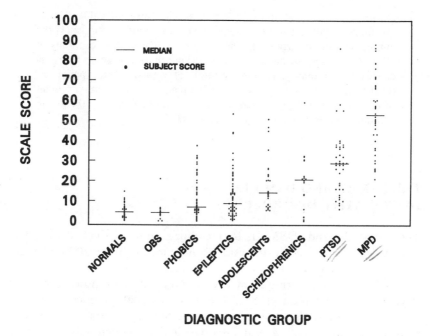

DIAGNOSTIC GROUP

Figure 1-1. Scatterplot of total Dissociative Experiences Scale (DES) scores for a number of group samples. OBS, patients with organic brain syndrome; PTSD, patients with posttraumatic stress disorder; MPD, multiple personality patients.

The Adaptive Functions of Dissociation

The adaptive nature of the dissociative process, particularly as a response of extreme trauma, has been identified both by victims of trauma (Bettelheim, 1979; Frankl, 1962) and by clinicians working with trauma victims (Frankenthal, 1969; Bliss, 1984a; Braun & Sachs, 1985; Kluft, 1984a; Spiegel, 1984). Frankel (1976), in his seminal work *Hypnosis: Trance as a Coping Mechanism*, outlines the evidence that dissociative/hypnotic mechanisms play an important role in dealing with day-to-day stress as well as protecting an individual against catastrophic trauma. Ludwig (1983) has enumerated seven adaptive functions served by the dissociative process:

> Dissociation represents the fundamental psychobiological mechanism underlying a wide variety of altered forms of consciousness, including conversion hysteria, hypnotic trance, mediumistic trance, multiple personality, fugue states, spirit possession and highway hypnosis. This

Very important

mechanism has great individual and species survival value. Under certain conditions, it serves to facilitate seven major functions: (1) the automatization of certain behaviors, (2) the efficiency and economy of effort, (3) the resolution of irreconcilable conflicts, (4) escape from the constraints of reality, (5) the isolation of catastrophic experiences, (6) the cathartic discharge of certain feelings, and (7) the enhancement of herd sense (e.g. the submersion of the individual ego for the group identity, greater suggestibility, etc.). (p. 93)

THE DSM-III AND DSM-III-R DISSOCIATIVE DISORDERS

The DSM-III and DSM-III-R recognize four distinct dissociative disorders: (1) psychogenic amnesia; (2) psychogenic fugue; (3) depersonalization disorder; and (4) multiple personality. In addition, there is a catch-all category covering atypical dissociative presentations (American Psychiatric Association, 1980a, 1987). In clinical practice, however, distinctions among these disorders may be blurred, with a given patient showing symptoms of several disorders either sequentially or simultaneously. Multiple personality patients may, for example, exhibit psychogenic amnesia, experience fugue episodes, and report periods of prolonged depersonalization (Putnam *et al.*, 1986). In addition to the DSM-III and DSM-III-R dissociative disorders, a number of other dissociated states (e.g., hypnoid states) and dissociative symptoms (e.g., abreactions) have been described over the years in the clinical literature.

Psychogenic Amnesia

Psychogenic amnesia is a sudden inability to recall important personal information that is too extensive to be explained by ordinary forgetfulness and is not associated with an organic mental disorder (American Psychiatric Association, 1980a). Most often the missing personal information involves the individual's identity and may include name, age, marital status, occupational information, and personal life history (Rapaport, 1971). The individual's fund of general knowledge is usually intact, in marked contrast to organic mental impairments, in which general information is the first to go and personal information is preserved till the end. Individuals with psychogenic amnesia are usually aware of the fact that they are unable to recall important personal information, though they may exhibit classic *la belle indifférence* toward their impairment.

Psychogenic amnesia has been classified into several types based on the disturbance in recall. "Localized" or "circumscribed" amnesia involves a failure to recall all events occurring during a circumscribed period of time (American Psychiatric Association, 1980a). The DSM-III describes this as the most common form of psychogenic amnesia, but few of these cases make it into the literature. "Selective" amnesia is a failure to recall some but not all of the events during a circumscribed period of time. "Generalized" amnesia involves a failure of memory for important personal information that spans the individual's entire life. This is the form that is most commonly reported in the clinical literature. "Continuous" amnesia involves an impairment of recall that encompasses the individual's entire past life and continues into the present.

There are no useful data on the incidence of any of the dissociative disorders. Psychogenic amnesia has been described as the most common dissociative reaction seen in hospital emergency rooms (Nemiah, 1981). Abeles and Schilder (1935) reported an incidence of 0.26% of all in-patients admitted to the Bellevue psychiatric service. The incidence of psychogenic amnesia is much higher in soldiers in combat, with rates of 5% and 8.6% reported for the Pacific and North African campaigns of World War II, respectively (Torrie, 1944; Henderson & Moore, 1944).

The onset of psychogenic amnesia is sudden and usually occurs immediately following a traumatic experience. The individual may experience unusual somatic sensations, dizziness, headache, or feelings of depersonalization. The course is usually brief and self-limited, typically lasting hours to days, and recovery is frequently spontaneous (American Psychiatric Association, 1980a; Abeles & Schilder, 1935). In rare instances, the amnesia may last for months (Abeles & Schilder, 1935; Kanzer, 1939; Kennedy & Neville, 1957). A hypnosis- or drug-facilitated interview frequently will yield the missing information and may provide an abreaction of the traumatic event. Abeles and Schilder (1935) reported that about a quarter of their cases had had at least one previous episode of amnesia.

Psychogenic Fugue

Psychogenic fugue involves a sudden, unexpected travel away from one's home or customary place of work, with an inability to recall the past, that occurs in the absence of an organic mental disorder (American Psychiatric Association, 1980a). There is often the assumption of a new identity.

Although the DSM-III and DSM-III-R state that this new identity is usually gregarious and less inhibited than the original identity, other authorities have observed that this secondary identity is often quiet and prosaic (Janet, 1890; Nemiah, 1981).

The travel of an individual in a fugue state may take the form of aimless wandering, but often appears purposeful and may include use of public transportation. A casual observer is not likely to notice anything unusual in the person's behavior. Charcot observed, "What is most wonderful in fugues, is that these individuals contrive not to be stopped by the police at the very beginning of their journey" (quoted in Rapaport, 1942, p. 201). In describing persons in a fugue state, Janet observed:

> In fact, they are mad people in full delirium; nevertheless, they take railway tickets, they dine and sleep in hotels, they speak to a great number of people. We are, it is true, sometimes told that they were thought a little odd, that they looked preoccupied and dreamy, but after all, they are not recognized as mad people . . . (quoted in Rapaport, 1942, p. 201)

In contrast to psychogenic amnesia patients, who are aware of their memory loss, fugue victims are usually unaware of their loss of self-referential information (Rapaport, 1971). Typically, individuals in a fugue state have no memory of their primary identity. When they recover their primary identity, they often have a reciprocal amnesia for the events of the fugue state.

Fugue episodes can occur in a variety of organic mental disorders, such as temporal lobe epilepsy (Mayeux et al., 1979), and in toxic or withdrawal states (Slater & Roth, 1974; Akhtar & Brenner, 1979). Therefore, a thorough medical and neurological evaluation is necessary. Fugues are also a common feature of MPD, and this possibility should always be considered in the differential diagnosis (Putnam et al., 1986). The incidence of fugues is unknown and considered to be common by some authorities (Slater & Roth, 1974) and rare by others (Berrington et al., 1956). It is generally acknowledged that the incidence markedly increases during times of war or natural disaster (American Psychiatric Association, 1980a; Putnam, 1985a). Psychogenic fugues usually have an acute traumatic precipitant that occurs immediately prior to the onset of the fugue (Putnam, 1985a).

Depersonalization Disorder

Depersonalization becomes a disorder when the individual experiences one or more episodes in which feelings of depersonalization cause social or occupational impairment (American Psychiatric Association, 1980a) or cause marked distress (American Psychiatric Association, 1987). The experience of depersonalization involves an alteration in the individual's sense of self so that the person feels unreal, as if he or she were in a dream, like a machine, dead, self-estranged, or otherwise significantly changed from his or her normal state. Sensory disturbances such as anesthesias, paresthesias, alterations in sense of body size or body parts, macroscopia or microscopia, or the experience of being outside of one's body and watching one's self from a distance or looking down from above are often present. The individual may also have passive-influence experiences, so that he or she feels controlled or that certain functions (e.g., speech) are not under the individual's control but have a "mind of their own."

The individual may report that memories have a dreamlike quality and at times cannot be distinguished from fantasy, so that the person becomes unsure of whether or not something actually occurred. While the individual is in a depersonalized state, past memories may be experienced as events that happened long ago to some other person. In the normal state, many individuals will have difficulty recalling events experienced during the depersonalized state or will comment on the dreamlike quality that these memories have.

Depersonalization is only considered to be a diagnosable disorder when it occurs in the absence of another disorder that includes feelings of depersonalization as part of its syndromal presentation (American Psychiatric Association, 1980a, 1987). As a symptom, depersonalization is found in a wide range of psychiatric and neurological conditions, including schizophrenia, depression, phobic and anxiety states, obsessive–compulsive disorder, substance abuse, sleep deprivation, temporal lobe epilepsy, and migraine headaches (Putnam, 1985a). Transient feelings of depersonalization are also commonly found in "normal" individuals, particularly adolescents (Roberts, 1960; Dixon, 1963; Sedman, 1966; Harper, 1969; Myers & Grant, 1970). Even Sigmund Freud reported personal experiences with feelings of depersonalization (Freud, 1941; Stamm, 1969). No single explanation accounts for the widespread nature of feelings of depersonalization, which are present in about 15–30% of all psychiatric patients irrespective of diagnosis (Putnam, 1985a). Nevertheless, as documented earlier in this chapter, depersonalization syndromes are frequently associated with a history of sustained traumas (e.g., concentration camp experiences).

Onset of a depersonalization disorder is usually abrupt, and recovery is generally gradual. Only about 10% of patients with depersonalization syndrome report persistent feelings of depersonalization

(Putnam, 1985a). Dizziness or fainting episodes are frequently associated with onset of depersonalization syndromes (Nemiah, 1981). Derealization, a feeling of unreality or detachment from the environment, is frequently present in addition to the sense of estrangement from self, although derealization may occur independently of feelings of depersonalization.

Dissociative Disorder Not Otherwise Specified

Dissociative disorder not otherwise specified is a residual category to accommodate the many dissociative phenomena that do not fit into the conventional DSM-III/DSM-III-R dissociative disorders but are characterized by a dissociative alteration in the normally integrative functions of identity, memory, or consciousness (American Psychiatric Association, 1987). In the DSM-III this category is called atypical dissociative disorder. The Ganser syndrome, a condition usually associated with symptoms such as amnesia, disorientation, perceptual disturbances, fugue, and conversion reactions, is included under this category in the DSM-III-R. Cocores *et al.* (1984) summarize the data indicating that the Ganser state is a dissociative disorder.

Multiple Personality

Multiple personality, renamed multiple personality disorder (MPD) in the DSM-III-R (American Psychiatric Association, 1987), is the primary subject of the rest of this book. In this complex and chronic condition, all of the elements of the other dissociative disorders may be found. Definitions and DSM-III/DSM-III-R diagnostic criteria for this disorder are discussed in Chapters Two and Three.

DISSOCIATIVE DISORDERS NOT INCLUDED IN DSM-III

Hypnoid States

Breuer (Breuer & Freud, 1895/1957) credits Moebius with first having identified the link between hypnoid states and hysteria. In their classic book *Studies on Hysteria*, Breuer and Freud (1895/1957) expanded on their thesis, first advanced in the "Preliminary Communication," that hypnoid states were the *sine qua non* of hysteria. Continuing in this vein, Freud (Freud & Breuer, 1893/1924) wrote:

> [I]ndeed, the more we occupied ourselves with these phenomena the more certain did our conviction become that splitting of consciousness, which is so striking in the well-known classical cases of *double conscience*, exists in a rudimentary fashion in every hysteria and that the tendency to this dissociation—and therewith to the production of abnormal states of consciousness, which may be included under the term *hypnoid*—is a fundamental manifestation of this neurosis. (p. 34)

> [T]here is one thing common to all these hypnoid states and to hypnosis, in spite of all their differences—namely, that the ideas which emerge in them are marked by great intensity of feeling but are cut off from associative connection with the rest of the content of consciousness. These hypnoid states are capable of association among themselves and the ideas belonging to them may in this way attain different degrees of psychical organization. (p. 35)

Freud, following his break with Breuer and the abandonment of his belief that actual childhood sexual trauma had occurred to his patients, rejected the idea of the hypnoid state as a necessary feature of hysteria (Ellenberger, 1970). Interest in hypnoid states declined in Europe following Freud's rejection of hypnosis and his adoption of free association as the therapeutic technique. In the United States, Morton Prince, William James, and their contemporaries continued to investigate these altered states and their role in psychopathology for another decade.

Psychoanalysts have continued to observe hypnoid states in some patients. Fliess (1953) has hypothesized that hypnoid states serve as a mechanism for the evasion of sexual affects. Brenman *et al.* (1952) suggest that fluctuations in hypnoid states act as a defense against aggressive impulses. Loewald (1955) equates the hypnoid state with "an early ego state" that is an essential part of the hysterical mechanism. Dickes (1965) classifies the hypnoid state as an ego defense and notes that these states arise as a defensive mechanism during a traumatic childhood. Silber (1979) concurs, reporting that hypnoid states originate in the context of childhood sexual trauma. Hypnoid or trance-like states have been identified as a powerful predictor of early MPD in children and adolescents by modern investigators (Elliott, 1982; Fagan & McMahon, 1984; Kluft, 1984b).

Somnambulism

Somnambulism was traditionally included on the early lists of dissociative disorders. Somnambulists were the focus of many discussions and stories during the late 18th and 19th centuries. They were reputed to be able to swim rivers, climb walls, walk across rooftops, or write poetry during their sleepwalking episodes (Ellenberger, 1970). It was generally believed that their lives would be endangered if they were awakened during these acts. The early magnetizer Puységur gained renown in part from his ability to artificially induce or stop somnambulism. Eric Carlson has published several fascinating accounts of early 19th-century som-nambulists, including Jane C. Rider (Carlson, 1982), who experienced a nocturnal hyperacuity of vision during her episodes, and Rachel Baker (Simpson & Carlson, 1968), who preached in the somnambulistic state.

Somnambulism has been redefined in recent times as a disorder of sleep and arousal (American Psychiatric Association, 1980a). This newer conceptualization comes in large part from the work of Kales and his collaborators (Kales *et al.*, 1966a, 1966b; Kales & Kales, 1974; Kales *et al.*, 1980). Kales *et al.* (1980) define somnambulism as "a state of dissociated consciousness in which phenomena of the sleeping and wak-ing states combine" (p. 1406).

Laboratory studies show that somnambulism occurs primarily dur-ing the first three hours of sleep and generally in stage 3 or 4 sleep. Typically the person sits up in bed, then gets up and moves around. Motor coordination is usually poor, and the person has an automaton-like quality (i.e., moves slowly and stiffly). The person's eyes are open, and his or her facial expression is blank. Complex behaviors such as dressing and eating have been observed in laboratory settings. These behaviors are usually out of context and indicate the person's lack of awareness of his or her surroundings. Somnambulists are difficult to awaken and regain awareness gradually. In most cases, the person is completely amnesic for the episode. There is rarely more than one epi-sode per night (Kales *et al.*, 1980).

Somnambulism is common in childhood; it typically disappears about age 10 and is rare in adulthood (Kales *et al.*, 1980). Sleepwalking that continues into adulthood generally has a later age of onset than sleepwalking that is outgrown. An increased familial incidence of sleep-walking has been reported by some investigators, and a genetic predispo-sition has been suggested (Kales *et al.*, 1980). A major life event is frequently associated with the onset of sleepwalking in adult somnambu-lists and is less often found in the histories of subjects who outgrew their sleepwalking (Kales *et al.*, 1980). Kales *et al.* (1980) found that adult somnambulists were more likely to exhibit psychopathology, particularly difficulties in handling aggression, than were subjects who outgrew the disorder.

Somnambulistic wanderings may, however, be part of the clinical picture of MPD. In two cases with which I am familiar, the patients first sought help for and were treated for somnambulism. Only later was it recognized that these patients were suffering from MPD. Their somnambulism was caused by the nocturnal emergence of alters, primarily child alters, who were abreacting childhood trauma or acting out forbidden impulses. Both of these patients displayed extraordinarily complex behavior during these sleepwalking episodes, including calling their therapists from phone booths, stealing objects, working in the yard, and building complex structures.

Possession States

Possession states are extremely common. They have been reported to occur in most cultures (Yap, 1960; Mischel & Mischel, 1958; Wittkower, 1970), and are also prevalent in a variety of forms in modern-day America (Pattison & Wintrob, 1981). Ellenberger (1970) has traced the roots of modern dynamic psychiatry to the early practice of exorcism for demonic possession.

Although certain aspects of possession states are culturally determined (e.g., the behavioral differences seen in syndromes such as *amok*, *latah*, *koro*, *imu*, *witiko*, *pibloktoq*, and *negi negi*), in all cultures they grow out of a religious or magical context in which all life events, such as illness, accident, good fortune, and misfortune, are experienced as closely interrelated (Pattison & Wintrob, 1981). Enoch and Trethowan (1979) have advanced the concept of "psychological causality," which they trace back in its Western form to the ancient Greeks' concept of a sacred disease, as the common denominator in possession states and their allied disorders. Psychological causality is the belief that events occur because someone or something that has become personified has willed its occurrence.

The history of possession and its treatment by exorcism has been extensively reviewed elsewhere (see Pattison & Wintrob, 1981, for an excellent bibliography). The classic psychiatric review was done by Oesterreich (1966), who felt that there were two main forms of possession: a "somnambulistic" or hysterical form, and a "lucid" or obsessional form. In the lucid form, the individual remains aware of himself or herself, but feels invaded and engaged in a struggle for control over his or her behavior. In the somnambulistic form, the individual has lost all consciousness of self and speaks with the "I" of the intruder (Ellenberger,

1970). After recovering consciousness, the person has an amnesia, partial or complete, for the events occurring during a somnambulistic possession experience. In contrast, a victim of lucid possession retains memory for the events occurring during the possession experience. A number of other typologies of possession have been offered (Pattison & Wintrob, 1981; Enoch & Trethowan, 1979).

Pattison and Wintrob (1981) point out that although the concept of possession by "other forces" is widespread, there is a continuum of abstraction upon which this can be expressed. At the concrete end of this continuum, an individual may be possessed by the "spirit" of a specific person, animal, god, demon, or other being; at the more abstract end, an individual may be considered to be possessed by thoughts, impulses, ideas, memories, or images. Possession may be experienced as malevolent or beneficial. It may be desirable or socially unacceptable.

An individual's first onset of a possession state is usually abrupt, chaotic, and sometimes violent (Kenny, 1981; Ravenscroft, 1965; Enoch & Trethowan, 1979; Mischel & Mischel, 1958). Ravenscroft (1965), in his vivid description of possession states in the Haitian Vodun culture, distinguishes between ceremonial and nonceremonial induction. In the former, the possession state is often facilitated by crowd excitement, chanting and singing, circular rhythmic dancing, drumming, darkness, candlelight or torchlight, and other ceremonial inducements. Nonceremonial inductions of possession states are frequently associated with personal crises or severe stress (Ravenscroft, 1965; Mischel & Mischel, 1958). Ravenscroft (1965) has noted that the death or estrangement of a significant other frequently occurs shortly prior to an individual's first possession state.

The individual often experiences an intitial sensation of dizziness or disequilibrium with the onset of possession (Mischel & Mischel, 1958; Ravenscroft, 1965). On occasion, the person may fall to the ground and writhe with convulsions. More often, the onset is rapidly followed by a dramatic transformation. Marked facial changes may occur, including changes in jaw position (e.g., protrusion), rearrangement of facial folds and creases, widening of the eyes, and dilation of the pupils (Mischel & Mischel, 1958; Oesterreich, 1966). The possessed individual's posture, gait, mannerisms, and behavior may also change dramatically. Changes in speech, including pitch, vocabulary, and presence of speech defects, are common. In cultures such as Haitian Vodun, where the individual is possessed by specific gods, other ceremonial participants can quickly recognize which god is present on the basis of the stereotypic behaviors displayed by the possessed individual, which are characteristic for each god (Mischel & Mischel, 1958; Ravenscroft, 1965).

Speaking in tongues, or "glossolalia," may occur. This usually involves speaking in a fabricated language or an unknown tongue, and has long been associated with possession states, religious ecstasy, and some mediumship experiences. Some authorities have identified two forms of glossolalia. The first occurs in conjunction with highly emotional group religious ceremonies such as Pentacostal services, though it has also been reported in the more staid denominations such as Episcopal, Lutheran, and Presbyterian (Enoch & Trethowan, 1979). The second form occurs in individuals engaged in quiet meditation, contemplation, and dedication. Most investigators see glossolalia as a form of dissociative reaction, though some have identified forms of secondary gain associated with the experience (Enoch & Trethowan, 1979; Jahoda, 1969).

Demographic data on the participants in possession states are scanty. Both Mischel and Mischel (1958) and Ravenscroft (1965) report that these states are much more common in women than in men. Possession states, while reported to occur in children on rare occasion, are most common in adults between the ages of 25 and 45 (Mischel & Mischel, 1958; Ravenscroft, 1965). Ravenscroft (1965) reports that first possession usually occurs in females between the ages of 17 and 22, while males typically experience their first possession between the ages of 22 and 28 years. The frequency of possession episodes declines after about age 45 and often ceases around age 60 (Ravenscroft, 1965).

Violent behavior toward self or others may occur, but more commonly the individual only flirts with violence, and is rarely hurt or injurious to others. Individuals may attempt to fight off the possession, sometimes by self-inflicted pain (Ravenscroft, 1965). Childish or regressed behavior, including incontinence and soiling, is frequent (Mischel & Mischel, 1958). Possessed persons often exhibit extraordinary levels of physical energy and activity and may dance in a frenzy for hours. A possession experience is often terminated by the individual's falling into a swoon-like state.

The relationship of possession states to mental disorders has interested a wide range of investigators, and many opinions and theories exist. As with other dissociative states, many authorities conceptualize possession states as existing on a continuum from essentially normal, culturally acceptable experiences to extreme forms of psychopathology (Pattison & Wintrob, 1981; Enoch & Trethowan, 1979).

Out-of-Body and Near-Death Experiences

Out-of-body experiences, usually defined as an experience in which the individual perceives his or her awareness or mind as being outside or separated from the physical body (Twemlow *et al.*, 1985), are not uncommon. This experience occurs fairly frequently in the chronic dissociative disorders, such as depersonalization syndrome and multiple personality. Several surveys, primarily of college students, indicate that at least a quarter of the sampled populations reported such experiences (Hart, 1954; Green, 1968; Palmer & Dennis, 1975). A survey by Shiels (1978) found that these experiences were found in over 70 non-Western cultures and showed a high degree of similarity. Out-of-body experiences are also often a component of near-death experiences occurring in individuals who suffer life-threatening trauma or are revived or resuscitated after respiration or heart beat have ceased (Twemlow *et al.*, 1985; Sabom, 1982; Greyson, 1985).

Out-of-body experiences in persons who are not psychiatric patients frequently occur when the individuals are feeling physically relaxed and mentally calm (Twemlow *et al.*, 1985). Such an experience has great vividness and reality and is not dreamlike. The individual usually reports that his or her mind or sense of awareness is experienced as separated from the body but in the same location as the body, and that there is a desire to return to the body (Twemlow *et al.*, 1985). In Twemlow *et al.*'s (1985) survey, about 10% of out-of-body experiences were associated with traumatic circumstances. In Sabom's (1982) review of near-death experiences, however, 30% of individuals reported viewing their bodies as if from the outside, and 54% reported transcendental experiences in which their consciousness entered another dimension or region.

A number of researchers have introduced classification schemes for out-of-body and near-death experiences (Twemlow *et al.*, 1985; Greyson, 1985; Schapiro, 1975–1976). Debate continues over whether or not all of these experiences share a core set of elements (Greyson, 1985). Work has also focused on the personality correlates of individuals with frequent out-of-body experiences (Irwin, 1980; Palmer & Vassar, 1974; Palmer & Lieberman, 1975). Various theories of etiology have been advanced; they fall into two main categories, separationist theories and psychological theories (Irwin, 1980). The separationists believe that a nonphysical element of existence (e.g., the soul, the psyche, the astral body) actually leaves the body and travels to another location. The psychological theories hold that out-of-body experiences are a special state of consciousness and that the experience of being outside of the body is essentially hallucinatory.

Unusual Psychiatric Syndromes

Capgras and Reboul-Lachaux first described in 1923 a syndrome in which the patient believed that a person, often a close relative, had been replaced by an exact double (Enoch & Trethowan, 1979). The double is usually a key figure in the individual's life, and in married persons it is frequently the spouse. The similarities of the Capgras syndrome to depersonalization and derealization phenomena have been commented on by several investigators (Enoch & Trethowan, 1979).

The *folie à deux* (or *folie à plusieurs*) syndrome is probably composed of several syndromes. The core feature is the transfer of mental symptoms, particularly paranoid delusions, from one person to another (Enoch & Trethowan, 1979). Dissociative forms have been reported (Kiraly, 1975). Cotard syndrome, *le délire de négation*, has also been considered to be a dissociative variant, though other authors believe it to be a paranoid form of involutional psychosis. In its extreme form, the primary symptom is a complete denial of the existence of self. In milder forms, this may be expressed as a sense of depersonalization-like change in self, or feelings of despair or self-loathing (Enoch & Trethowan, 1979).

FACTORS THAT INFLUENCE THE FORM OF DISSOCIATIVE REACTION

If we accept the observation that many dissociative reactions have their origin as an adaptive response to overwhelming trauma, then we can inquire into why one form of dissociative reaction occurs (or is chosen) over another form for a particular traumatic precipitant. Although a number of theories or models exist that attempt to account for the genesis of one specific form, MPD, no theory has attempted to account for the range of forms that traumatically induced dissociative disorders can take. A review of the literature suggests that several factors may play a role in influencing the form of traumatically induced dissociative reaction (Putnam, 1985a).

Age

Several lines of circumstantial evidence suggest that the age of the individual at the time of the trauma, when coupled with certain other factors, may play a crucial role in determining the form of dissociative reaction (Putnam, 1985a). The demographic data on victims of dissociative disorders are scanty, but indicate that some types of dissociative reactions are more likely to be seen in specific age groups (Putnam, 1985a; Bernstein & Putnam, 1986). A second line of evidence comes from data indicating that the age or developmental stage during which sustained trauma occurs plays an important role in determining whether or not an individual develops MPD. In addition, data from several types of studies indicate that a history of childhood trauma is also a strong correlate of adult hypnotic susceptibility (Putnam, 1985a).

Gender

The role of gender, if any, in predisposing an individual toward a specific type of dissociative reaction (or even dissociative reactions in general) is extremely difficult to assess. Many of the published studies and case collections were subject to forms of sampling biases that may have overrepresented either sex. The published case collections of multiple personality patients have all exhibited a significantly higher incidence of females. The magnitude of this difference has steadily declined as more cases have been reported; however, female to male ratios as high as 8:1 or 9:1 have been observed (Allison, 1974a; Putnam et al., 1986). Some experienced therapists have reported much lower ratios of between 4:1 and 2:1 (Kluft, 1984a; Bliss, 1984a). A number of clinicians have specu- lated that the apparently higher incidence of female MPD cases is caused, at least in part, by a significant sampling bias. Female MPD patients, with their tendency to direct their violence toward themselves in the form of suicide attempts and gestures or self-mutilation, are more likely to be seen in the mental health system; males, with their tendency toward more externally directed violence, are more likely to be encountered in the criminal justice system (Bliss, 1980; Greaves, 1980; Boor, 1982; Putnam et al., 1984). The single survey of a criminal population published to date indicated a surprisingly high incidence of MPD among rapists and sex offenders (Bliss & Larson, 1985). The speculations about this apparent association between gender and incidence of MPD are discussed more completely in Chapter Three.

SUMMARY

This chapter has surveyed the history of scientific and clinical inquiry into dissociation, starting with the seminal contributions of Pierre Janet and tracing the waxing and waning of belief and interest in dissociative disorders over the last century. What emerges is a near-unanimity of opinion by authorities that the dissociative process occurs along a con- tinuum ranging from minor, "everyday" examples (e.g., daydreaming) to psychiatric disorders (e.g., multiple personality). Pathological forms of dissociation are characterized by a major disturbance of memory and a profound disturbance of the individual's sense of self, and are often a response to overwhelming physical and/or psychological trauma. The dissociative response may initially be adaptive, but becomes maladaptive and pathological when it persists beyond the trauma context. Finally, the chapter has surveyed the range of clinical dissociative disorders, postponing the discussion of MPD, and has concluded with an examination of factors (e.g., age and sex) that may contribute to the form of dissociative response.

CHAPTER TWO

History and Definitional Criteria of Multiple Personality Disorder

Multiple personality disorder (MPD) is the ultimate dissociative disorder. As a syndrome, MPD contains all the principal elements of the other major dissociative disorders. Individuals with MPD will, at times, manifest psychogenic amnesia, fugue episodes, and profound depersonalization (Putnam *et al.*, 1986). Multiple personality is a chronic disorder and does not appear to be self-limited in the same fashion as the other DSM-III/DSM-III-R dissociative disorders. Without proper treatment, MPD appears to be a lifelong process, though it may manifest itself differently over the lifetime of an individual (Kluft, 1985a).

Multiple personality is also one of the most amazing and unusual mental conditions known. The existence of apparently separate and autonomous alter personalities, exchanging control over an individual's behavior, elicits intense fascination in some and protests of disbelief from others. The existence of these entities raises questions about fundamental assumptions of the unity of personality and the structure of consciousness. The wide variety of symptoms commonly found in MPD includes most of the types of symptoms found in all of the other psychiatric disorders combined.

The history of MPD parallels the history of modern psychiatry (Ellenberger, 1970). All of the eminent figures associated with the early development of modern psychiatry were forced to come to grips with the questions raised by MPD. Benjamin Rush, the father of American psychiatry, was among the earliest pioneers to study and lecture on MPD (Carlson, 1981). Jean-Martin Charcot and his many famous associates in the Société de Psychologie Physiologique, such as Babinski, Bernheim, Binet, and Janet, used dissociative phenomena in general and MPD in particular as the centerpiece for theories of psychopathology and the mind. In the United States a similar process occurred, with luminaries such as William James and Morton Prince theorizing about the nature of consciousness and the organization of the mind, based on their personal experience with MPD patients.

Even Freud, who ultimately rejected hypnosis as a therapeutic technique and substituted a psychodynamic formulation based on repression rather than dissociation, began his life's work by inquiring into the nature of double consciousness (Breuer & Freud, 1895/1957). Despite the hiatus of interest in dissociation and multiple personality that followed the widespread acceptance of Freud's theories, MPD and the dissociative process have recently resumed their role as central features in recent models and theories of the organization of consciousness (Hilgard, 1977; Fischer & Pipp, 1984). Every theory or model that seeks to explain the organization and structure of human consciousness and behavior must account for the phenomena found in MPD.

THE HISTORY OF MULTIPLE PERSONALITY DISORDER

The Earliest Cases

The archetypes of MPD, shamanistic transformation and possession states, lie as far back in time as religious belief and behavior can be traced. Images of shamans, changed into animal forms or embodying spirits, can be found in Paleolithic cave paintings and contemporary Eskimo carvings. Researchers of shamanism point to the near-universality of themes and the commonality of traditions over time and across seemingly irreconcilable ethnic and cultural lines as evidence that shamanism expresses a fundamental process of the human psyche (Halifax, 1982; Harner, 1982).

The concept of demonic possession dominated Western thinking for many centuries, and it was only after a significant decline in the acceptance of possession as an explanation for disordered behavior that cases of multiple personality began to be recognized (Ellenberger, 1970). Oesterreich (1966) identified two forms of possession, the lucid and the somnambulistic, which have been described in Chapter One. Ellenberger (1970) has observed that these two forms of possession parallel two of the major manifestations of multiple personality. He speculates, "The phenomenon of possession, so frequent for many centuries, could be considered as one variety of multiple personality" (p. 127). It would not be surprising, considering the grim picture of medieval life provided by such authorities as Barbara Tuchman (1978), if the incidence of MPD were not substantially higher in those times than in these.

Paracelsus is credited by Bliss (1980) as having described the first case of MPD, in 1646, involving a woman who was amnesic for an alter personality who stole her money. In 1791, Eberhardt Gmelin reported on the case of "exchange personalities" (Ellenberger, 1970). He treated a 20-year-old German woman who would suddenly "exchange" her personality, language, and manners with a personality who spoke perfect French and behaved like an aristocratic lady. As the French personality, the woman retained memory for all that had happened in her French state, whereas she was amnesic for this same behavior in her German personality. Gmelin was able to switch her back and forth between these two personalities with a wave of his hand.

Benjamin Rush, signer of the Declaration of Independence, chief surgeon of the Continental Army, and author of the first American textbook on psychiatry, collected case histories of dissociation and multiple personality for his lectures and writings on physiological psychology (Carlson, 1981, 1984). Rush theorized that the mechanism responsible for the doubling of consciousness lay in a disconnection between the two hemispheres of the brain—the first of many such speculations on the subject of hemispheric laterality and multiple personality. The single most influential early case was that of Mary Reynolds, first published by Dr. Samuel Latham Mitchell in 1816 and later popularized in the United States by the Rev. William S. Plumer for *Harper's New Monthly Magazine* in 1860, and in Europe by Robert Macnish in his 1830 book *The Philosophy of Sleep* (Carlson, 1984).

In many ways, however, Despine's case of Estelle is more illuminating (Ellenberger, 1970). In 1836, Despine undertook the treatment of an 11-year-old Swiss girl whose symptoms evolved over time from an initial paralysis and exquisite sensitivity to touch to an overt dual existence with a second personality who was able to walk, loved to play in the snow, and could not tolerate the presence of her mother. The sight of certain objects (e.g., cats) could send her into a state of catalepsy. Estelle exhibited marked discrepancies in behavior, food preferences, and interpersonal relations in her two different states. The 60-year-old Despine developed a close rapport with his young patient and was able to effect a cure through psychotherapy implicit in the variety of hydrotherapeutic and magnetic treatments he employed. His detailed monograph, published in 1840, first set forth principles for the psychotherapy of MPD that are recognized as valid today (Kluft, 1984b).

The Ascent of Multiple Personality: 1880–1920

During the period from 1880 to about 1920, there was a great flourishing of interest in multiple personality (Ellenberger, 1970; Taylor & Martin, 1944; Sutcliffe & Jones, 1962). A relatively large number of cases were reported, particularly in France and the United States. Dissociation and multiple personality became subjects of intense interest for many of the great physicians, psychologists, and philosophers of the era. The clinical approach toward these cases was characterized by detailed reporting (often entire volumes were devoted to a single patient) and an active experimental stance toward dissociative phenomena, together with elaborate theorizing about the nature of consciousness and the relationship between dissociated personalities and normative experiences such as dreaming and hypnosis. It was also a time of great international medical conferences and meetings, many of which devoted extensive time to sessions on dissociation.

Several cases recorded during this epoch stand out for the quality or importance of the observations. Eugène Azam (1822–1899) studied Félida X over a period of 35 years and published her case in 1887 with a preface by Charcot (Azam, 1887). Born in 1843, Félida X lost her father in infancy and had a difficult childhood. From age 13 on, she manifested a second personality, who would emerge after Félida sank into a lethargic state for several minutes. The second personality was gay and vivacious and suffered none of the physical ailments that plagued Félida. In her first personality she was amnesic for the behavior of the second, whereas the second personality remembered her whole life history. On occasion, a third personality, who suffered from attacks of anxiety and hallucinations, would emerge. At one point, the first personality presented with a pregnancy that she could not explain, and the second personality emerged and took responsibility. A strikingly similar example of an unexplained pregnancy in MPD has been reported by Solomon and Solomon (1984). Over time the second personality became predominant, but she continued to have brief relapses into the first personality. Each personality considered itself to be Félida's normal state and the other to be abnormal.

Janet reported on several cases, including the celebrated Léonie. Following the first experiments that brought Janet his initial recognition (described in Chapter One), he resumed working with her and discovered an alter personality. This alter, known by her childhood name of Nichette, was a child personality. Janet also worked with Lucie, whose second personality, Adrienne, relived in fits of terror a traumatic childhood incident. Janet helped her by providing a corrective abreactive experience, and the second personality disappeared (Ellenberger, 1970).

Janet's third patient, Rose, is sometimes cited as a case of MPD, though there is less evidence for the diagnosis (Sutcliffe & Jones, 1962). Rose suffered from a variety of somnambulistic states; in some she was paralyzed, but in others she could freely walk.

The case of "Christine Beauchamp," reported in great detail by Morton Prince in _The Dissociation of a Personality_ (1906), is one of the most famous of all MPD cases, rivaled only by Mary Reynolds, Eve (Thigpen & Cleckley, 1957), and Sybil (Schreiber, 1974). Prince began his work with "Miss Beauchamp" in 1898 when she was a 22-year-old preparatory school student seeking help for headaches, fatigue, and an "inhibition of will." He tried hypnosis to ease her plight and discovered two different personalities, referred to as "B II" and "B III." The former was an intensification of the presenting personality, "B I," but the latter was very different. B III called herself Sally and was childlike, with an impish love of practical jokes, which she played on B I. Sally stuttered, lacked B I's manners, and could not speak French. She was scornful and contemptuous of B I and sought to cause her problems by indirect influence (e.g., forcing B I to utter inappropriate words) or by overtly sabotaging B I's affairs.

A fourth personality, B IV or the Idiot, emerged later in the course of therapy. This personality was extremely regressed and associated with a traumatic event at age 18. Miss Beauchamp was known to have had a painful childhood. When she was 13 her mother died, and during adolescence she suffered a series of unspecified traumas that caused her to run away from home. Prince synthesized B I and B II and "hypnotized" B III out of existence. The resulting "Miss Beauchamp," now known to have been Clara Norton Fowler, was reportedly cured. She subsequently married one of Prince's associates, Boston neurologist Dr. George Waterman (Kenny, 1984).

Walter Franklin Prince (no relation to Morton Prince) also described a classic case of MPD in great detail (W. F. Prince, 1917). Prince presents a 50-page "meager outline" of the case, drawn from 1,900 pages of notes taken over 3 years of daily observation. Doris Fisher came from a deprived childhood and was physically abused by her father. Prince associates the origin of two alters with her being dashed to the floor by her father in a fit of fury. Prince goes on to describe many phenomena that are classic for MPD patients, including child alters, auditory and visual hallucinations, abreactions with tearing at her body, and "shrinking from imaginary blows" and a wide variety of sensory disturbances. He also noted that the "primary personality" never went to sleep, only the secondary alters. Prince described the switching behavior classically noted in MPD patients:

There was a certain motor index which always preceded a change of personalities in this case; whether it has been noted in any other is not to the writer known. This was a sudden jerk or oscillation of the head from the neck, varying from an almost imperceptible twitch to a jerk which shook the whole body. It was more pronounced in the transition from a lower to a higher personality, and most of all, generally speaking, when the transition was from M. to R. D. (W. F. Prince, 1917, p. 89)

Prince observed that switches occurred whenever a personality became tired. Switches were also associated with "Pain, grief, fear, wounded sensibilities, disagreeable memories, self-reproach, or any other species of painful emotion, in proportion to its suddenness and intensity, or even a pleasurable emotion if too tumultuous or swift of approach" (p. 90). On occasion, he observed more than 50 switches in a day. Eventually one of the personalities, Sick Doris, was absorbed by Real Doris; another was integrated into Real Doris; and a third, Sleeping Real Doris, "disappeared." The phenomena carefully detailed in Walter F. Prince's case report are a microstudy of MPD.

The rich case descriptions of this period readily lent themselves to the speculations and theories advanced by many prominent clinicians of the time. Two major categories of models emerged: "dipsychism," the concept of the duality of the mind, and "polypsychism," the concept of the mind as a cluster of subpersonalities (Ellenberger, 1970). Dessoir was the foremost advocate of dipsychism with his book *The Double Ego* (Ellenberger, 1970). He saw the human mind as consisting of two distinct layers, each with its unique characteristics, which he referred to as "upper consciousness" and "lower consciousness." Polypsychism, a term coined by the magnetizer Durand de Gros, describes the models in which the human mind was divided into subsections, each with its own subego. All of these subegos were under the central control of an "ego-in-chief" which is our usual consciousness (Ellenberger, 1970). The models elaborated by William James, Morton Prince, Boris Sidis, Frederick Myers, and others to account for dissociation were all variants of either dipsychism or polypsychism. It was these early models, theories, and speculations, primarily based on observations of extreme cases of dissociation, that paved the way for Freud's "discovery" of the unconscious.

The Decline of Interest in Multiple Personality Disorder: 1920–1970

Reviewers of multiple personality all comment on the waxing and waning in the numbers of case reports over the last two centuries (Taylor &

Martin, 1944; Sutcliffe & Jones, 1962; Greaves, 1980). The period from about 1920 to the early 1970s represents the nadir of MPD as a clinical entity. The early to mid-1920s saw a number of important or interesting cases described in rich detail, such as Goddard's (1926) Norma. C. C. Wholey (1926) presented a case to the annual meeting of the American Psychiatric Association as a movie, which survives to this day. This silent film illustrates swooning-type switches, personality-specific differences in pain sensitivity among alters, and opposite-gender and child alters—all clinical phenomena commonly reported in present-day MPD patients (Putnam *et al.*, 1986). A few cases continued to be reported in reputable journals during the 1930s and 1940s but added little new information other than the author's sense of novelty, which served to reinforce the prevailing perception of the extreme rareness of the condition.

The most important case of this period was Eve, first reported in 1954 by Thigpen and Cleckley (1954) and later expanded by them into a best-selling book, *The Three Faces of Eve* (1957), which in turn generated a hit movie by the same name starring Joanne Woodward. The case of Eve is noteworthy more for the attention that it attracted than for any new information or formulations. Perhaps the most important aspect of this case is the fact that Thigpen and Cleckley reported being able to substantiate through other sources some childhood stories indicating that at least one of Eve's alter personalities, Eve Black, was present by 6 years of age. In a classic childhood MPD scenario, an amnesic Eve White, desperately protesting her innocence, was whipped for misbehavior committed by Eve Black. Eve Black expressed her pleasure at "coming out" to commit the offense and then withdrawing to leave Eve White to experience the pain and punishment.

Two thorough review articles written during this period sought to establish criteria for the disorder and to determine whether or not MPD was a real entity (Taylor & Martin, 1944; Sutcliffe & Jones, 1962). The critical and conservative tone of these reviews conveys much about the skeptical climate surrounding MPD during this period. Both sets of reviewers defined diagnostic criteria and excluded a number of cases that failed to meet their definitions. Although both concluded that MPD was a real clinical entity that could not be discounted as fad or fraud, they set a stance of defensive skepticism that later authors were forced to adopt for purposes of credibility. Many of the articles and reports on MPD over the next two decades focused on proving that MPD existed rather than on contributing new clinical knowledge. The study of multiple personality is only now beginning to extricate itself from the consequences of this defensive position and to rise above the frequent and often ignorant challenges to "prove" that MPD exists. It is curious, in these times when syndromes appear or disappear with each new edition of the *Diagnostic and Statistical Manual of Mental Disorders* (DSM), that MPD, one of the oldest psychiatric entities on record, remains continually called upon to prove its existence while other newly defined disorders are routinely accepted.

When one looks back over this period of decline and defensive justification of MPD, it appears as if a number of factors were responsible for creating a widespread climate of disbelief and skepticism. The decline of interest in dissociation as a clinical and laboratory phenomenon, discussed in Chapter One, paralleled the increasing suspicion of MPD and undoubtedly contributed to the outright rejection of the disorder in some circles. Stinging public criticism leveled at some of the prominent MPD investigators, particularly Morton Prince, may also have served to dampen the enthusiasm of others for reporting cases (Ellenberger, 1970). Some critics, although less personal in their attacks, continued to hammer on the theme that multiple personality was an artifact of hypnosis. William Brown, for example, in his retort to Bernard Hart's presidential address to the medical section of the British Psychological Society, said: "There is much to be said for the view that the phenomena of multiple personality may be in the main artefacts, due to the hypnotic methods of investigation and treatment employed by their observers" (Hart, 1926, p. 260). Many others favoring the psychoanalytic approach contributed additional criticisms in the same vein (Ellenberger, 1970). There is no doubt that the rise of the psychoanalytic therapeutic model, and the competition between this model and earlier theories formulated by Janet and others, provided a major impetus for many of the objections to hypnosis and MPD.

An additional factor that may have played a substantial role in the decline of MPD cases during this period has been identified by Rosenbaum (1980). He notes that the diagnosis of schizophrenia, although originally introduced by Bleuler about 1908, "caught on" in the United States during the late 1920s and early 1930s. In reviewing the *Index Medicus* for cases, Rosenbaum notes that there were more cases of multiple personality than schizophrenia reported during the period 1914–1926. Beginning about 1927, however, there is a sharp increase in the number of reported cases of schizophrenia, matched by an equally dramatic decline in the numbers of multiple personality reports. Rosenbaum notes that Bleuler included multiple personality in his category of schizophrenia:

> It is not alone in hysteria that one finds an arrangement of different personalities one succeeding the other. Through similar mechanisms

schizophrenia produces different personalities existing side by side. As a matter of fact there is no need delving into those rare though most demonstrable hysterical cases, we can produce the very same through hypnosis. (Bleuler, quoted by Rosenbaum, 1980, p. 1384)

It is likely that many multiple personality patients were diagnosed as having schizophrenia during this period. Certainly, the lay public's understanding of "schizophrenia," which likewise evolved over this period, is that it is a form of "split personality" usually conceptualized along the lines of multiple personality (Bernheim & Levine, 1979). The finding that MPD patients are often misdiagnosed as suffering from schizophrenia has been replicated several times (Putnam *et al.*, 1986; Bliss, 1980; Bliss *et al.*, 1983; Bliss & Jeppsen, 1985).

It was late in this same period that the psychopharmacological revolution began with the introduction of Thorazine, followed by a host of other neuroleptic medications. The introduction of these potent medications began the movement away from the psychoanalytic treatment model toward the current biological/medical treatment paradigm. This paradigm places less emphasis on direct contact between patient and clinician as part of the therapeutic process. The resulting decrease in patient–clinician interaction may also have contributed to the decreased recognition of MPD patients, who often require a lengthy period of intimate therapy before revealing their amnesias and other dissociative experiences.

The Re-Emergence of Multiple Personality as a Separate Disorder: 1970–Present

During the 1970s, a foundation was laid upon which the current resurgence of interest in and knowledge of MPD rests. The dedication and hard work of a small number of clinicians, initially in an isolated and independent fashion but later with increasing cooperation and mutual support, re-established MPD as a legitimate clinical disorder. The old and forgotten knowledge from the time of Janet and Morton Prince was resurrected and much new information added. Laboratory investigations were begun again, and MPD became a suitable subject for doctoral dissertations, heralding a growing acceptance in the academic community (Boor & Coons, 1983). The culmination of this decade of effort came with the publication in 1980 of the DSM-III, which officially re-established the legitimacy of multiple personality and created a separate

diagnostic category for the dissociative disorders (A₁
Association, 1980a).

The new era began with the publication of Ellenbₑᵣ
extensively researched and enlightening history of the origins and ᵤ
opment of dynamic psychiatry. This impressive work of scholarship goes
far beyond a detailed historical account and presents a fascinating synthesis of the events, themes, and personalities responsible for shaping
modern psychiatry. Ellenberger devotes considerable attention to dissociation and multiple personality, both as important historical issues in
psychiatry and as clinical entities. It is in the richly detailed historical
context recreated by Ellenberger that one can best appreciate the considerable influence dissociative phenomena have had on modern thinking
about mental processes.

During the 1970s, Arnold Ludwig, Cornelia Wilbur, and their colleagues in the Department of Psychiatry at the University of Kentucky
published an important series of MPD case reports and papers on
dissociation (Larmore *et al.*, 1977; Ludwig *et al.*, 1972; Ludwig, 1966).
The case of Sybil, however, is the one most often credited with reintro-
ducing the public and the mental health professions to the syndrome of
multiple personality (Schreiber, 1974). *The Three Faces of Eve*, while
well known, gives a misleading picture of MPD and ironically may have
helped to obscure the clinical features of the disorder. The book *Sybil*,
with its graphic treatment of the amnesias, fugue episodes, child abuse,
and conflicts among alters, served as a template against which other
patients could be compared and understood. Like those of other famous
multiples before her, the case of Sybil became the subject of extensive
media attention and widespread popular recognition. Cornelia Wilbur's
long psychoanalytic therapy, supplemented by hypnosis and other therapeutic interventions, ultimately produced a successful resolution that has
served as an example for many multiples and their therapists. Although
Dr. Wilbur's paper reporting on the case of Sybil was refused by the
medical journals because of the strong prevailing disbelief in the existence of such cases at that time, Schreiber's (1974) account is both
detailed and accurate enough to serve as mandatory clinical reading for
students of MPD.

As the 1970s continued, case reports of multiple personality became
increasingly commonplace, with many of the authors taking their cue
from Ludwig *et al.* (1972) and administering standardized tests to their
patients' different alters as a form of proof of the syndrome's existence.
However, the publication and widespread adoption of the DSM-III
(American Psychiatric Association, 1980a) conferred a legitimacy upon

MPD that no other form of "proof of existence" could. The 1980s to date have seen an even more rapid growth in the numbers of cases reported, with collections of 50 or more MPD patients increasingly commonplace. In addition, a number of other related areas of interest have rapidly developed, including a literature on the experimental psychophysiological investigation of MPD; the recognition of child and adolescent forms of MPD; a variety of treatment interventions ranging from hypnosis to group therapy; and, of course, the ever-present, centuries-old literature of theory and speculation on the nature of MPD in particular and human personality in general. Future historians will be better positioned to identify the causes for the rediscovery of MPD. A number of factors and trends, however, appear to have converged at this time and are, at least in part, responsible for the dramatic renewal of interest in this age-old disorder.

The increasing interest in careful psychiatric diagnosis and nosology, which was spurred in large part by researchers' seeking to refine their study populations for purposes of determining drug specificity or identification of biological traits, led to the widespread adoption of criterion-based diagnostic classification systems. MPD patients, with their atypical mixtures of symptoms (e.g., persistent accusatory auditory hallucinations in the absence of delusions or a formal thought disorder), no longer easily fitted into these newly tightened diagnostic categories. MPD, which had long been swept into other diagnostic categories, was again highlighted as a separate and distinct disorder. The DSM-III, in particular, served to enhance the recognition of MPD in several ways. The more rigorous definitions for other disorders such as schizophrenia often served to exclude MPD patients from these catgories. The establishment of specific criteria for multiple personality, together with a good text discussion of the dissociative disorders, provided many clinicians with their first exposure to the disorder beyond the erroneous stereotype evoked by *The Three Faces of Eve*. And, as noted above, the official seal of approval conferred by the DSM-III encouraged many clinicians who had quietly treated cases to share their knowledge more openly.

During this same period, there was a parallel renewal of interest in hypnosis and dissociative models of the mind. The work of Ernest Hilgard, who formulated a "neodissociative" theory of consciousness, was particularly influential in rekindling interest in this field (Hilgard, 1977). Some of the experimental phenomena of deep hypnosis, such as the "hidden observer," first identified by Hilgard and his colleagues, have become the subject of intense interest and controversy in recent years. The data generated by hypnosis researchers have stimulated the MPD community and vice versa.

DEFINITIONAL CRITERIA FOR
MULTIPLE PERSONALITY DISORDER

Clinical Features of Multiple Personality over Time

It is instructive to read through the literature of single case reports spanning the history of multiple personality. After one has read any 10 randomly selected case reports, a "once you read one case report, you've read them all!" effect sets in. As a clinical syndrome, MPD is remarkably constant across time. The thinking and clinical acumen of Pierre Janet, Morton Prince, William James, and other early investigators seem highly relevant because their observations are so simliar to what one sees today. When viewed from this historical perspective, most of the symptoms and other phenomena associated with the core disorder have remained unchanged since the earliest case descriptions, though a few have not.

Although some of the authors of these single case reports were aware of the reports of earlier clinicians, most seem not to have been particularly well informed; they merely described, often with a degree of marked astonishment, what they witnessed occurring in their patients. Typically the patient, usually a female, was observed to undergo a sudden dramatic transformation and to present a side of herself that was greatly at odds with her previous behavior. Often this other aspect was childlike and differed from a depressed adult personality in speech, mannerisms, affect, food and other preferences, as well as in such physiological phenomena as pain sensitivity or somatic symptoms. The transitions among personalities were usually rapid and often appeared related to environmental stimuli. In some patients they might be associated with syncopal episodes or brief periods of sleep (i.e., "swoon" switches). There was usually an amnesic barrier separating the personalities, although the barrier might be polarized so that information about one personality was available to the other but not vice versa.

Thomas Mayo (1845) described a patient he treated in 1831 thus:

> She appeared to pass alternately, and in succession through two different states of mental existence, or rather, I might say, her normal state was exchanged for an abnormal one. . . . The phenomena of her abnormal state were those of extreme excitement, entirely dissimilar to her natural habit, which was dull and quiet. Under this state she made considerable progress in needle-work, and in many points of intellectual acquirement, far beyond the energy and ability of her normal condition. She became also lively and spirited in conversation. At the same time she lost her consciousness of her relation to her father and mother, and former associates, calling them by wrong names. She was,

however, at no time incoherent. On the subsidence of her abnormal state, her recollections of her father, mother, and friends, in their just relation to her, would return, and she would resume her quiet and dull character . . . (p. 1202)

More than half a century later, R. Osgood Mason (1893) wrote about his patient, Alma Z, who was under his care for 10 years:

Instead of the educated, thoughtful, dignified, womanly personality, which was usual, worn out with long-continued illness and pain, there appeared a bright, sprightly, child personality, with a limited vocabulary, ungrammatical and peculiar dialect, decidedly Indian in character, but as used by her most fascinating and amusing. The intellect was bright and shrewd, her manner lively and good natured, and her intuitions were remarkably correct and quick, but strangest of all she was free from pain, could take food and had comparatively a good degree of strength. . . . She possessed none of the acquired knowledge of the primary personality . . . (p. 594)

Two decades later, Walter F. Prince (1917) described the differences between two of Doris's personalities:

Sick Doris (S. D.) was characterized by woodenness of expression and a dull eye, when her face was in repose. Her glance was apt to be furtive, and her voice was monotonous and colorless. . . . She was reserved, half-independent and half-deprecatory, and nervous. . . . Her sense of humor was not responsive to any but the most obvious jokes, she thought in terms of the literal and concrete, and metaphorical and abstract expressions often baffled her. . . . She suffered from pains in her hip and internal organs. . . . It was startling to see the stolid, mature face of S. D. dissolve into the laughing, mischievous countenance of a young tomboy. The very shape of the face altered, and her voice was strikingly different, strident at times, at others almost infantile, full of inflections and vocal coloring. In point of view, mental habits and tastes, she was in every way juvenile, and she had some extraordinarily naive notions which are not usually carried beyond the age of five or six. (pp. 83–84)

Sixty years later, Rosenbaum and Weaver (1980) summarized the differences between two alter personalities of their patient, Sara K, who had been intermittently followed since her presentation in 1941:

Maud walked with a swinging, bouncing gait contrasted to Sara's sedate one. Whereas Sara was depressed, Maud was ebullient and happy even though suicidal. Suicide and death meant nothing to Maud. Sara stayed in her room all day and talked to no one, whereas Maud was interested in the ward, the personnel, and the patients.

Maud dressed differently. Sara had two pairs of slippers. One was a worn pair of plain grey mules; the other a pair of gaudy, [striped], high-heeled, open-toed sandals. Sara always wore the mules. Maud used gaudy makeup. Sara used none. Sara's IQ was 128, Maud's was 43. Sara did not smoke, Maud had a compulsion to smoke. Sara's sensory system was normal, but Maud had no skin sensation except touch. Maud did not know the meaning of "pain" or "hurt." Maud had no conscience, no sense of right and wrong. . . . Maud never slept and could not comprehend what sleep was. Maud was never present over-night, she would lie in bed until she changed into Sara, although Sara never changed to Maud at night. (Rosenbaum & Weaver, 1980, p. 598)

The principal types of alter personalities seen in the MPD patients of today—the depressed and depleted host or presenting personality and child alters—were repeatedly observed by clinicians over the last century and a half. Marked differences in speech, affect, mannerisms, behavior, sensory phenomena, and other somatic phenomena almost always differentiated the alter personalities. A thorough review of the case report literature will confirm that the psychiatric and medical symptoms experienced by present-day MPD patients, such as headaches, auditory hallucinations, and gastrointestinal disturbances, were commonly described by clinicians throughout the history of MPD (Putnam & Post, 1988).

Some clinical features of MPD have, however, changed over time. The most striking of these is the difference in the numbers of alter personalities reported for the earlier cases and the numbers found in modern patients. Many of the very earliest cases are dual personalities, a condition that is rarely encountered in modern patients. When more than one alter was present, usually no more than four distinct personalities were identified. An interesting trend toward increasing numbers of identified alters has appeared recently. A review of 38 case reports, meeting retrospectively applied DSM-III criteria, found an average of 3.5 alter personalities, with a range of 1–8 (Putnam & Post, 1988). Ralph Allison (1978b) reported a mean of 9.7, with a range of 1–50, and Eugene Bliss (1980) found a mean of 7.7, with a range of 2–30. Putnam et al. (1986) reported a mean of 13.3 alters for 100 independently diagnosed MPD patients, and Kluft (1984a) found an average of 13.9 alters in 33 of his MPD patients. Kluft, after adding additional cases, has recently revised his average number of alters to more than 15 alters per patient (R. P. Kluft, personal communication, 1985). Therapists reporting cases with 50 or more alters in a single patient are not unheard of, and most experienced therapists will have seen at least one or more of these complex patients.

Part of the explanation may be that modern therapists are much more willing to seek out and identify alters who do not declare themselves overtly. In reading between the lines of the earlier case reports, I am struck by the possibility that the authors were missing some alters. They often reported observing "states" that the patient would go into, in addition to the overt switches among the identified personalities. In these "states" the patient would show marked differences in behavior, often suggestive of abreactive personality fragments. The answer to this riddle is not completely obvious, however, and this trend should be monitored over time.

A second feature of multiple personality that appears to have evolved over time is the slowly emerging association of the disorder with traumatic childhood experiences. The existence of a traumatic origin, such as a parental death, for the creation of some of the alter personalities was described by Janet and Morton Prince, though the specific traumas cited are relatively mild compared to those noted in modern cases (Ellenberger, 1970; Prince, 1906). Walter F. Prince (1917) did cite some specific physical abuse episodes for his patient Doris. Goddard (1926) was the first to report sexual abuse as a possible precipitant, but strongly implied that he believed this to be a fantasy. Morselli (1930) was the first to report a history of incest in his patient, Elena F. Shortly thereafter, Lipton (1943) reported a history of prolonged incest with both father and brother in his patient, Sara K. Until the late 1970s, however, the majority of case reports did not include a history of clearly identified childhood trauma as part of the case history, though many of the early cases did identify childhood environments characterized by extremely authoritarian, religious, or perfectionistic standards (Boor, 1982).

The increasingly documented association of MPD and child abuse is probably a strong function of the recent increase in awareness of child abuse. One should remember that the "battered child syndrome," which first stimulated present-day concern about child abuse, was first described in 1962 (Kempe et al., 1962). The reported incidence of child abuse has risen dramatically over the last decade by as much as 900% in some samples (Browne & Finkelhor, 1986). The frequency with which modern-day therapists report histories of child abuse in their MPD patients, compared to the earlier clinicians, probably reflects in large measure a greater concern with child abuse in general and the increasingly well-known association between MPD and child abuse in particular.

Diagnostic Definitions of Multiple Personality

Authors of early case reports offered elaborate descriptions of their patients in order to establish the presence of the disorder. Frequently the patient described was compared to a well-known case such as Mary

Reynolds, Félida X, or "Miss Beauchamp." By the 1890s, however, a sufficient number of cases had accumulated to allow some generalizations to be drawn. In 1895, R. Osgood Mason described the characteristic features of multiple personality as follows:

> In each of these cases, from some physical cause, such as sickness, debility or shock, loss of consciousness occurred, and when consciousness returned it was found to be a consciousness altogether different from that which existed before: the patient looked, talked and acted altogether like a different person, and this new consciousness or self claimed to be an entirely independent person. (p. 420)

Morton Prince, who articulated the view held by most investigators that multiple personality was merely an extension of the dissociative process, declared in 1906:

> Multiple personality, of course, is the same thing as dissociated or what is also termed disintegrated personality, where the normal individual alternately becomes disintegrated and healthy, changing back and forth from disease to health; or, from the point of view of this study, becomes alternately a hysteric and healthy. Where there are more than two personalities, we may have two hysteric states successively changing with each other, and, it may be, with the complete healthy person. (p. 172)

Prince's viewpoint, while neatly placing multiple personality at the end of a dissociative continuum, forces the therapist to decide which of the personalities is the "healthy one" (Crabtree, 1986)—a disastrous situation from a clinical perspective. A decade later, Charles W. Stone (1916) defined cases of dual personality in this manner:

> Each personality carries along its own mental continuity, has its own character, and its own memory, which do not fuse into a concrete whole with those of the primary or other personalities. There may be an impassable gap between them. When one appears the other may be absent. The primary personality may not know what the secondary personality does, yet the secondary personality may know what the primary has done. The secondary personality may differ in character, ambitions, aims, and even in educational accomplishments from the primary, because it becomes endowed with volition, intelligence, and other mental processes, acting independently of the similar processes of the original personality. (p. 672)

Over time these early highly descriptive definitions became more abstract, so that Taylor and Martin (1944), while stating that their definition was imprecise enough that "no two students in combing the literature would draw up an identical list of cases," defined multiple personality as follows: "A case of multiple personality we take to consist of two or more personalities each of which is so well developed and integrated as to have a relatively coordinated, rich, unified, and stable life of its own" (p. 282).

Sutcliffe and Jones (1962), in their critique of the history and causes of the disorder, emphasized that "the significant alterations of personality characterizing the syndrome are loss of self-reference memories and confusions and delusions about particular identity in time and place" (p. 231). Ludwig *et al.* (1972), however, provided the definition that most authorities used until the advent of the DSM-III. They defined multiple personality as

> the presence of one or more alter personalities, each presumably possessing differing sets of values and behaviors from one another and from the "primary" personality, and each claiming varying degrees of amnesia or disinterest for one another. The appearance of these alter personalities may be on a "coconscious" basis (i.e., simultaneously coexistent with the primary personality and aware of its thoughts and feelings) or separate consciousness basis (i.e., alternating presence of the primary and alter personalities with little or no awareness or concern for the feelings and thoughts of each other), or both. (Ludwig *et al.*, 1972, pp. 298–299)

Ludwig *et al.* noted that there is some confusion in the literature about how to "count" the number of alter personalities, with some authors including trance states necessary to elicit alters and others including personalities achieved by the merger of alters. They concluded that as long as an investigator can specify criteria for regarding an alter as distinct and can provide objective evidence that it meets these criteria, it can be counted as a separate personality.

All of these definitions were eventually supplanted by the DSM-III diagnostic criteria, which borrowed liberally from earlier sources. The DSM-III established the following criteria as necessary for the diagnosis of multiple personality:

> A. The existence within the individual of two or more distinct personalities, each of which is dominant at a particular time.
> B. The personality that is dominant at any particular time determines the individual's behavior.
> C. Each individual personality is complex and integrated with its own unique behavior patterns and social relationships. (American Psychiatric Association, 1980a, p. 259)

In clinical practice, the criteria established by the DSM-III have generally worked well. The first criterion requires that the clinician determine that the patient has two or more "distinct personalities" that alternate in dominance. The specification of what constitutes "distinctness" is left to the clinician's judgment, but usually this is readily apparent and manifests itself by an array of differences in appearance, affect, cognition, speech, mannerisms, behavior, and often observable physiological responses or sensitivities. The second criterion is that "the personality that is dominant at any given time determines the individual's behavior." This is usually the rule, but instances of mixed dominance, struggles for control, and rapid switching (i.e., the "revolving-door syndrome," in which dominance cannot be clearly attributed to a given personality) do occur.

The third criterion—that *each* personality "is complex and integrated with its own unique behavior and social relationships"—is not completely fulfilled in some cases of multiple personality. This criterion requires that the complexity and consistency of a personality be manifested in social relationships, something that many secretive alters actively avoid. Personality fragments, defined as entities with a persistent sense of self and a characteristic and consistent pattern of behavior, but with a limited (compared to a personality) range of function, emotion, or history, are common (Kluft, 1984c). Many of these fragments appear only in highly specific contexts (e.g., guardian personalities who protect the body from physical injury) and would fail to meet criterion C. Thus, many patients who would benefit from being treated as cases of multiple personality could be denied this approach if this last criterion is strictly interpreted.

The DSM-III-R (American Psychiatric Association, 1987) eliminates the last criterion and defines multiple personality disorder as follows:

A. The existence within the individual of two or more distinct personalities or personality states (each with its own relatively enduring pattern of perceiving, relating to and thinking about the environment and one's self).

B. Each of these personality states at some time, and recurrently, takes full control of the individual's behavior. (p. 106)

This revision is an attempt to broaden the diagnostic criteria so that patients who may not initially meet the DSM-III criteria, but who would benefit clinically from the therapeutic approach applied to MPD, can be diagnosed and treated earlier in their life course. Time will tell whether or not these suggested revisions will prove workable.

SUMMARY

The dramatic transformations of self seen in MPD have always been a part of the human condition, though in earlier times they were associated with shamanistic ritual and demonic possession. Multiple personality emerges as one of the first mental disorders recognized during the Enlightenment. The history of interest and belief in this condition parallels that of dissociation and hypnosis described in Chapter One, with a waxing and waning of case reports over the last two centuries. The early cases bear a striking resemblance to modern ones in most aspects. As clinical knowledge accumulated, a series of syndromal definitions were refined that increasingly stressed the alternation of control over the individual's behavior by separate and distinct states of consciousness, each with a unique and enduring sense of self and a characteristic set of perceptions and behaviors.

CHAPTER THREE

Etiology, Epidemiology, and Phenomenology

ETIOLOGY

MPD appears to be a psychobiological response to a relatively specific set of experiences occurring within a circumscribed developmental window. Effective treatment of MPD requires an understanding of its traumatic precipitants and the initially adaptive role of dissociation in mitigating overwhelming trauma during childhood. Although there are competing theories of the genesis of MPD, the most compelling and clinically useful model is based on evidence that repeated childhood trauma enhances normative dissociative capacities, which in turn provide the basis for the creation and elaboration of alter personality states over time.

Historical Review

The first explanations of multiple personality assumed a supernatural etiology such as spirit possession or reincarnation (Ellenberger, 1970; Berman, 1974; Stern, 1984). These explanations were popular during the period from about 1800 to the turn of the century, and, with a few exceptions (e.g., Allison, 1978c; Stevenson & Pasricha, 1979), have largely disappeared. During the period from about 1880 to the mid-1920s, physiological explanations, often involving what would now be termed a "hemispheric disconnection syndrome," were invoked in conjunction with the then newly discovered lateralization of cerebral functions such as speech (Ellenberger, 1970; Myers, 1886; Mitchell, 1888; Kempf, 1915; Carlson, 1981, 1984). Such explanations continue to hold interest for some modern theorists (Braun, 1984d; Brende, 1984).

During the half century from about 1920 to 1970, a period associated with a marked decline in the numbers of reported cases (see

Chapter Two), psychological explanations (e.g., role playing and iatrogenic creation by hypnosis) were the commonly offered explanations (Taylor & Martin, 1944; Sutcliffe & Jones, 1962; Berman, 1974; Stern, 1984; Ellenberger, 1970). These theories remain in modified forms today (Spanos et al., 1985). State-dependent learning, first proposed as an explanation for multiple personality by Ribot (1910) in 1891, is often incorporated into many of these psychological or hypnotic models of dissociation and MPD as an explanation for the amnesias and directional awareness that characterize these conditions (Ludwig et al., 1972; Braun, 1984d; White & Shevach, 1942; Kluft, 1984a; Putnam, 1986a).

The major change in all theories of the etiology of MPD over the last decade is the recognition of the role played by traumatic experiences in the genesis of MPD and other dissociative disorders (Putnam, 1985a). With rare exceptions (e.g., Spanos et al., 1985), all current theories of the etiology and nature of MPD revolve around the traumatically induced nature of dissociative states of consciousness.

Childhood Trauma

The linkage between childhood trauma and MPD has slowly emerged in the clinical literature over the last 100 years, although this association is obvious to any clinician who has worked with several cases. The slow recognition of the relationship between MPD and childhood trauma was probably due in part to the fact that few early clinicians worked with more than one case, and in part to the lack of stringent diagnostic criteria, which led to an overlap of this population with other disorders (e.g., epilepsy, psychogenic fugue, and organic amnesias) (Coons, 1984).

The earliest case reports of multiple personality were limited to descriptions of the patients' behaviors and did not speculate on etiology. Starting in the early 1900s, a few reports implicated traumatic life experiences, such as a parental death, in the development of MPD (M. Prince, 1906; W. F. Prince, 1917; Cory, 1919). Goddard (1926) was the first to mention sexual abuse in connection with his case; however, he strongly implied that he did not believe his patient's report of incest, which he considered a "*hallucinosis incestus patris*" acquired in "a home for wayward girls" (p. 185). Morselli's (1930) patient, Elena F, recovered memories of her father's incestuous assaults during the course of violent abreactions in therapy. These memories were later confirmed by independent sources (Ellenberger, 1970). Taylor and Martin (1944), in their review of MPD written at about midcentury, noted the role of "severe conflicts" in the origin of MPD, but did not elaborate.

It was not until the 1970s, that the first reports clearly connecting MPD to childhood trauma began to appear in single case histories. Among the first and best-known was the case of Sybil, treated by Cornelia Wilbur and dramatized by Schreiber (1974). The number of cases in which childhood trauma was alleged to be a significant precipitating factor has steadily increased, in parallel with the increasing recognition of the disorder (Greaves, 1980; Bliss, 1980; Boor, 1982; Wilbur, 1984a; Saltman & Solomon, 1982; Coons & Milstein, 1984).

The National Institute of Mental Health (NIMH) survey of 100 MPD cases found that 97% of all MPD patients reported experiencing significant trauma in childhood (Putnam et al., 1986). Incest was the most commonly reported trauma (68%), but other forms of sexual abuse, physical abuse, and a variety of forms of emotional abuse were reported. Figure 3-1 shows the types of childhood trauma retrospectively reported by MPD patients in the NIMH survey.

Most patients reported experiencing three or more different types of trauma during childhood. For example, some combinations of sexual abuse and physical abuse was reported by two-thirds of the NIMH survey patients. Coons and Milstein (1984) report a history of sexual abuse in 75% of their 20 MPD patients and a history of physical abuse in 50%, with an overall 85% incidence of child abuse in their sample.

To date, it has not been proven that childhood trauma *causes* MPD. In most reports, including the NIMH survey, there is no outside verification that any trauma actually occurred. An independent verification of alleged abuse, which often occurred 10 or more years prior to being reported in therapy, is almost impossible for the average therapist to obtain. R. P. Kluft (personal communication, 1986) has reported being able to verify through independent sources some of the traumas reported by his patients. Bliss (1984a) also reports being able to establish the veracity of retrospective reports of abuse in a subset of his MPD patients. Current work with child multiples, in whom the trauma can often be more easily documented, should soon provide the data necessary to establish an unequivocal association between MPD and childhood trauma. In the meantime, no therapist who has worked with more than two or three multiples doubts the existence of a causal relationship between MPD and childhood trauma, primarily child abuse.

Child Abuse

Sexual abuse is the most frequently reported type of childhood trauma in MPD patients (see Figure 3-1). The most commonly reported form of sexual abuse is incest (Putnam et al., 1986; Saltman & Solomon, 1982).

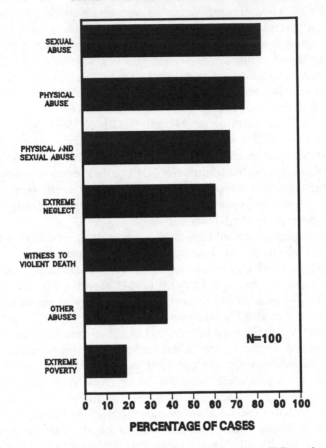

Figure 3-1. Types of childhood trauma reported by 100 MPD patients in the NIMH survey. Adapted from Putnam *et al.* (1986).

In most instances, this is father–daughter incest or stepfather–stepdaughter incest, though mother–daughter, mother–son, and older sibling–younger sibling incest have also been reported. The active incestual involvement of both parents and/or siblings with the MPD victim appears to be a more common occurrence than with child sex abuse victims who do not have MPD, but the data are scanty and may be misleading. Single episodes of sexual molestation or rape during childhood were reported by 15% of MPD patients in the NIMH survey (Putnam *et al.*, 1986). In addition to the various combinations of oral, genital, and anal sexual contact, enemas, douches, and other "hygiene" preparations and utensils are frequently used in sexually and physically abusive ways with these patients.

In comparing the descriptions of sexual abuse that I have heard from MPD patients with those of other sex abuse victims, I am struck by the quality of extreme sadism that is frequently reported by most MPD victims. Bondage situations; the insertion of a variety of instruments into vagina, mouth, and anus; and various forms of physical and sexual torture are common reports. Many multiples have told me of being sexually abused by groups of people, of being forced into prostitution by family members, or of being offered as a sexual enticement to their mothers' boyfriends. After one has worked with a number of MPD patients, it becomes obvious that severe, sustained, and repetitive child sexual abuse is a major element in the creation of MPD.

Some form of physical abuse was reported by approximately three-quarters of MPD patients in the NIMII survey (Figure 3-1). Such abuse may range from beatings with hands or fists and kicking to bizarre forms of torture. Assaults with implements, burning by matches or steam irons, and cuttings with razor blades or glass are commonly reported by MPD patients. Many patients report that the physical abuse would be inflicted in ritualized ways by their abusers, who often offered explanations that they were "cleansing" or "purifying" the children in some fashion. Some multiples report being used in "Black Masses" and other Satanic rituals. Again, it is my impression that the abuse suffered by multiple personality patients tends to be far more sadistic and bizarre than that suffered by most victims of child abuse.

Confinement abuses seem to be exceptionally common in the retrospective accounts of MPD patients. This form of abuse involves the repeated confinement of a child through various means, such as tying the child up; locking the child in closets, cellars, or trunks; stuffing the child in boxes or bags; or even burying the child alive. Wilbur (1984a) has reported a case in which her patient was buried alive with a stove pipe over his face to provide air. The abuser then urinated down the stove pipe onto the child's face. I have seen two patients who reported being repeatedly buried for long periods as punishment. I believe that confinement abuses, which repeatedly subject a terrified child to prolonged periods of isolation and sensory deprivation, may specifically contribute to the development of a chronic dissociative process such as MPD.

Various forms of emotional abuse are reported by multiples. Ridicule, demeanment, and denigration were often systematically inflicted upon them as children. Even when actual physical abuse was not inflicted, the children may have been ceaselessly intimidated by threats of violent punishments or other abuses. Valued possessions and even pets may have been destroyed in front of the children as an example of what was going to happen to them. In some instances, MPD patients report that although they were not directly abused themselves, they were made to witness the physical and/or sexual abuse of siblings. The children may also have been secluded and forbidden to have playmates or other nonschool contact with peers. They may have been denied an opportunity to learn or practice skills or basic health care.

Nonabusive Traumas

One finding from the NIMH survey that surprised us was the number of MPD patients who, during childhood, reportedly witnessed the violent death of a relative or close friend (Putnam *et al.*, 1986). In many of these instances, a child was present when one parent killed the other. Some MPD patients report seeing an abused sibling die at the hands of a parent. The data on family psychopathology of MPD patients are scanty, but strongly suggest that these patients grew up in highly disturbed homes where domestic violence was common (Putnam *et al.*, 1986; Braun, 1985).

I have seen several cases of MPD in children and adolescents who came from war zones, such as Cambodia and Lebanon. In each case, the child had witnessed the massacre of several family members through military or terrorist actions. One adolescent multiple, for example, reported seeing her parents blown to bits in a minefield and trying to piece their bodies back together. This same child later witnessed her grandfather being shot to death and a sibling being beheaded. Another child reported seeing her family crushed to death when a tank ran over their car.

In rare instances, sustained pain or debilitating injury seems to have provided the traumatic stimulus necessary to provoke chronic dissociation. In one case, the patient was confined to a series of body casts for several years and underwent repeated surgery. The deprivation, isolation, chronic pain, and discomfort, together with the depersonalization produced by being unable to move his body, were traumatic experiences that this patient divided up among his alters. Near-death experiences (e.g., drowning and resuscitation) have also been associated with the subsequent development of MPD (Kluft, 1984b).

A Developmental Model of Multiple Personality

Over the last two centuries, dissociative disorders have spawned a large number of theories to account for the disturbances of self and memory seen in these conditions. Many of the eminent figures in psychology and psychiatry of the last century used multiple personality as the centerpiece for their particular organizational model of the mind. Today, MPD continues to stimulate theorizing and modeling on a wide array of fronts (Andorfer, 1985; Bliss, 1986; Braun & Sachs, 1985; Brende, 1984; Kluft, 1984a; Putnam, 1986a; Spanos *et al.*, 1985). The following is my contribution to the genre.

Normative Substrates

I think that the evidence suggests that we are all born with the potential for multiple personalities and over the course of normal development we more or less succeed in consolidating an integrated sense of self. We are not born as multiple personalities, because personality is acquired and manifested over time; rather, at birth, our behavior is organized into a series of discrete states. Behavioral states of consciousness have, in fact, emerged as the essential ordering principle for all infant studies (Wolff, 1987). Starting with the work of Prechtl and his colleagues (Prechtl *et al.*, 1973; Prechtl & O'Brien, 1982), infant consciousness researchers have evolved an agreed-upon taxonomy of newborn infant behavioral states (Wolff, 1987). The transitions between infant behavioral states exhibit psychophysiological properties that are highly similar to those observed across switches of alter personalities in MPD (Putnam, 1988c).

As the child grows, additional behavioral states are added and the transitions between states are smoothed out, so that it becomes increasingly difficult to identify discrete behavioral states in children older than a year (Emde *et al.*, 1976). In adults, discrete behavioral states are most clearly manifested in certain psychiatric conditions, such as the affective states seen in mood disorders or the anxiety states seen in the anxiety and phobic neuroses. Again, the switches between affective states and the onset–offset of anxiety states exhibit many of the psychophysiological principles observed in infant behavioral state transitions and the switches of MPD alter personality states (Putnam, 1988c).

One can postulate that among the many developmental tasks that we face in the course of growing up are consolidating self and identity across behavioral states and learning to modulate transitions among behavioral states. We see evidence of progress in these developmental tasks as children manifest increasing attention spans (i.e., the ability to sustain a given state longer) and a more unified sense of self across contextual changes, the adolescent identity crisis notwithstanding.

A second normative process that most authorities believe contributes to the development of MPD is the propensity of children to enter into a specific kind of state of consciousness, the dissociative state (Put-

nam, 1985a). Dissociative states are characterized by significant alterations in the integrative functions of memory for thoughts, feelings, or
actions, and significant alterations in sense of self (Ludwig, 1983; Nemiah, 1981). The tendency to enter spontaneous dissociative states is
thought to be related to the capacity to enter voluntary hypnotic states
(Bliss, 1980, 1986; Hilgard, 1977; Kluft, 1984a; Zamansky & Bartis,
1984). Eve Carlson and I found a very high correlation between scores on
our Dissociative Experiences Scale, which measures spontaneously occurring dissociative experiences, and on the Stanford Hypnotic Susceptibility Scale, Form C (Carlson & Putnam, 1988).

Studies on the hypnotic susceptibility of children indicate that, as a
group, children are significantly more hypnotizable than adults (Ambrose, 1961; Gardner & Olness, 1981; London, 1965; London & Cooper,
1969). Some cross-sectional studies suggest that there is a curvilinear
relationship between hypnotizability and age. Hypnotic capacity rises
during childhood, peaks at about age 9–10, and declines during adolescence to stabilize at adult levels (Gardner, 1974, 1977; Place, 1984;
Williams, 1981). Thus, if hypnotizability is associated with a propensity
to use dissociation to cope with stress, then children, with their higher
level of hypnotizability, may be more likely to or more easily able to
invoke dissociative states as defenses against overwhelming trauma.

A third normative developmental substrate that may play a role in
the genesis of MPD is the capacity of children for fantasy in general, and
the ability to project "personality" into objects and situations in particular. Imaginary companionship is a personification of this ability. Most
investigators regard it as a normal developmental phenomenon, though
there is some disagreement over the ages during which it is most common
(Harriman, 1937; Hurlock & Burstein, 1932; Nagera, 1969). There is also
some disagreement over the purpose(s) of imaginary companionship, but
among the suggested functions are dealing with fears (Baum, 1978),
serving as a scapegoat or as an auxiliary superego (Nagera, 1969), and
acting as a form of transitional object (Benson & Pryor, 1973).

The relationship of imaginary companions to MPD is tantalizing
but ambiguous. Alter personalities sometimes report that they first arose
as imaginary companions but later took on a life of their own when the
child was unable to cope with abuse or some other trauma. Lovinger
(1983) believes that imaginary companions become alter personalities
when the child is not able to complete specific developmental tasks
because of a traumatic environment. These tasks include development of
self-criticism; maintenance of self-esteem and love; creation of a division
between drives and urges; development of reason and judgment; and the
borrowing of parental attitudes toward behavior. Braun and Braun

(1979) and Bliss (1983) have suggested that alter personalities evolve from imaginary companions originally created to help the child through the deprivation associated with abuse. Myers (1976) has described the reactivation in adulthood of imaginary companions created to deal with childhood traumas.

The Role of Trauma

The severe, sustained, and repetitive trauma that occurs during the early to middle childhood of most victims is thought to promote the development of MPD through several interconnected mechanisms. The first is a disruption of the developmental tasks of consolidation of self across behavioral states and the acquisition of control over the modulation of states. The recurring trauma (generally child abuse) instead creates a situation in which it is adaptive for the child to heighten the separation between behavioral states, in order to compartmentalize overwhelming affects and memories generated by the trauma. In particular, children may use their enhanced dissociative capacity to escape from the trauma by specifically entering into dissociative states. Dissociative states of consciousness have long been recognized as adaptive responses to acute trauma, because they provide (1) escape from the constraints of reality; (2) containment of traumatic memories and affects outside of normal conscious awareness; (3) alteration or detachment of sense of self (so that the trauma happens to someone else or to a depersonalized self); and (4) analgesia.

In most MPD cases, the abuse is inflicted on the child by a parent or other caretaking figure. One of the most important tasks of a caretaker, particularly in early childhood, is helping the infant or toddler to enter and sustain a behavioral state that is appropriate for the circumstances. One only has to watch good parents feeding a toddler in public to see how they help their child achieve and maintain an appropriate state and how they suppress inappropriate states or help the child recover from disruptions of state. It is easy to speculate that the bad parenting accompanying abuse fails to aid the child in learning to modulate behavioral states.

The Elaboration of Alter Personalities

There appear to be several forms of MPD-like dissociative reactions in traumatized children. Using their heightened fantasy capacities, children quickly endow dissociative states with psychological and physical attributes associated with feelings and body images evoked by the trauma.

Some children, particularly younger children, appear to have external-ized "imaginary companionship" systems of alter personalities who are experienced by the child as outside influences. Often these externalized systems are composed of cartoon characters, superheroes, animals, an-gels, dwarfs, genies, or even machines. The choice of metaphor for a given child's system is often easily traceable in therapy. Some children with externalized alter personality systems appear to internalize the systems during puberty. Other children appear to have systems of inter-nalized alter personalities from the beginning.

One can conceive of these dissociated states, each imbued with a specific sense of self, being elaborated over time as the child repeatedly re-enters a given state to escape from trauma or to execute behaviors that he or she is unable to perform in normal consciousness. Each time the child re-enters a specific dissociative state, additional memories, affects, and behaviors become state-dependently bound to that state, building up a "life history" for the alter personality. The number of different alter personalities in adult MPD victims is significantly correlated with the number of different kinds of trauma suffered in childhood (Putnam *et al.*, 1986), suggesting that a child enters into different dissociative states depending upon the circumstances. The transitions between alter personality states (switches) closely resemble those seen between infant behavioral states, because the normal integrative and state-modulating mechanisms have failed to develop fully, leaving the MPD victim depen-dent on more developmentally primitive mechanisms.

Thus we all start out in infancy with our behavior organized into a series of discrete states, but with time and healthy caretakers' help, we learn to modulate our behavioral states and to extend our sense of self across different contexts and demands to develop what we experience as a unified personality. Victims of MPD, however, travel another develop-mental route. Rather than integrating a self across a variety of behavioral states, they create multiple "selves" by elaborating a series of dissociative states into alter personalities. In the context of the trauma, this is a life-saving solution for an otherwise powerless child. It becomes maladaptive, however, in an adult world that stresses continuity of memory, behavior, and sense of self.

EPIDEMIOLOGY AND DEMOGRAPHICS

Epidemiology is the study of the occurrence and distribution of an illness. To date, there have been no large-scale studies of the epidemiology of MPD or of any of the other DSM-III dissociative disorders. The only dissociative phenomena that have received systematic surveys of incidence and/or prevalence are feelings of depersonalization and hypnotic susceptibility. Many of the patients included in surveys of feelings of depersonalization would probably not meet DSM-III/DSM-III-R criteria for depersonalization disorder. The data on these two dissociative phenomena suggest that both exist along a continuum of intensity or capacity for depth and are widely distributed in normal subjects and psychiatric patients (Putnam 1985a; Bernstein & Putnam, 1986). The little information that we do have on the incidence, prevalence, and distribution of MPD is based on descriptive clinical lore, anecdotes, and a few extrapolations based on the numbers of MPD cases diagnosed in circumscribed settings.

Several "guesstimates" of the number of MPD cases in the United States have been offered (Braun, 1984a; Horevitz, 1983; Coons, 1984). These and similar unpublished estimates suggest that the number of MPD cases in the United States may well number in the thousands Eugene Bliss (Bliss et al., 1983; Bliss & Jeppsen, 1985; Bliss & Larson, 1985) and his colleagues are the only investigators who have attempted to sample psychiatric and criminal populations for patients meeting criteria for MPD.

All of these "guesstimates" and Bliss's surveys suffer from significant methodological limitations that preclude any large-scale generalizations about the overall incidence or prevalence of MPD. These scanty data do, however, suggest that although MPD has been generally viewed by the mental health professions as an extremely rare condition, it may be more prevalent than is generally realized. It is hoped that screening for MPD and other dissociative disorders can be incorporated into some of the large mental health epidemiological studies planned for the future.

The data available on the demographics of patients with MPD are more substantial and show some interesting trends. There are three major sources for these data: (1) statistics derived from reviews of case reports in the literature; (2) statistics from case series reported by individual clinicians; and (3) surveys of cases in treatment with different therapists. In general, there is a high degree of agreement among these different sources of data as to the gender ratios, age at time of diagnosis, presenting symptoms, and past psychiatric history (Putnam, 1986b).

Gender

The overwhelming majority of cases of MPD recorded to date occur in women, with the female-to-male ratios commonly running 5:1 or better

(Allison, 1978b; Bliss, 1980, 1984b; Bliss & Jeppsen, 1985; Solomon, 1983; Coons & Sterne, 1986; Putnam *et al.*, 1986; Stern, 1984). A few investigators have reported ratios as low as 2:1 or 3:1 (Horevitz & Braun, 1984; Kluft, 1984a). The question arises as to why this disorder appears to be more common in women. A number of different explanations have been tendered. MPD may be a genetic disorder with sex-linked characteristics. Cultural determinants may, according to some authors, influence women to "choose" this expression of psychological defense or psychopathology rather than another form (Berman, 1974). The higher incidence in women may also reflect the fact that females are at higher risk for physical and sexual abuse over a longer period of time than are males. Or, because of a sampling bias, we may be missing many male cases of MPD and the actual gender ratio may be closer to 1:1.

Male MPD patients may be escaping detection because they exhibit a form of MPD that differs from the "classic" presentation that is largely derived from experience with female patients. There appear to be some differences between male and female MPD patients (see Chapter Five). It is also possible that male MPD cases are missed because they are not seen in the mental health system, but are being handled in other ways. As noted earlier (see Chapter One), the most commonly expressed speculation is that because male MPD patients are more likely to express their violence outwardly, as compared to the more often self-directed violence of female MPD patients, the males are ending up in the criminal justice system rather than the mental health system (Wilbur, 1985; Putnam *et al.*, 1984; Bliss, 1983). The Bliss and Larson (1985) study found a high rate of MPD and dissociative experiences among convicted sexual offenders, suggesting that there may be a considerable population of MPD victims in the criminal justice system. A more systematic exploration of this possibility should be undertaken.

Age

There is also a remarkable degree of agreement among various sources of information as to the average age of MPD patients at the time of diagnosis. A review of the literature found a mean age at diagnosis of 28.5 years (Putnam & Post, 1988). A number of case series reported an average age at diagnosis between 29.4 years and 34.5 years (Allison, 1978a; Bliss, 1980; Coons & Sterne, 1986; Horevitz & Braun, 1984; Kluft, 1984a; Putnam *et al.*, 1986).

Although there is strong evidence that MPD begins in childhood, it appears as if most patients with MPD are not diagnosed until their third or fourth decade, although many will already have an extensive psychiatric history with a plethora of misdiagnoses prior to the diagnosis of MPD. Intriguing cross-sectional data on the life course of MPD patients presented by Kluft (1985a) suggest that the clinical presentation of MPD varies with age and that the most floridly "multiple" clinical presentations typically occur during the third and fourth decades. This may explain the remarkable uniformity of age at diagnosis reported across a variety of patient samples.

Ethnic and Socioeconomic Status

The data on ethnic and socioeconomic status are scanty, but sufficient to allow one to conclude that MPD occurs across all major racial groups and socioeconomic settings. Although most cases involve whites, black (Ludwig *et al.*, 1972; Solomon, 1983; Stern, 1984; Coons & Sterne, 1986) and Hispanic (Allison, 1978a; Solomon, 1983) MPD victims have been described. About 13% of the cases that I have evaluated have been blacks, and about 2% involved Orientals (primarily victims of the Cambodian holocaust). Cross-cultural case reports are scarce, but cases do exist in non-Western settings (Alexander, 1956; Varma *et al.*, 1981). The data on socioeconomic status indicate that MPD can be found in all walks of life (Coons & Sterne, 1986; Stern, 1984; Solomon, 1983; Putnam *et al.*, 1986).

SYMPTOM PROFILE

Introduction

Recognizing and diagnosing MPD can be a difficult task. For a variety of reasons, including a widespread professional skepticism about the very existence of MPD, most clinicians do not receive sufficient information about this disorder during their formative training years. Multiple personality, while not as rare as previously supposed, is uncommon, and consequently clinical exposure to it is limited for most professionals. MPD is seldom included on the standard lists of differential diagnoses for the major psychiatric disorders, so that it rarely comes to mind when clinicians are considering which conditions to rule out in a patient. For these and other reasons, the possibility that a patient may be suffering from MPD often simply does not occur to many clinicians.

There is a patient profile, however, that should suggest MPD. The core features of this profile are that these patients typically suffer from a profusion of psychiatric, neurological, and medical symptoms; have received a host of diagnoses; and are refractory to the standard treatments for these diagnoses (Putnam *et al.*, 1984, 1986; Kluft, 1985a). Bliss (1984b) has described this phenomenon as a "superabundance of symptoms," and Coons (1984) has characterized it as a "multiplicity of symptoms." Unfortunately, this profusion of symptoms, which may be suggestive of a wide range of psychiatric disorders, usually obscures the underlying dissociative pathology, so that these patients often spend years in treatment for conditons they do not have.

The following discussion serves to highlight the most commonly reported symptoms in MPD patients. In order to detect MPD in a patient, it is important to look beneath the superficial expression of a given symptom for possible dissociative dynamics underlying the process. For example, a presenting complaint of "depression" from a multiple may on first evaluation appear to be a run-of-the-mill neurotic depression. The dynamics contributing to the patient's experience of helplessness and hopelessness are, however, very different. The MPD patient may feel powerless to influence or change his or her life, because he or she is continually confronted with painful evidence that his or her behavior is *not* under "conscious" control.

Psychiatric Symptoms

Depressive Symptoms

The single most common presenting symptom in MPD patients is depression (Allison, 1978b; Coons, 1984; Bliss, 1984b; O'Brien, 1985; Putnam *et al.*, 1986). Presenting symptoms suggestive of depression were seen in 88% of the cases in the NIMH survey (Putnam *et al.*, 1986) and comprised the single most common presentation in case series reported by Bliss (1984b) and Coons (1984). In addition to depressed mood, several other symptoms commonly reported in MPD patients would superficially appear to reinforce the diagnosis of a major affective disorder. About three-quarters of presenting MPD patients will describe themselves as having "mood swings" or sudden changes in the way they feel or behave (Coons, 1984; Bliss, 1984b; Putnam *et al.*, 1986). Frequently there is a history of one or more suicide attempts or gestures, and suicidal or self-destructive ideation is present (Bliss, 1980, 1984b; Coons, 1984; Putnam *et al.*, 1986). The typical "host" personality initially presenting for treatment usually has low self-esteem, is overwhelmed and anhedonic, and generally expresses a negative outlook toward life. MPD patients may also report difficulty in concentrating, fatigue, sexual difficulties, and crying spells.

Insomnia or other sleep disturbance is a commonly noted feature of MPD (Putnam *et al.*, 1986). Careful inquiry, however, will reveal that this sleep disorder is not the difficulty falling asleep or early-morning awakening seen in anxiety disorders or depression. Rather, it is the type of sleep disturbance noted in posttraumatic stress syndromes, with recurrent nightmares and terrifying hypnagogic and hypnopompic phenomena. Unfortunately, most MPD patients will not voluntarily report the cause of their sleep disturbance, and many therapists fail to ask for more information.

Taken together, the symptoms just described are superficially suggestive of a major affective disorder. A careful history taken with the possibility of a dissociative disorder in mind, however, can often uncover evidence of atypical features that help differentiate the depressive symptoms seen in MPD from those found in major depression. In MPD, the depressive symptoms are rarely sustained for any length of time. The patient may be able to provide a history of periods of feeling good or even happy, interspersed among the periods of depression. The mood swings are too frequent to be due to any but the most rapidly cycling bipolar disorder. Typically, the patient may experience several "mood swings" within a day, and even doing so several times within an hour is not uncommon. Sometimes the patient may not provide any history of precipitous shifts in mood, but family members may comment on this, sometimes as directly as this: "Doctor, some days she's just a different person!" Vegetative signs tend to be short-lived or absent in MPD patients with depressive presentations, as opposed to patients with a major depressive disorder.

Dissociative Symptoms

Multiple personality is the ultimate dissociative disorder, and all MPD patients suffer from a variety of dissociative symptoms. They do not, however, usually first present with complaints directly referrable to dissociation. On the contrary, in many cases it requires several months or more of contact before the patient will begin to discuss these symptoms with the therapist. Amnesia or "time loss" is the single most common dissociative symptom in MPD patients (Coons, 1984; Bliss, 1984b; Putnam *et al.*, 1986). The NIMH survey study found that the most commonly reported dissociative symptoms in MPD patients were as follows: amnesias (98%), fugue episodes (55%), feelings of depersonalization

(53%), and sleepwalking (20%) (Putnam *et al.*, 1986). Bliss (1984b) describes essentially the same dissociative profile, led by amnesias (85%), dazed states (83%), depersonalization (54%), derealization (54%), and fugue states (52%).

There seem to be several converging dynamics that keep patients from volunteering information about their dissociative symptoms. The most important reason is that the dissociative experiences themselves produce a disturbance of memory and recall that often prevents a patient from easily recalling the experiences. As Dr. Bennett Braun has pithily observed, "You can have amnesia for your amnesia." Even if the patient is not completely amnesic for all of his or her dissociative episodes, the dissociative process still produces a distortion of recall so that memories of a dissociative episode (e.g., a fugue) may have a distant, detached, and dreamlike quality that makes the patient question whether or not the experience actually occurred.

When patients can directly remember dissociative episodes, they are often reluctant to report them for other reasons. They may be concerned that they will be considered "crazy" and discounted or even committed to a hospital. MPD begins in childhood, and dissociative experiences are not new for these patients. In fact, they have been "losing time" and finding themselves in strange places with some regularity all of their lives. They may not consider these experiences to be unusual, and therefore do not offer them as presenting complaints. MPD patients may also attribute their dissociative experiences to another cause—for example, drug or alcohol blackouts. These other explanations are attractive because they allow the patients to explain these experiences to themselves and others in a more socially accepted fashion. To test for the presence of dissociative symptoms, the diagnosing clinician must systematically inquire about a specific range of experiences that are the consequences of dissociative psychopathology. These special questions about dissociative history and mental status are covered in Chapter Four.

Anxiety and Phobic Symptoms

Symptoms suggestive of phobic, anxiety, or panic disorders are often present in MPD patients and may be part of the initial clinical picture (Coons, 1984; Bliss, 1984b; Putnam *et al.*, 1986). Again, the dynamics underlying these symptoms may be peculiarly dissociative and must be looked for. Attacks of anxiety in the host personality often accompany the switching to other alter personalities. The host may experience somatic symptoms such as dyspnea, palpitations, sensations of choking or smothering, feelings of unreality, paresthesias, faintness, and trembling prior to and during a personality switch. The "cued" aspect of alter personality switches may also give rise to phobic-like behavior, in that certain places, objects, social situations, words, or other emotionally charged stimuli may trigger switches to frightened alter personalities or elicit flashbacks of traumatic memories (Putnam, 1988c). Many MPD patients learn to avoid these triggers and thus behave in a phobic manner toward them.

Substance Abuse

Substance abuse is frequently seen in MPD (Coons, 1984; Putnam *et al.*, 1986). Polydrug abuse was noted in a third of the patients in the NIMH survey (Putnam *et al.*, 1986). Sedatives and hypnotics appear to be the medications most commonly abused by multiples (Coons, 1984; Putnam *et al.*, 1986). Alcohol and stimulant abuse was reported in about a third of the NIMH survey cases. Hallucinogens do not appear to be popular with MPD patients. Coons (1984) has found that drug abuse often begins with abuse of analgesics prescribed for the frequent headaches noted in MPD patients.

Since nondissociative polydrug abusers share many of the symptoms and complaints reported by MPD patients (including depression, sleep disturbances, poor self-esteem, anxiety attacks, multiple somatic complaints, and, importantly, blackouts), the evaluating clinician must carefully determine whether or not substance abuse is *always* associated with blackout episodes. Unfortunately, many MPD patients would rather admit to the more socially acceptable drug or alcohol blackouts than admit that they do not really know the reason why they "lose time."

Hallucinations

The majority of MPD patients will experience auditory and/or visual hallucinations, though they will seldom admit to these experiences early in therapy (Bliss *et al.*, 1983; Coons, 1984; Putnam *et al.*, 1986). Auditory hallucinations typically include voices that berate and belittle the patient (usually the host personality) or command the patient to commit self-destructive or violent acts. The voices may discuss the patient in the third person, commenting on his or her thoughts or actions, or may argue among themselves. The patient may hear crying, screaming, or laughter. Typically, the crying sounds like an infant or small child in distress. There may also be voices that give solace, support, or advice (Putnam et al., 1984).

Almost always, the voices are described as being "heard" within the patient's head or experienced as "loud thoughts." They are usually heard clearly and distinctly (Coons, 1984). These features can help to distinguish them from the auditory hallucinations found in schizophrenic patients, which are more often (but certainly not always) experienced as emanating from outside of the person and are often heard indistinctly. The hallucinatory voices of MPD patients often carry on lengthy discussions that seem coherent and logical to the patient. This "secondary-process" quality can help to distinguish them from the more "primary-process" voices reported by schizophrenic patients. If, as is generally the case, the presenting personality is unaware of the existence of other alter personalities, hearing these voices can be a terrifying experience.

The visual hallucinations reported in MPD are a curious blend of hallucination and illusion and frequently include changes in the patient's perceived body image. MPD patients often report seeing themselves as different people when they look into a mirror. They may see themselves as having hair, eyes, or skin of a different color, or as being of the opposite sex. In some instances, these alterations of perception of self are so disturbing that the individuals may phobically avoid mirrors. They may describe seeing themselves sequentially change into several different people while looking into a mirror. MPD patients may also hallucinate their alter personalities as separate people existing outside of their bodies. This experience is common enough that it has been incorporated into David Caul's internal group therapy treatment techniques (Caul, 1984); these techniques are discussed in Chapter Ten.

MPD patients may report autoscopic hallucinations, such as seeing themselves as if they were watching a movie or looking down at themselves from above. These out-of-body experiences are usually accompanied by feelings of profound depersonalization and are similar to experiences described in near-death situations by some individuals. Disembodied faces floating in air or projected onto other people are reported frequently by MPD patients. They may hallucinate blood, hideous scenes, or other evidence of violence at times. This last form of hallucination may occur in therapy and is typically associated with the emergence of material related to past traumatic experiences. Olfactory and tactile hallucinations are reported in 5–12% of cases and are more common in MPD patients with temporal lobe abnormalities as documented by electroencephalograms (EEGs) (Putnam, 1986a). MPD patients, however, will often experience many "somatic memories" associated with abusive or traumatic experiences that can be mistaken for tactile hallucinations.

Thought Disorder

At times, MPD patients may appear to have a profound thought disorder. This is caused by a dissociative phenomenon known as "rapid switching" or the "revolving-door crisis," which occurs when no single alter personality is able to gain and maintain control over the patient's behavior. The revolving-door phenomenon often follows and further contributes to a personal crisis by producing a marked psychosis-like picture. The patient appears to be extremely affectively labile, typically cycling rapidly through a wide range of inappropriate emotions. The patient will appear to have signs of a major thought disorder, including blocking, thought withdrawal, and "word salad" speech. In a revolving-door crisis, the patient may exhibit extreme ambivalence, doing and undoing some act in a psychotic or perseverative fashion.

What is happening is that the patient is failing to stabilize in a single alter personality state long enough to carry on coherent and integrated behavior. A series of alters are whizzing by, and the lability, incoherence, and ambivalence manifested by the patient represents the sum total of his or her often incompatible affects and behaviors. Rapid cycling may represent a struggle among alters for control of behavior, each attempting to displace the others; or it may be caused by an abandonment of control, during which the major personalities have surrendered executive control and other alters, often unwillingly, are being thrust into this vacuum. Probably the most important feature that distinguishes this presentation from a true thought disorder is that it is usually transient and can be related to a specific crisis. MPD patients do not show a true sustained thought disorder, such as is often found in schizophrenia (Coons, 1984; Putnam et al., 1984). A more extensive discussion of revolving-door crises follows in Chapter Eleven.

Delusions

Experienced therapists differ on whether or not MPD patients suffer from delusions. Sutcliffe and Jones (1962) characterized the syndrome as a delusion of identity in time and place. Others have termed this phenomenon a "quasi-delusion" (Coons, 1984) or a "pseudodelusion" (Kluft,

1984c). Bliss (1984b) reported that paranoid delusions occurred in roughly a third of his cases, and the NIMH study found delusions reported in 20% of surveyed cases (Putnam *et al.*, 1986). The crux of this issue, however, is the definition of a delusion and how this is applied to the convictions of independence and autonomy held by some alter personalities. Many alters exhibit a fixed belief that they are separate and can physically harm another personality without injury to themselves. My opinion is that the intensity and incontrovertibility of this manifestly false belief often qualify it as a delusion.

MPD patients may present with apparent delusions of being controlled. There is a valid basis to this experience, as many host personalities are passively influenced by other alters and at times find themselves, against their will, behaving in a manner that is repugnant to them. The alterations in body image that often accompany the transitions among personalities (e.g., feeling and seeing one's self as a small child) can be misinterpreted as somatic delusions by therapists unaware of the alter personalities.

Often, what appears to be a delusion turns out to have a basis in fact when the therapist begins to understand the dynamics of the patient's dissociative psychopathology. Although some MPD patients undoubtedly have ideas that qualify as delusional, one rarely finds that these delusions are of the type frequently seen in paranoid disorders, where the patient believes that some external agency (e.g., the government, the Russians, aliens from Mars, etc.) is persecuting them or sending them messages through the media or in other ways. The delusions of MPD are most often those of passive-influence experiences, which have a basis in fact, or delusions of separateness secondary to the excessive narcissistic investments of some alters in their individuality.

Suicidal and Self-Mutilative Symptoms

Suicidal behavior is extremely common in MPD patients (Greaves, 1980; Bliss, 1980, 1984b; Coons, 1984; Putnam *et al.*, 1986). Both Bliss (1980, 1984b) and the NIMH survey (Putnam *et al.*, 1986) found that at least three-quarters of MPD patients had made one or more serious suicide attempts. Self-mutilation—typically cutting with glass or razor blades, or burning with cigarettes or matches—occurs in at least a third of MPD patients (Putnam *et al.*, 1986). The percentage of self-mutilators is probably much higher, because this behavior is often not reported to therapists and is rarely spontaneously discovered except by physical examination. The mutilation may also take bizarre forms, such as insertion of broken glass or other foreign objects into the vagina (Riggall, 1931; Bliss & Bliss, 1985).

Catatonia

Catatonic behavior may occur at times with MPD patients (Putnam *et al.*, 1984). The NIMH survey found this symptom present in about 14% of cases (Putnam *et al.*, 1986). A number of MPD patients have described to me going into a catatonic state when they were overwhelmed by outside stimuli that triggered massive recall of traumatic experiences. They have also described using the catatonic state as a form of healing experience that filtered out or slowed down overwhelming stimuli to a tolerable level.

Transsexualism and Transvestism

Patients with MPD may compose a sizeable percentage of cases of transsexualism and transvestism. To date, however, there are only a few case reports of transsexuals with MPD-like features (Green & Money, 1969; Money, 1974; Weitzman *et al.*, 1970; Money & Primrose, 1968; Lief *et al.*, 1962). It is not clear from the accounts whether these patients would meet full syndromal criteria for MPD. A sizeable percentage of multiples have alter personalities who perceive themselves to be of the opposite sex from the patients' biological gender (Putnam *et al.*, 1986). In several cases with which I am familiar, an alter personality has sought a sex-change operation or has mutilated the person's genitals in a crude attempt to change the body's sex. A careful survey of dissociative symptoms should be conducted with transsexuals and transvestites to determine whether unrecognized MPD is a primary motivation for these behaviors in a subgroup of this population.

Neurological and Medical Symptoms

Headache

The single most common neurological symptom reported in MPD is headache (Bliss, 1980, 1984b; Coons, 1984; Greaves, 1980; O'Brien, 1985; Putnam *et al.*, 1986; Solomon & Solomon, 1982). The headaches are usually described as extremely painful and often associated with visual disturbances such as scotoma. Several patients have described these headaches to me as "blinding." Usually these headaches are not relieved by standard analgesics, frequently necessitating the use of potentially addicting pain medication (Allison, 1978a; Coons, 1984). Dynamically, a number of therapists have associated the presence of headaches with conflicts and struggles for control among alter personalities (Coons, 1984; Solomon & Solomon, 1982). In the laboratory, we have noticed that headaches frequently accompany "forced" switching such as that which occurs during research studies (Putnam, 1984b). A high incidence of headache is also part of the clinical picture of other dissociative disorders such as depersonalization syndromes and fugue episodes (Shorvon, 1946; Davidson, 1964; Kirshner, 1973). As Greaves (1980) has observed, there is something important about the connection between headaches and dissociation that is worthy of note and further study.

MPD patients often suffer a variety of other neurological complaints, the most disturbing of which involve syncope or other loss of consciousness and/or seizures or seizure-like behaviors. Little is known about these symptoms except that they occur in a substantial percentage of patients and appear to be related in some fashion to the psychophysiological mechanisms of dissociation. Seizures or seizure-like behaviors were reported in 21% of the single case reports reviewed (Putnam & Post, 1988) and in a series of MPD/dissociative patients studied at the Beth Israel Behavioral Neurology Unit (Mesulam, 1981; Schenk & Bear, 1981). Bliss (1980) reports that "convulsions" occurred in 18% of his first series of cases, and the NIMH survey found that seizure-like episodes, frequently accompanied by nonspecific bitemporal slowing of the EEG, were noted in 10% of cases (Putnam, 1986a; Putnam et al., 1986). The relationship of dissociative behavior and temporal lobe phenomenon is clearly documented with respect to fugue episodes; like headache, this phenomenon deserves future clinical and scientific investigation (Akhtar & Brenner, 1979; Mayeux et al., 1979; Putnam, 1986a).

A variety of sensory disturbances have been reported to occur in MPD patients; most of these sensory abnormalities have a "hysterical" quality. Numbness and tingling or paresthesias are relatively common, typically involving the limbs (Bliss, 1980, 1984b; Putnam et al., 1986). Visual disturbances, ranging from "hysterical" diplopia to complete blindness, are reported in about a fifth of MPD patients (Bliss, 1980; Putnam et al., 1986). Not infrequently, these visual disturbances are limited to a subset of the alter personalities, and later in therapy can be psychologically linked to specific experiences. Psychogenic deafness is not infrequent in this population (Bliss, 1980; Putnam et al., 1986).

Motor disturbances in MPD likewise exhibit a "hysterical" character. Classic functional limb paralysis is reported in at least 10% or more of patients (Bliss, 1980, 1984b; Putnam et al., 1986). Disturbances of gait, paresis, and other forms of motor weakness are not rare, and may lead to extensive neurological evaluation before their functional nature is recognized (Brende & Rinsley, 1981; Putnam et al., 1984; Bliss, 1980, 1984b).

Aphonia was noted in 10% of the NIMH cases and a third of Bliss's (1980) patients. Phenomena resembling tardive dyskinesia may also occur; these primarily oral/facial twitching movements can frequently be associated later with rapid switching of alter personalities.

MPD patients often exhibit medical symptoms referrable to the cardiorespiratory system. Typically, these symptoms are similar to those seen in anxiety or panic attack patients and include dyspnea, palpitations, chest pain, and choking or smothering sensations (Bliss, 1980; Putnam et al., 1984, 1986). Gastrointestinal symptoms, particularly functional bowel disorders, are very common in MPD patients (Bliss, 1980; Putnam et al., 1986). Unexplained nausea and/or abdominal pain is also a common symptom and later can usually be related to specific abusive experiences. Pain involving the reproductive system is reported in at least a third of cases, and again often can later be associated with viscerally remembered past trauma. Self-induced or factitious illness has been reported in MPD patients and should always be kept in mind, particularly with unusual dermatological reactions or unexplained fevers (Wise & Reading, 1975; Shelley, 1981).

Changes in the Symptom Profile over Time

We know little about the life course of multiple personality or any of the other dissociative disorders. We also know little about the day-to-day symptoms, experiences, and behavior of these unusual patients. For the moment, this second point is best addressed by the biographical and autobiographical accounts appearing in the popular press. Loewenstein et al. (1987) have applied experiential sampling techniques to the study of the daily switching pattern in MPD, and such studies promise interesting results for the future. The little we do know about the life course or natural history of MPD comes from a 15-year follow-up by Cutler and Reed (1975) and a 38-year follow-up by Rosenbaum and Weaver (1980) on single cases, and from the cross-sectional analysis of presenting symptoms as a function of age by Kluft, using his large case series (Kluft, 1985a).

The dearth of good longitudinal data is a problem that plagues all of medicine and is only now being systematically addressed in psychiatric research. In the absence of better information, cross-sectional data across different age groupings are the best substitute. Kluft (1985b), drawing on his experience with well over 100 cases, found that, in general, clinical presentation did vary as a function of the patient's age. Kluft found that only a few MPD patients (6.2%) presented with florid evidence of alter personalities. The most "open" cases were patients presenting in their 20s, and by their 30s most patients had taken on a clinical presentation of depression with features of anxiety and mild obsession. He found that patients in their 40s were essentially similar but appeared to be driven by "some inner sense that if they did not seek help soon, any chance of changing their pathological adaptations would be lost" (1985b, p. 224). He observed that, with one exception, patients in their 50s presented with depression, anxiety, and passive-influence experiences. He reported finding some patients with classic MPD in their 60s, but noted that in many older patients, "there is a progressive diminution of the external manifestations, an atrophy of individual differences, and a spontaneous integration of some components during and after middle age" (1985b, pp. 227–228).

These spotty longitudinal and cross-sectional data support a clinical impression that dissociative disorders in general and MPD in particular, while still present in older patients, tend to diminish in intensity with time. Although this process should not be mistaken for a cure, it may be considered indicative that MPD undergoes an evolutionary change over the life course of an individual and may take a variety of forms over the years. In my experience, a number of older MPD patients reach some form of reconciliation among their alter personalities that permits them to live more comfortably while still remaining multiples. These patients, however, often had turbulent adult histories filled with personal suffering and anguish, and most probably could have been significantly helped by earlier diagnosis and treatment.

Past Life History of Patients

Psychiatric History

A number of features occur frequently enough in the past history of MPD patients that they should serve to increase the index of suspicion for the disorder. The diagnosis of MPD is rarely made on a patient's first encounter with the mental health system (Bliss et al., 1983; Kluft, 1985a; Putnam et al., 1986). Thus, one historical feature that many MPD patients share is a past psychiatric history characterized by multiple previous diagnoses. A corollary of this observation is that MPD patients will also have a past history of nonresponsiveness to the standard treatments for these diagnoses and disorders (Putnam et al., 1984; Kluft, 1985a). Past psychiatric diagnoses commonly acquired by MPD patients include depression, schizophrenia, schizoaffective disorder, manic–depressive illness, a variety of personality disorder diagnoses (most prominently borderline personality disorder), and temporal lobe or other forms of epilepsy (Bliss *et al.*, 1983; Putnam *et al.*, 1986).

Medical History

Similar patterns also commonly characterize the medical histories of MPD patients. They often receive extensive medical and neurological workups for atypical or unexplained symptoms, as well as for the neurological and medical symptoms discussed above. As with the psychiatric disorders, MPD patients often prove refractory to the standard treatments for their diagnosed medical disorders. There may be a history of unusual responses or adverse reactions to medications or anesthetics (Putnam, 1985b). There may even be indirect evidence of alter identities manifested by the use of different names in the old records or by very different and conflicting histories or other information.

Social History

There is a dearth of data about the day-to-day life of MPD patients, but the clinical stereotypes and anecdotal historical information suggest that these patients typically have an occupational history marked by frequent job changes, though the jobs themselves are often responsible and sometimes high-level positions. Some multiples are, however, itinerant, traveling the country in prolonged fugues and briefly establishing residency or entering treatment in a number of communities. In some cases, I have noted a periodicity to their wanderings, so that I know when to expect to hear from them again.

History of Victimization as an Adult

Revictimization in adulthood is part of the legacy of childhood abuse (Browne & Finkelhor, 1986; Russell, 1986). Coons and Milstein (1984) found a significantly higher rate of rape in 17 MPD patients, compared to an age- and sex-matched control group of nondissociative patients. About half of the NIMH survey sample of MPD patients reported being raped or forcibly sexually assaulted as adults (Putnam *et al.*, 1986). A preliminary survey of victims of two or more separate rape attempts suggested an extremely high incidence of major dissociative symptoms in this group (Putnam, 1988b). The role of the dissociative process in predisposing victims to repeated victimization needs to be explored more fully.

SUMMARY

Severe, repetitive, often sadistic childhood trauma has become widely recognized as playing a major role in the development of MPD. A developmental model has been outlined, emphasizing the interaction between recurrent trauma and such normative childhood capacities as high hypnotizability, spontaneous dissociation, and a capacity for imaginative involvement and fantasy; the child uses these capacities adaptively for protection against the trauma. The traumatized child repeatedly enters into contextually determined dissociative states of consciousness that acquire a history of experiences and affects and a state-dependent repertoire of behaviors. Over time, these states are elaborated into alter personalities.

A clinical profile of MPD in adults emerges that is characterized by initial presentations with symptoms superficially suggestive of depression and/or anxiety. Dissociative symptoms, such as amnesias, fugues, or depersonalization, are rarely volunteered until well into the course of treatment. In many cases, MPD patients are treated for other psychiatric disorders and typically are unresponsive to standard therapies. In addition, substance abuse and/or a psychosis-like picture may complicate diagnosis. Self-destructive behaviors are frequent, as are migraine-like headaches. As with most psychiatric illnesses, longitudinal data are lacking and the life course of MPD is largely unknown, though a history of frequent changes in employment and repeated victimization in adulthood are common.

CHAPTER FOUR

Diagnosing Multiple Personality Disorder

A clinician who suspects that his or her client may be suffering from MPD can make use of a number of strategies to confirm or exclude this diagnosis. A diagnosis of MPD can only be made when the clinician determines that the patient does have separate and distinct alter personalities meeting the DSM-III/DSM-III-R criteria discussed in Chapter Two. The task of identifying and eliciting suspected alter personalities can be difficult and anxiety-provoking for both therapist and patient. This chapter discusses several strategies for determining whether or not a patient is suffering from MPD.

MPD is a chronic dissociative condition, as opposed to transient and generally self-limited dissociative conditions such as psychogenic amnesia or psychogenic fugue states. Consequently, one can expect to find evidence of the dissociative process in the patient's day-to-day life experiences and in patient–therapist interactions. The first step in the diagnostic process is to determine whether the patient is having dissociative experiences. Initially, this is best pursued by a thorough history. Often, however, the history is ambiguous or at best suggestive and requires additional diagnostic interventions to clarify what is actually occurring with the patient. This chapter begins with discussions of history taking and interview interactions in cases where dissociative pathology needs to be ruled in or out. Next, the chapter examines a number of specific diagnostic interventions that can yield additional information. A discussion of two specific diagnostic techniques, hypnotic screening and drug-facilitated interviews, is postponed until Chapter Nine, which covers hypnotic and abreactive therapeutic interventions.

TAKING A HISTORY FROM PATIENTS

Difficulties

During initial interviews of patients who later proved to have MPD, I have noticed a recurring pattern: I find that it is difficult to obtain a coherent history. When I finish taking the history and start to write it down, it becomes apparent that much of the information is inconsistent or even contradictory and that it is difficult to establish a clear chronological sequence of events. This reflects the fact that MPD patients have great difficulty in providing a clear and chronological life history, because memories of their life history are divided up among a number of alter personalities.

In most instances, the initial historical information will be obtained primarily from the host personality, who often has the least access to early historical information and experiences frequent gaps in the continuity of his or her existence. The host personality, discussed further in Chapter Five, is the alter that usually presents for treatment (Putnam *et al.*, 1986). The host suffers the consequences of the behavior of other alter personalities, but has little or no knowledge of the events that lead up to the situations. For example, a host personality may find himself or herself in an emergency room undergoing gastric lavage for an overdose. Since another personality actually took the overdose, the host may have no memory of taking the pills. When asked about this episode at a later date, the patient/host may remember the incident only vaguely and may be unable to provide much detail. MPD patients often say such things as "I must have been depressed; *they* tell me I took a whole bottle of pills." Frequently, a patient will be unable to determine whether a given episode occurred before or after another event.

Two features that characterize the chief complaint and past history of an MPD patient are frequent inconsistencies and the lack of a clear chronology. The inconsistencies become most apparent if the clinician returns at a later date to gather more information about a specific event. I have had the experience of obtaining three or four different and contradictory accounts of specific episodes from a patient. When this happens, a clinician may wonder whether the problem is his or her own or the patient's. Neophyte therapists often conclude that they must have misunderstood or incorrectly remembered what such patients had told them previously. I tell residents that when they begin to wonder just who has the memory problem, they or their patients, they should think about the possibility of MPD.

Information provided by MPD patients during this early phase of evaluation is usually vague and lacking in substantive detail. A patient may say "I can't remember" repeatedly or otherwise indicate that he or she has a "terrible" memory. MPD patients usually do *not* describe their difficulties with recall as amnesia or provide other information to suggest that they are having amnesic episodes. Instead, they pass off the missing information as the result of a poor memory. If they have received electroconvulsive therapy (ECT) in the past, they frequently attribute their memory difficulties to this.

Unfortunately, many clinicians accept these explanations and fail to pursue these memory difficulties any further. When faced with a patient who apparently has significant difficulties in recall of personal history, it is important to determine the cause of this difficulty. The withholding of information by MPD patients is usually attributable to a number of different mechanisms. The personality being questioned may be amnesic for the particular event, or the personality may be aware of more information but may be denying recall because of internal system pressures. A patient may, on occasion, confabulate information to fill in an otherwise unacceptable gap in memory or to placate the interviewer (Kluft, 1985c, 1986a). Patients are often reluctant to reveal what they do know about their condition for fear that they will be considered "crazy."

Many multiples have developed compensatory behaviors to help them deal with missing information and gaps in memory. These may be activated to aid in evading difficult questions or to distract the interviewer. In addition, the personality system may be actively eluding diagnosis by lying about information, or, more commonly, by omitting important details and providing information suggesting one avenue of inquiry and closing off another. It has been my experience that when multiples try to mislead therapists they usually do it through omission rather than by outright lying, though the latter does occur. It is important to listen carefully to what these patients say. They can be masters at appearing to say one thing while actually saying another. When I review something that I have been told by a multiple, I make a point of mentally translating it into as concrete a statement as I can, in addition to dealing with it on a more abstract level. An important double meaning can often be found in the concrete interpretation.

Another common ploy used by multiples is to pretend to know more than they do. A multiple may be baffled by something that has happened or may have no memory of a previous conversation with the interviewer, but will behave as if he or she knows exactly what is going on and will answer any questions in a manner that tends to deflect the interviewer from discovering the deficits in the patient's knowledge. It is important not to make assumptions. Working with multiples is not easy, and a therapist often gets his or her first taste of these difficulties during the evaluation process.

Useful Inquiries

A clinician who suspects that a patient may be suffering from a chronic dissociative condition such as MPD should explore a number of specific areas in the history and mental status examination. For heuristic purposes, these questions are grouped into four categories: amnesia or "time loss"; depersonalization/derealization; life experiences; and Schneiderian primary symptoms. In actual practice, I sprinkle these questions into my history taking, intermixing categories and questions as the situation dictates.

Questions about Amnesia or "Time Loss"

In questioning patients about MPD, it is often wise to begin obliquely. I typically begin this part of the history by asking the patient about experiences of "time loss." Often I do not initially define "time loss," and if they report such experiences I ask for several examples. If they do not acknowledge these experiences, I define the term with an example such as this: "An example of what I mean by "time loss" would be the experience of looking at a clock and seeing that it was, say, 9:00 in the morning, and the next thing that you are aware of is that it is, say, 3:00 in the afternoon, and you have absolutely no recollection of what has happened between 9:00 A.M. and 3:00 P.M. Has anything like that ever happened to you?" If the patient admits to having had such experiences, I ask for examples.

It is important to hear a number of specific examples before deciding whether or not a patient is actually having experiences of time loss. Many normal people will have occasional microdissociative episodes associated with either a monotonous situation (e.g., driving on an empty interstate highway) or a period of intense concentration or preoccupation (e.g., taking an important examination or reading an exciting novel). In the case of MPD patients or of chronic dissociators who do not have MPD, episodes of time loss are frequent, occur in a variety of settings, and are not exclusively associated with monotony or intense concentration. In addition, there is usually no obvious secondary gain from this time loss. Unfortunately, while all multiples will have one or more personalities who lose time (usually including the host or personality seeking treatment), not all multiples will initially admit to the experience of losing time.

If the examples provided by the patient suggest that he or she has had unaccounted-for periods of time, it becomes important to establish whether these episodes occurred in the absence of drug or alcohol use. It is usually best to take the specific examples provided by the patient and determine whether they were preceded by any drug or alcohol use. The association of intoxicants and time loss does not necessarily rule out a dissociative disorder, but it does complicate the differential diagnosis considerably.

If the patient denies any experiences of time loss, I will still include some of the following questions in my interview. If the patient has admitted to some experiences suggestive of time loss, I will ask about experiences in which the patient finds evidence of having done something that he or she does not remember doing. Most patients who acknowledge periods of time loss can provide examples of performing complex tasks for which they have no memory. One patient, a certified public accountant, would report that he often lost 3 or 4 hours, only to find completed work sheets on his desk at the end of the day. His boss and coworkers never commented on any peculiar behavior during these episodes of lost time, but he was highly distressed because several times he "came to" in an empty office and wondered how his coworkers could have left without his noticing. Again, the examples of time loss provided by dissociating patients usually include many prosaic examples, such as those described above, without any obvious secondary gain.

I will ask patients whether they have ever found themselves dressed in clothing that they did not remember putting on. I may even ask such patients to close their eyes and tell me what they are wearing. Most people can tell you what they are wearing because at some point they made a conscious decision to put it on. A multiple, however, may have a number of personalities with very different tastes in clothing, hairstyle, and makeup. Consequently, the host personality may find herself or himself dressed in clothing that he or she did not and would not choose. I will often ask female patients whether they ever find clothing in their closet that they would never wear. Many of them will admit to this and often add comments like "It's two sizes too small anyway," or "I would never wear anything that revealing." Female multiples usually will have similar experiences with makeup and hairdos. Finding mysterious wigs, false eyelashes, jewelry, perfumes, and shoes are among the perplexing experiences shared by many female multiples. In males, the same type of experience exists but may be more prominent for such possessions as weapons, tools, or vehicles.

Questions along the same line include finding possessions that the patients do not remember buying. Specific examples often provided by MPD patients include finding items in their shopping baskets at the supermarket or on their trays at a cafeteria that they did not choose. One should also ask about finding notes, letters, photographs, drawings, or other personal items for which a patient cannot account.

Similar types of experiences occur with people and relationships. I will probe this area by asking questions such as this: "Do you find that you are approached by people who insist that they know you, but you do not remember them or the situations that they describe?" We all have had experiences like this at some time; multiples, however, have this sort of thing happen repeatedly. They may report that people will address them by different names or insist that they know them from someplace, despite their denials. The clinician should be sure to find out the names by which patients are addressed at these times, as this information may indicate the existence of alters who, in fact, do know these people.

MPD patients will have had experiences of being told that they did or said something that they cannot remember, but that made a significant impression on their family members, friends, or coworkers. Often these interactions involve anger or other strong emotions that the host personality cannot tolerate. One patient, for example, repeatedly had the experience of arriving at her job, only to find out that "she" had quit in a stormy scene the day before. Relationships may also end as abruptly and, for the unaware host, in a manner as painfully baffling.

Another area of genuine perplexity for many multiples is the fact that they do not remember many of the important events in their lives. They may *know* that they graduated from high school or college on a certain date, or that they were married, gave birth, won an award, or experienced some other noteworthy event, but they do not actually *remember* the experience. As Bennett Braun observes, in such cases it is very important to make the distinction for the patient between the knowledge that such an event occurred and the act of remembering the actual experience.

A person can have knowledge that an event occurred because he or she has been told about it, but have no actual memory for the experience. For our purposes, memory for an event constitutes the recall of visual or other images of the experience that would place one in the situation. I might ask a question about this type of experience as follows: "Are there important events or experiences in your life, such as weddings or graduations, which you have been told about by other people, but you cannot remember at all?" One of my MPD patients, for example, responded by saying that she could not remember any of her birthdays or Christmases from childhood to the present. Again, as with all of these inquiries, it is important to get specific examples and examine them in detail to determine whether the patient has understood the intent of the question and whether other complicating factors, such as drugs or alcohol, cloud the issue.

Fugue-like experiences are common in MPD (Putnam et al., 1986). These may range from minifugues, in which the patient loses only brief amounts of time and travels short distances, to extensive fugues, in which the patient may "wake up" in another state or country. In most cases, it is the host personality who "comes to" and is baffled by the situation. I inquire about this type of experience by asking patients whether they ever have the experience of finding themselves some place and not knowing how they got there. Normal people may "space out" at times when they are preoccupied, find themselves in another room of their house, and wonder what they are doing there. Multiples, however, are more likely to find themselves in another part of town or driving in a car with no memory of getting in or idea of where they are going. As one patient summed it up, "I'm tired of finding myself on a corner watching the 'Walk' and 'Don't Walk' signs and not remembering how I got there." If the patient reports more than one extensive fugue-like episode, there is a high probability that he or she has MPD.

Questions about Depersonalization/Derealization

Depersonalization and derealization experiences are an important symptom of dissociative disorders in general and are common in MPD in particular (Putnam et al., 1986; Bliss, 1984b). These symptoms, however, may also be present in other psychiatric or neurological conditions, such as schizophrenia, psychotic depression, or temporal lobe epilepsy. Transient feelings of depersonalization are also common in normal adolescents. Depersonalization may also constitute part of a near-death experience in normals who have been severely traumatized (Putnam, 1985a). Therefore it is important to keep a differential diagnosis in mind when inquiring about symptoms of depersonalization/derealization.

I usually begin my exploration of this area by asking patients whether they have ever had the experience of watching themselves as if they were looking at another person or watching themselves in a movie. I am looking for "out-of-body" experiences, which occur in at least half of all multiples. In many cases, it is the host personality who is observing another personality perform some action. Patients will often describe this as watching themselves from a distance, but feeling that they had no control over what they were doing. They may feel as if they are off to one side, looking down from above, or watching from deep within themselves. This is usually a very frightening experience for an MPD patient, although non-MPD individuals who have this experience in near-death situations often report a feeling of detachment or tranquility. In my experience, many multiples will acknowledge having out-of-body experiences, but have difficulty in providing specific examples. This difficulty seems to be in part a function of how disturbing the experience is to recall. The out-of-body experience is most common in MPD and normals undergoing transient dissociative reactions as a result of life-threatening trauma, and is relatively rare in schizophrenia and other psychiatric illnesses, though it may occur ictally in epileptics.

I ask about other forms of depersonalization/derealization, such as feeling unreal, feeling oneself to be mechanical or dead, feeling as if everyone or everything else in the world is unreal, and so on. These experiences, however, are not uncommon in schizophrenia, psychotic depression, phobic or anxiety syndromes, or even obsessive–compulsive disorders; therefore, positive answers must be evaluated within the context of the larger differential diagnosis.

Questions about Common Life Experiences

A person with MPD is going to have certain kinds of life experiences that other people rarely have. After listening to over 100 patients tell me about life with MPD, I have extracted a number of life experiences common to multiples and unusual for those who do not have the disorder. Comparison of my results with those of seasoned MPD therapists suggests that the following life experiences are commonly encountered by patients with MPD.

The experience of being called a liar is common for multiple personality patients. Apparent pathological lying or disavowing of observed behavior is one of the best diagnostic predictors in child and adolescent multiples (Putnam, 1985c). Adult MPD patients will often recount that they acquired a reputation as liars in childhood. I will ask patients whether they have often had the experience of being accused of lying when they believed that they were telling the truth. This may happen to all of us at some time or other, but MPD patients will have this experience frequently in childhood and fairly often as adults. Consequently, some MPD patients will become obsessed with the "truth" as adults. It may also explain in part why these patients are so exquisitely sensitive to any departure from truth by the therapist.

Multiples are perceived by other people as lying when they deny doing things that they were seen to do. In most instances, this is because the personality that is denying the behavior is amnesic for the actions of another personality who actually performed the action. The clinician should try to garner a number of specific examples for the reasons cited above, and also because they may be useful at a later date in therapy to explain heretofore unexplainable phenomena to the host personality.

When evaluating a patient for possible MPD, it is particularly useful to take a structured childhood history. At least two important types of information can be gathered in this way. The first is evidence of large amnesic gaps in the person's memory for childhood, a common finding in MPD victims. The second is the occurrence of certain types of life experiences common for multiples during childhood and adolescence. I have found that a person's year-by-year school history is the easiest and most universal structure that can be used to rapidly organize this information and to detect significant gaps in memory.

I generally begin by asking patients how far back they can remember and at what age they feel that the memories of their childhood begin to become more or less continuous. Many people will have fragmentary memories from age 2 or so, but typically memories do not start to become more continuous until age 6 or older. By about third or fourth grade (age 8 or 9), most normal people should be able to give a year-by-year history of where they lived, where they went to school, who their important friends were, and what was happening in their homes. I usually go through patients' childhoods grade by grade, asking them where they lived, where they went to school, who their teachers were, a couple of best friends' names, and what was going on at home. I also ask about any unusual experiences or events during each year.

Intermixed with the grade-by-grade history, one can ask patients about their experiences of being called liars, of erratic school performance (e.g., failing one marking period and getting A's the next), of getting back tests and homework that they did not remember doing, or of discovering that they had taken courses that they could not remember. Another common experience MPD patients have in childhood is feeling that everyone else in their class was told something that they were not (Kluft, 1985a). Many MPD patients will have large gaps in the continuity of their childhood memories, and statements such as "I can't remember seventh through ninth grade" or "I can't remember anything before I was 16" are not uncommon.

Flashbacks, intrusive images, dreamlike memories, and nightmares are common occurrences in MPD victims and are part of the constellation of symptoms that MPD shares with posttraumatic stress disorder.

The flashbacks are triggered by environmental stimuli in a manner similar to that described for flashbacks associated with posttraumatic stress disorder. I will ask a patient about having the experience of remembering a past event in a way that was so vivid and so real that it seemed as if it were really happening again. A clinician may have to ask several similar questions to uncover the existence of this phenomenon in a patient. An MPD patient who is having flashbacks may or may not admit to this experience. The flashbacks are very disturbing, and the host personality often deals with them (like so many other frightening experiences) by denial. Usually the existence of flashback phenomena is reported at a later point in therapy. It is worthwhile, however, to look for them early in the evaluation of a patient suspected to have MPD. The existence of flashback phenomena that are not associated with drug use is strong evidence that the patient is suffering from some form of major dissociative pathology.

Intrusive mental images also occur in MPD patients. A common example is the intrusion of visual or sensory memories of childhood sexual abuse during intercourse with a spouse or lover. In many instances, these intrusive images are so frightening and compelling that the patient's sex life is seriously impaired. These experiences are akin to flashbacks, but differ in that the patient can tell that they are mental images and are not actually happening. The image is often stereotyped and occurs repeatedly, although the patient may not recognize it as a memory. One of my patients, for example, described the repeated experience of seeing or imagining a dark, unrecognizable figure leaning over her while she was having sex with her husband. The image was frightening, and she often "froze" when it occurred, effectively terminating intercourse. Later in therapy, the image resolved itself into a memory of her incestuous stepfather leaning over her bed at night. Similar phenomena have have been reported by victims of incest and childhood sexual abuse who do not have MPD.

Multiples will report having vague, dreamlike memories that they cannot place in context. These snatches of memory may be associated with strong emotional responses that seem to be inappropriate to the content. Patients will often preface reports of these memories with comments such as "I don't know whether this really happened or I made it up." I will ask patients whether they are troubled by memories of events that they are not sure really happened or that they may have just dreamed happened.

The high frequency of sleep disturbance seen in MPD has been mentioned in Chapter Three, together with a caution about not mistaking this "insomnia" for the types of sleep disturbances found in depression. MPD victims, like other victims of severe trauma, suffer from a sleep disorder characterized by severe and often repetitive nightmares, multiple awakenings from deep sleep, and hypnagogic/hypnopompic phenomena. I generally inquire carefully about nightmares in my initial evaluation. Most MPD patients seem willing to talk about nightmares, even when they are reluctant to admit to other terrifying experiences such as flashbacks or intrusive images. I will ask about content, which is usually not well remembered, and whether or not they wake up out of bed, screaming, or convinced that something terrible is happening to them. Somnambulism is not uncommon in adult victims of MPD. MPD patients also frequently have the experience of waking up in the morning and finding evidence that they were busy during the night, although they do not remember anything. They may find drawings, notes, poems, relocated furniture, discarded clothing, or other evidence that they have been up and busy. If this is a common life experience for a patient, there is an excellent chance that he or she has MPD.

Another common life experience for MPD patients is finding that they possess knowledge or skills that they have no memory of having acquired. I will ask patients whether they ever have had the experience of discovering that they know how to do something, such as speaking a foreign language, playing a musical instrument, or performing job skills, that they cannot remember learning. The converse of this process is also common in MPD—that is, the sudden and inexplicable loss of skills, abilities, or knowledge that the patients previously possessed. One patient, a respiratory therapist, would periodically find that she could not remember how to run her equipment. During these episodes, she would hide in the ladies' room or feign an illness and leave work. Her erratic behavior led to the loss of several jobs.

Questions about Schneiderian Primary Symptoms

Kluft (1984c, 1987) has pointed out that patients with MPD often satisfy many of Schneider's first-order symptoms for schizophrenia. MPD patients will report hearing voices talking, arguing, or screaming in their heads. The voices may be pejorative and critical or supportive. They may comment on the patient's thoughts or actions. The patients may also have passive-influence phenomena, such as the experience of their bodies' being controlled by an outside force or thought withdrawal. A common expression of passive-influence phenomena is automatic writing. "Made" thoughts, feelings, and impulsive actions are also common experiences. Kluft (1984c) suggests that patients who have made suicide attempts may be more likely to have these experiences. MPD patients, however, rarely express feelings of thought diffusion (i.e., the spreading of one's thoughts to others), audible thoughts, or delusional perceptions.

The mental status examination should include questions relevant to these symptoms. Many multiples are fearful of acknowledging the existence of voices early in the course of therapy, lest the therapist think that they are "crazy." The clinician can begin by asking patients whether they ever find themselves talking out loud when they are alone, and, if so, whether they ever get some sort of an answer. Many host personalities already have some form of communication with the other alters when they present for treatment, although they are usually not aware of what is actually happening. The experience of the host personality is that he or she gets into arguments with himself or herself.

INTERVIEW INTERACTIONS WITH PATIENTS

If a patient is suffering from MPD, he or she will display signs and symptoms of this condition during the course of evaluation and treatment. The trick is to recognize and follow up these manifestations of MPD. Most multiples can suppress switching or other dissociative phenomena for short periods of time. Sustained interactions or periods of intense stress, however, are likely to evoke dissociation in the patients that will be detectable to a knowledgeable observer. It is important to maintain a high index of suspicion regarding the possibility of covert switching occurring during sessions with a patient.

I discuss the various physical and psychological changes associated with personality switching in Chapter Five. The processes of actually detecting these changes in a patient involve a willingness to consider the possibility that the lability, changeability, or dichotomous behavior on the part of the patient is caused by switches of alter personalities, rather than by "mood swings," "splitting," or some other "unified personality" interpretation. A clinician will not find MPD if he or she is not willing to look for it. Also, looking for MPD cannot create the disorder in a patient if it is not already there.

There are two major ways of detecting possible personality switching that may be going on during sessions with the patient. The first is the recognition of physical signs of switching. These signs are discussed in Chapter Five and most prominently include facial changes, such as upward eye rolls, rapid blinking, or twitches or grimaces. Changes in voice and speech are common (Putnam, 1988c). Careful observation over time will reveal that these physical changes are consistently associated with a set of psychological reponses (i.e., an alter personality).

The second major indicator of personality switches occurring within a session with the patient is the presence of intrainterview amnesia. This occurs when an alter personality emerges who does not have access to the state-dependent memories of a prior alter and therefore does not know what has happened prior to his or her emergence. Many multiples have developed strategies to cover missing memories and will attempt to conceal their amnesia. These strategies are generally aimed at diverting the interviewer's attention away from the missing information and into some area in which the alter feels more comfortable. The interviewer should be attentive to significant shifts in the train of thought or a dramatic refocusing of attention.

For example, I worked with a patient who, in the middle of discussing an important or painful experience, would suddenly fixate on some object in the room (e.g., a painting on the wall or the title of a book on a shelf) and begin to make conversation about this object. Attempts to bring her back to the preceding line of thought, to connect the two topics, or to interpret this behavior as a resistance produced no results. It became increasingly apparent that she did not remember what we had just been discussing. Initial attempts to find out about possible amnesia were met with comments such as "I don't want to talk about that [the unspecified preceding topic] any more." When I persisted and asked her to specifically tell me what we had just been discussing, she eventually admitted that she could not remember. A series of these interactions occurred over several sessions before she was able to acknowledge her experience of time loss in and out of therapy.

Another manifestation of intrainterview amnesia can be a pattern of admitting to symptoms, behaviors, or experiences and then subsequently denying these acknowledgments. This pattern of "doing and undoing" is common in MPD. It may be the result of amnesia for previous statements and actions, or may be attributable to opposite values and views of the world expressed by different alter personalities.

A clinician who suspects intrainterview amnesia can initially approach the issue indirectly in a manner similar to the queries about time loss experiences described above. It may become necessary, however, to confront the patient directly and ask him or her to specify in detail the information for which the clinician believes the patient may be amnesic. When faced with direct evidence of time loss within a session, some patients may become frightened. It is important to cushion the impact of such an interaction by letting such patients know that this is a symptom of their problem, that it probably happens to them in other circumstances, and that one of the goals of treatment will be to alleviate these episodes.

From time to time, multiples will slip (perhaps on purpose) and make self-references in the first person plural or the third person. The use of "we" in a collective manner, rather than the editorial sense, is a particularly common observation (Greaves, 1980). Patients may also say "he" or "she" in reference to their own behavior. Kluft (1985a) believes, however, that the use of "we" statements is more characteristic of MPD patients after diagnosis and socialization to treatment than before.

Another commonly reported observation is that MPD patients have an exaggerated startle reflex. Certainly, some non-MPD psychiatric patients (e.g., posttraumatic stress disorder victims) will also display a heightened startle reaction, but most multiples will demonstrate frequent startle responses to minor stimuli. Another manifestation of this process is an erratic habituation to a noxious stimulus; for example, patients may initially react to a repetitive loud noise with repeated startle responses, then appear to "tune it out," only to react again at a later point to the same stimulus as if it were new. This behavior often indicates that a switch has occurred and a new, unhabituated alter is present.

DIAGNOSTIC PROCEDURES

Mental Status Examination

Table 4-1 summarizes the principal findings associated with the mental status examination in MPD.

The Use of Sequential Tasks and Observations

The diagnosis of MPD is not likely to be made during the first contacts with a patient. We (Putnam et al., 1986) found that the median length of time in treatment with the therapist who made the diagnosis of MPD was 6 months after initial presentation, with a number of cases continuing for several years before a diagnosis was made. The MPD patients in the NIMH survey averaged 6.8 years from initial presentation in the mental health system for symptoms referrable to MPD to diagnosis (Putnam et al., 1986). Therefore, the diagnosis of MPD is more likely to be made after an extended period of interaction and observation with the patient (Putnam, 1985b).

Table 4-1. Mental Status Examination in Multiple Personality Disorder

Area	Characteristics
Appearance	Style of dress, grooming, general appearance, and mannerisms may change dramatically from session to session. Marked changes in facial appearance, expression, posture, and mannerisms may occur within a single session. Handedness and habits such as smoking may change within a short space of time.
Speech	Changes in rate, pitch, accent, loudness, vocabulary, and the use of idiosyncratic expressions or profanity may occur within a brief period of time.
Motor processes	Rapid blinking, eyelid fluttering, marked eye rolls, tics, twitches, startle reactions, or shudders and facial grimaces often accompany the switching of alter personalities.
Thought processes	Thought processes may appear to be nonsequential and illogical at times. Associations may appear to be loose, and patients may appear to block or lose their train of thought. This is most prominent with rapid switching or "revolving-door" crises. Thought disorder does not persist beyond a crisis, however.
Hallucinations	Auditory and/or visual hallucinations may be present, including pejorative voices, voices commenting or arguing about the patient, or command hallucinations. Voices are most frequently experienced as *within* the patient's head. Positive or secondary-process voices may be present.
Intellectual functioning	Short-term memory, orientation, calculations, and fund of knowledge are generally intact. Long-term memory may show spotty deficits.
Judgment	Patient may display rapid fluctuations in appropriateness of behavior and judgment. These shifts often occur along an age dimension (i.e., shifts from adult to childlike behavior).
Insight	The personality presenting for treatment frequently (i.e., about 80% of the time) is not aware of the existence of alternate personalities. Patients show a marked inability to learn from past experiences.

One way of collecting longitudinal information on suspected MPD patients is to give them some form of sequential daily task on which performance can be studied over time. The keeping of a diary or similar task has proven useful in detecting cases of MPD. Kluft (1984c) instructs his patients to write down whatever thoughts come into their minds for a 30-minute period each day, and to bring these writings to the session. I have also found this technique to be a useful tool for permitting alter personalities to declare themselves. The biggest problem that I have had with this technique is getting the patients to bring the material to a session. In many instances patients are embarrassed, ashamed, or frightened by what they find written down and are reluctant to show this to the therapist. In most cases I have had to insist on compliance with this task and repeatedly remind the patients. It is desirable to have all of the entries made in a single notebook for ease of comparison.

The alter personalities may announce themselves by signing their contributions to the diary or through dramatic changes in style, spelling, grammar, and content. Handwriting changes are often observable, and after enough specimens are collected a correlation can usually be made between the handwriting features and the style and content of the diary entry. This technique will provide the therapist with a convenient entry into the alter personality system by giving a preview of some of the alter's thoughts, feelings, and concerns. Often personalities hostile to the host or others will use this as an opportunity to make nasty comments or threats. Later, during the course of therapy, a modification of this diary task, the "bulletin board," can greatly facilitate the process of increasing cooperation and communication within the multiple's system.

The Use of Extended Interviews

Several years ago, Richard Kluft shared with me his diagnostic technique of deliberately extending an evaluation interview with a suspected MPD patient for several hours. I have found this to be an extremely successful tactic with some patients. Kluft observed that it is difficult for an MPD patient to keep from switching at some point during the stress of a prolonged interview session. A typical extended session lasts about 3 hours, though it may be necessary to spend a large part of the day with some highly secretive MPD patients. During this interview, which is exhausting and stressful for both parties, it is important to continue to probe aggressively for dissociative experiences and to be alert for intra-interview amnesia and other evidence of covert switching.

Psychological Testing

There are no definitive psychological or physiological tests for MPD at this time. Over the years, many different types of psychological measures have been administered to MPD patients, but usually only one or two patients have been tested on any given measure, making it impossible to generalize the results. The only two measures that have been repeatedly administered to MPD patients are the Minnesota Multiphasic Personality Inventory (MMPI) and the Rorschach test. Some general observations about the performance of MPD patients have been made and replicated for these two measures.

The MMPI

Three studies have administered the MMPI to 15 or more MPD patients (Coons & Sterne, 1986; Solomon, 1983; Bliss, 1984b). A number of consistent results were reported across all three of these separate studies. Characteristic MMPI profiles in MPD include an elevated F, or validity, scale and an elevated Sc, or schizophrenia, scale (Coons & Sterne, 1986; Solomon, 1983; Bliss, 1984b). Critical items on the Schizophrenia scale that are frequently endorsed by MPD patients include item 156, "I have had periods in which I carried on activities without knowing later what I had been doing," and item 251, "I have had blank spells in which my activities were interrupted and I did not know what was going on around me" (Coons & Sterne, 1986; Solomon, 1983). Coons and Sterne (1986) found that 64% of their patients endorsed item 156 initially and 86% endorsed this item on retest an average of 39 months later. They found that 64% endorsed item 251. They note that with the exception of auditory hallucinations, critical items related to psychosis were not frequently endorsed.

An elevated F scale, which produced technically invalid profiles in many instances, was consistently found by all three studies (Coons & Sterne, 1986; Bliss, 1984b; Solomon, 1983). Solomon (1983) has interpreted this as a "cry for help" and notes that it was associated with suicidality in his sample. All three studies also noted that the MPD patients appeared polysymptomatic on the MMPI and that many exhibited profiles commonly regarded as indicative of borderline personality disorder.

Although this MMPI profile may be of value in suggesting the possibility of MPD, there are no findings that could be considered as pathognomonic of MPD. Coons and Sterne (1986) retested their sample an average of 39 months after the first administration and reported little change in a given patient's profile over time, even when the patient had had extensive treatment. Normalization of the MMPI with treatment has been reported in two single case studies with repeated testing (Brassfield, 1980; Confer & Ables, 1983).

The Rorschach Test

A lesser number of MPD patients have been administered the Rorschach. Wagner and Heise (1974), in examining the responses of three MPD patients to the Rorschach, noted two common features: (1) a large number of diversified movement responses, and (2) labile and conflicting color responses. Wagner *et al.* (1983) expanded these observations, based on a fourth case of MPD. Danesino *et al.* (1979) and Piotrowski (1977) endorse Wagner and Heise's (1974) original observations, based on their interpretation of two other MPD cases. Lovitt and Lefkof (1985) take issue with the Wagner *et al.* (1983) decision rules. They used a different Rorschach scoring protocol, Exner's Comprehensive System, to study three MPD patients. Although claims are being made for the specificity of the Rorschach in identifying MPD and other major dissociative psychopathology (Wagner *et al.*, 1983; Wagner, 1978), the number of cases put through these protocols is far too few to permit generalizations at this time. The discrepancies between Wagner *et al.*'s (1983) decision rules and the findings of Lovitt and Lefkof (1985) must also be resolved before the Rorschach can be used as more than an impressionistic screening device for major dissociative psychopathology.

The Physical Examination

Psychiatrists tend to neglect the use of the physical examination in their practice, particularly in outpatient settings. There are many reasons for this, and the use of the physical examination is a matter of judgment on the part of the therapist. In MPD, however, there are several reasons why a physical examination or at least a neurological examination of the patient is important and may aid in the diagnosis.

The single most prominent pathophysiological feature in MPD is amnesia manifested as memory difficulty. The differential diagnosis of memory problems demands that organic disorders, including closed head injury, tumor, cerebral vascular accidents, or dementing illnesses (e.g.,

Alzheimer disease, Huntington chorea, or Parkinson disease), be ruled out. A good neurological examination is required in many instances to screen for these possibilities.

A physical examination may also be useful in detecting evidence of self-mutilation. The sites of self-mutilation in MPD are often hidden from casual examination and commonly include the upper arms (hidden by long sleeves), back, inner thighs, breasts, and buttocks. Self-mutilation frequently takes the form of delicate self-cutting with razor blades or fragments of glass. The former will leave telltale thin scars like pencil lines. In many cases that I have seen, the scars are layered from the repeated cuttings and look like Chinese characters or chicken scratches. Another common form of self-mutilation is burning with cigarettes or matches plunged into the skin. These will leave circular or punctate scars. Evidence on physical examination of repeated self-mutilation is highly suggestive of a dissociative disorder such as MPD or depersonalization syndrome.

Another source of scarring in MPD is injury caused by abuse in childhood. In most cases, evidence of earlier injury is not conspicuous. I have, however, seen several cases where the results of childhood abuse were still prominent in adults. If I discover a scar (even an obvious postsurgical scar) during a physical examination, I always make a point of asking about its history. Some multiples are unable to account for surgical scars, and thus provide one more example suggesting amnesia for important life events.

MEETING THE ALTER PERSONALITIES

The diagnosis of MPD can only be made after the clinician has met one or more alter personalities and determined that at least one alter is distinct and takes full control of the individual's behavior from time to time (American Psychiatric Association, 1980a, 1987). I discuss the issue of how distinct and separate an alter has to be to distinguish it from a mood or an "ego state" later in this chapter. The question for the moment is this: How does the clinician go about meeting alter personalities in a patient suspected to suffer from MPD?

A review of the literature and the NIMH survey data both suggest that in about half of all cases the meeting is initiated by one or more alters who "come out" and identify themselves as being different from the patient (Putnam *et al.*, 1986). It is fairly common for an alter to approach the therapist in person, by phone, or by letter and identify himself or herself as being a friend of the patient's. In many instances the therapist has never even suspected that the patient has MPD. In my experience, when spontaneous revelation of the diagnosis occurs shortly after first contact, the patient is either in crisis or has been diagnosed before.

If, after taking a history and performing a mental status examination and specifically looking for time loss, depersonalization/derealization, characteristic life experiences, and Scheiderian first-rank symptoms, the clinician suspects that the patient may be suffering from MPD, there are a number of ways to attempt to elicit alter personalities.

My first approach is one of indirect inquiry. I broach the subject gently, often first asking the patient whether he or she has ever felt like more than one person. The patient often answers something like this: "I don't know who I am. I feel like I am a lot of people. Maybe there really isn't a me." Such people often feel as if they could be anybody, depending on the circumstances, and lack a sense of enduring individual identity. Occasionally, I get a response such as "Yes, there is another part of me and her name is Martha." When I do not get such a direct acknowledgment, I often follow up with a question such as "Do you ever feel as if there is some other part [side, facet, etc.] of yourself that comes out and does or says things that you would not do or say?" or "Do you ever feel as if you are not alone, as if there is someone else or some other part watching you?" If the patient makes a positive or ambiguous response to these questions, it is important to ask for specific examples. In particular, I am looking for either a name or an attribute, function, or description that I can use as a label to elicit this other part directly.

Suppose, for example, that the patient admits to a number of dissociative symptoms and says that at times he or she feels as if he or she is another person or as if there is another person present, and that the other part is vaguely described as hostile and angry or depressed and suicidal. Then the clinician can ask whether it would be possible to meet with this other part: "Can this other part come out and talk with me?" This question may produce signs of distress in a multiple. Some host personalities feel that they are barely able to suppress the appearance of undesirable alters and do not wish to have their therapist inviting them to come out. Not uncommonly, if the host has knowledge of the alters, the host will feel in competition with them for the therapist's attention and is not interested in introducing them. The therapist may be told in a variety of ways that this is not possible or desirable.

At this point, therapists new to MPD may become nervous. "How do I get these personalities, if indeed there really are any, to come out?" "What will happen if they do come out, are they dangerous?" "What if I am wrong and there really aren't any personalities; will I create some by asking for them?" These and other questions are commonly raised by therapists who suspect that they may be dealing with a multiple but as yet have not met any alter personalities overtly.

The basic way to meet suspected alter personalities is to ask for them. In many instances, it is possible to ask for them directly and to have one or more come forth. In some cases, however, hypnosis or a drug-facilitated interview may be useful to facilitate the emergence of an alter. As noted earlier, the discussion of hypnotic and drug-facilitated techniques is postponed until Chapter Nine.

Asking for Suspected Alter Personalities

If a therapist strongly suspects that a patient may have MPD but has not spontaneously met a recognizable alter personality, there comes a time when he or she may have to ask directly to meet an alter personality. This moment is probably harder for the therapist than for the patient. It can make one feel foolish, but often it is necessary. The first question is that of "who" to ask for. If the patient is actually a multiple, then in most cases the personality that the therapist knows as the patient is probably the host personality. As will be discussed in Chapter Five, the host is frequently the personality who presents for treatment, is usually depressed and overwhelmed by the circumstances of her life (this may be less true for a male), and is actively avoiding or denying evidence of the existence of other personalities. In cases where the personality presenting for treatment is not the host, then this personality is more likely to be aware of the multiplicity and to aid in disclosing it.

The alter that the therapist wants to ask for is usually the one that he or she has the most information about. If the therapist has been asking about dissociative experiences and getting positive answers and specific examples, these will have begun to provide some information about what is transpiring during these experiences. Perhaps, for example, the patient has described losing several jobs because of angry outbursts that he or she cannot remember. Then the therapist may speculate that if these unremembered episodes are caused by MPD, there is probably a personality who comes out and says or does angry things at work. The therapist can then ask for this personality by description: "I would like to talk directly to that part [aspect, point of view, side, etc.] of you that came out last Wednesday at work and told your boss to stuff it." The more directly a suspected alter is specified, the better the chances of eliciting its emergence. A proper name is generally the most powerful stimulus, but a repeated description of an attribute or function (e.g., "the dark one," "the angry one," "the little girl," "the administrator") is also useful. The tone of this request to meet with another part should be that of an invitation, not a demand.

I try to avoid using the word "personality" when I am working with a patient at this stage. Most patients (both those with MPD and those without), however, are aware that this type of question is in some way associated with multiple personalities. I initially stick to descriptions such as "part," "side," "aspect," or "facet" because this is one of the major themes of the treatment approach—namely, that the personalities are a "part" of a whole person. Later, when the bounds of the therapy are better established and the patient as a whole has achieved some degree of comfort with the diagnosis, I use the term "personality" more freely.

Usually the alter does not pop out the first time the therapist asks. It is often necessary to repeat the request several times. If nothing appears to have happened, the therapist should take a moment to observe the effect of the request on the patient. Ideally, the therapist has been alert for behavior suggestive of a switch. If nothing that appears to indicate a switch has occurred, does the patient appear to be made uncomfortable by the request? In my experience, most patients who do not have MPD are not seriously distressed by requests to meet a nonexistent part. They simply wait it out or say something such as "I don't think that there is anything there, Doctor." Multiples, on the other hand, often show significant discomfort with persistent attempts to elicit an alter. This will be evident in their demeanor, and they may appear to be extremely distressed at times. In some cases, the patients may enter an unresponsive trance-like state.

The degree of discomfort may become so pronounced that the therapist may feel as if the request should be withdrawn. The patient may hold his or her head, grimace, complain of headache or other pains, or give some other indication that the request is causing intense somatic distress. This discomfort is attributable to an internal struggle of some type. The host or another personality in the system may be attempting to prevent the emergence of the particular personality that the therapist is asking to meet; two or more personalities may be attempting to emerge simultaneously; or the system may be attempting to shove the requested, but reluctant, alter "out" to meet the therapist. Even if the patient is showing evidence of significant distress with this request, I would urge persistence. How long to persist is a judgment call. Not all alters emerge at the first request, and of course, the patient may not have MPD.

If the patient undergoes a dramatic transformation and says, "Hello, my name is Marcy," the therapist has passed the first obstacle. If a patient of mine appears distressed or may have switched but I am not sure, I often ask "What are you feeling now?" The patient may answer with something such as "Upset," "Frightened," or "Angry." I then ask,

"Does this feeling have a name?" Not infrequently a multiple will reply with a proper name (e.g., "John").

If a similar response is not forthcoming, then the therapist should spend some time examining with the patient his or her own perceptions about what was going on while the therapist was requesting to meet this personality. In cases of multiples who did not initially switch when requested, I have heard them describe "fading out," becoming distant and detached, feeling smothered, having a sense of terrible internal pressure, or feeling that a fog was closing in on them while I was making my request. Similar descriptions from a patient are highly suggestive of dissociative pathology and indicate that the therapist should persist, perhaps in another session, to elicit an alter. A second attempt should include an invitation to "any" other personality who may wish to meet the therapist, in addition to requesting to meet one or more alters whose existence the therapist infers from the patient's examples.

If a patient does not appear to feel anything and denies any internal response to the therapist's requests, then he or she may not have MPD. A strong alter personality or group of alters who wish to conceal the multiplicity, however, can do so successfully for prolonged periods of therapy, and most therapists experienced in the treatment of MPD will have one or more such cases. Therefore, the therapist should not irrevocably rule out the diagnosis of MPD, based on failure of an alter to come forward on request. In either event, the therapist should not feel chagrined about having made this request. In my experience, patients who do not have MPD tend to view this as one of those things that doctors do, like tapping people on the knee with a little rubber hammer. MPD patients, however, now know that the therapist suspects their multiplicity and even wishes to deal with it. This is, by and large, a positive result of this intervention and may well be responded to by the "spontaneous" emergence of an alter in the next few sessions. Sometimes the personality system just needs some time to process and respond to what may be the first attempt to approach it *as* a system.

If a patient continues to provide strong evidence that he or she is having frequent dissociative episodes, but the therapist is unable to elicit an alter personality by direct request, then it is worth considering the use of hypnotic probes or a drug-facilitated interview.

Forms of Communication with the Alter Personalities

The simplest case is one in which an alter personality emerges, identifies himself or herself, and proceeds to talk with the therapist. This is probably also the most common situation and occurs sooner or later in most MPD treatments. Alters may initially communicate with the therapist in other ways. They may speak, even though they are not "out" (i.e., in overt control of the body). These vocalizations are eerie and may be extremely frightening for the patient. In one case, for example, the first alter I met was named "Dead Mary" and vocalized through the terrified host personality. Dead Mary initially spoke of her hatred toward the patient and said that she wanted to "char her flesh to black ash"; later, upon direct emergence, she proved to be much less malignant than she sounded. The host personality's response to these vocalizations was one of pure horror. My studied response was to treat these vocalizations as a matter of course and to speak with Dead Mary in an interested and polite manner. In time, this approach prevailed and a useful dialogue was begun. Productive dialogue is, of course, the goal of contacting the alter parts of the patient.

Another form of contact is through inner vocalizations. The patient may "hear" the alter personality speak as an inner voice within, often as one of the "voices" that the patient has been hearing for years. The patient then can relay these internal responses to the therapist. In this case, the alter's responses are filtered by another personality (usually the host), with possible distortions. In situations where I have not been able to elicit an alter directly, I will ask the patient whether he or she has heard or felt any sort of internal response to my request. Dialogues based on the relaying of inner vocalizations are tenuous at best, but may be required to build enough trust to permit more direct contact.

Automatic writing—that is, the patient's writing of responses without apparent volitional control—is another means of communicating with an alter personality. Milton Erickson reported a case in which the treatment was conducted through automatic writing (Erickson & Kubie, 1939). If the patient has been able to keep a diary and reports finding entries that he or she does not remember writing, the therapist may be able to communicate with the author through automatic writing if attempts to directly meet this alter are unsuccessful. Automatic writing is slow, subject to a variety of problems, and not a useful way to conduct extensive therapy. It will, however, afford the therapist an initial window into the personality system that may prove useful later in treatment.

Ideomotor signaling, a technique that is most usefully coupled with hypnosis, may also provide a means of limited communication with unseen alter personalities. In ideomotor signaling, an agreement is made that some sign (e.g., raising the right index finger) is equivalent to some statement (e.g., "yes," "no," or "stop"). Braun reports being able to work with up to two lines of personalities using this technique (Braun, 1984c). Ideomotor signaling techniques are discussed in greater detail in Chapter Nine.

CONFIRMING THE DIAGNOSIS

When the therapist has met an entity that identifies itself as being different from the presenting patient (personality), this does not yet confirm the diagnosis of MPD. That awaits determining that the alter and any others that may subsequently appear are really separate, unique, and relatively enduring entities rather than transient ego-state phenomena. The therapist will need to determine, as best he or she can, the extent to which the alters are active outside of the therapy setting and the role that they have played in the patient's life history. The therapist will also need to assess the consistency of the alter personalities over time. True alter personalities are amazingly consistent and enduring entities that remain "in character" over time and across a wide range of situations.

All of the evidence to date suggests that MPD develops during a crucial window of vulnerability in childhood or early adolescence. Eventually, the therapist should be able to trace the origin of some of the patient's alter personalities back to this period or earlier. In other dissociative conditions, such as psychogenic fugue states, the elaborated secondary identity typically does not have a history of being active prior to its emergence during the fugue.

It will take some time to confirm the diagnosis of MPD, and both therapist and patient will probably go through a cycle of alternating acceptance and rejection of the diagnosis during the first part of therapy. This is to be expected. As discussed earlier in connection with the use of psychological testing in MPD, there are as yet no definitive tests to prove the existence of MPD in a patient. In many ways, the ultimate confirmation of the diagnosis lies in the response to treatment. If working with the patient as a multiple produces significant improvement in a person who has been refractory or minimally responsive to other therapeutic interventions, then "the proof is in the pudding."

Sharing the Diagnosis with the Patient

Even if the diagnosis has not been fully confirmed, the meeting of an alter part of the patient is a significant development and needs to be processed.

The patient may or may not have lost time during the appearance of the alter. The therapist should first determine how much of the experience is immediately available to the patient's recall. I often simply ask how much of the experience he or she was aware of and what can be remembered. It is important to ask also about what the patient felt at the time the alter was out and about the patient's current state of mind. After processing this information, I then summarize any missing elements and provide my own impressions. I try to do this in a matter-of-fact, professional manner.

The patient will be experiencing a number of concerns and fears at this moment. Foremost, in my experience, is the fear that this development will somehow change or terminate the therapy and that the therapist will abandon the patient as have so many other important people in his or her life. The host personality may also be grappling with the terror of finding that he or she is not alone in the body, or with the concern that it may no longer be possible to suppress the other personalities and all hell will break loose. The therapist cannot alleviate these anxieties, but can begin working with the personality system to help titrate the host's and any other personalities' fears to an acceptable level. I think that it is important for the therapist not to exaggerate the importance of the appearance of an alter, but to treat this as something that can be incorporated into the ongoing therapy and therapeutic relationship.

The therapist should not try to "prove" the diagnosis to the patient or others at this point. In particular, showing the patient videotapes or other documentation of the alters immediately after meeting them is likely to precipitate an adverse reaction. The therapist can ask the other parts of the patient for their advice on how to share the information with the patient. This is the beginning of enlisting the cooperation of the system of personalities to help the patient as a whole. The therapist should not expect too much at this point, but if an alter offers good advice, then this may be incorporated.

An important caution, however, is to avoid becoming involved in keeping secrets from one or more personalities. The request by one alter that the therapist keep information secret from another alter is a classic MPD dynamic that seeks to put the therapist in the middle of an internal conflict. A clinician who succumbs to this setup will quickly be placed in a seriously compromised position that will force him or her to betray the secret at some point. If the system does not want a specific personality to know some fact, such as the diagnosis, it will have ways of keeping that information secret.

There are two maxims to keep in mind while working with an MPD patient. The first is that everybody (meaning all of the alters who are not overtly present) is *always* listening in on the therapy. Although this is not strictly true all of the time, the therapist should temper all interventions, interpretations, comments, and asides as if it is, and should not say anything to any personality that another one should not hear. The second maxim is that MPD has originated as a survival mechanism for the patient, and for the most part it will continue to operate in this manner. Consequently, the therapist can let the multiple's system do the work of filtering out information that is intolerable to specific alters. The result of these two principles is that the therapist should formulate all remarks with the personality system as a whole in mind and should allow the system to determine who hears what.

The Patient's Reactions to the Diagnosis

If the patient does not have MPD, then the repercussions of having elicited a transient ego-state phenomenon are not likely to seriously disturb the patient. It is more of a curiosity or unusual experience that will not have a significant impact on daily functioning or the patient's sense of self. In the case of a multiple who has been hiding this secret, often behind the facade of the host personality, the revelation of the multiplicity may feel like a devastating failure. Yet at the same time there may also be a profound sense of relief that the secret is out, and hope that previously unspeakable things can now be said and dealt with. Each patient, of course, will be unique, but the response of a newly diagnosed multiple provides a cautionary tale—a preview of what much of the therapy is going to be like with this particular patient. The core work of treatment with victims of multiple personality is the uncovering and working through of secrets. The vast majority of these patients are victims of incest or other forms of sexual abuse, physical abuse, and emotional abuse. They are filled with secrets, which they keep even from themselves. The response of a particular patient to the uncovering of this first secret affords a glimpse into the patient's future responses to the uncovering of further secrets.

For a clinician, this situation is also a test of him or her as a therapist and, more specifically, as the *patient's* therapist. The personality system will be watching closely to see how the therapist responds. This is another aspect of the cautionary tale—testing. In therapy with multiples, *everything* is a test. Their need to test the therapist over and over, to determine whether he or she can be trusted with their secrets, is one of the reasons why multiples are among the most difficult of all psychiatric patients to treat. The fact that recovering and working through these secrets result in a profound change in their psychological state makes them among the most responsive to treatment of any psychiatric patient group. I do not think that a therapist can ever completely pass one of their tests. Fortunately, however, most multiples seem willing to give the therapist a second chance over and over again. The most important rule is to be honest with them.

Patients will have both immediate and long-term reactions to the diagnosis. In the weeks following the first appearance of an alter, there may be suicide gestures or attempts on the part of one or more alters or the host. It is worth reviewing the patient's medications with this in mind. Fugue episodes are not uncommon. I have had more than one newly diagnosed patient, frightened and bewildered, call me from a phone booth several states away. These sorts of incidents are upsetting for both patient and therapist. It is important, however, not to exaggerate them or become too involved in dealing with the specifics of a given situation and fail to move on to the next important steps of the treatment. These fleeing responses can be understood as serving, in part, to divert both therapist's attention and patient's attention away from the implications of the diagnosis.

Long-term responses to the diagnosis may include attempts by the patient to find out everything there is to know about MPD. Many of the patients that I have seen (although not all by any means) are above average in intelligence and capable of amassing a large armamentarium of facts on MPD. Unfortunately, since so little is actually known about this condition, many of these facts are incorrect at best. I try neither to encourage nor to discourage this search for information, and to answer any questions about "MPD in general" in a general manner. Then I will ask about how the question applies to the patients' situation. One of the strong factors motivating this search for knowledge is the patients' desire to make some sense of their lives. They want to know why they lose time and why they do not seem to inhabit the same world as the rest of us. This wish to make sense of what has happened and what is happening to them is one of the driving forces in therapy and should be nurtured. One should be alert, however, for attempts to use this knowledge to compete with or undermine the therapist. Should this happen, a clear interpretation of the resistance is necessary.

At some point, many MPD patients will experience a "flight into health," during which they deny that the MPD is active or even that it ever existed. They may seek to disprove that they are or ever were multiples, and even say that they faked it or made it up. This may happen within the first few weeks after meeting the first alter and may be repeated at other points later in therapy, often after some significant new revelation.

In those situations where the newly made diagnosis of MPD has precipitated serious life-threatening responses on the part of the patient, the common dynamic seems to be the fear of abandonment by the therapist. Often the therapist says or does something that leads the patient to believe that the therapist is going to stop seeing him or her. In some instances, this is an accurate perception. Many therapists new to MPD feel that they are in over their heads and seek to transfer their patients to a more "knowledgeable" therapist. In some cases, the therapist is simply using the diagnosis as an oportunity to get rid of a difficult and treatment-refractory patient. Almost without exception, multiples are exquisitely sensitive to abandonment, whether actual or merely contemplated.

ATYPICAL PRESENTATIONS

The general descriptions and discussions up to this point have primarily focused on "typical" cases of MPD. The profiles of these cases are drawn from clinical data amassed by therapists working primarily with female patients in outpatient psychiatric settings. Multiples can present in many other contexts, and as we learn more about this condition we will probably modify significantly what we consider to be a "typical" case. The following examples are meant to suggest the range of situations in which MPD patients may also present.

Chronically Hospitalized Patients

While working at St. Elizabeths Hospital in Washington, D.C., I have had the opportunity to visit, consult, and supervise on a variety of chronic inpatient wards, as well as at the John Howard Pavilion for the criminally insane. Occasionally, we have found a chronically hospitalized inpatient, usually with the diagnosis of schizophrenia, who in fact met DSM-III criteria for MPD. One common feature that seems to characterize all of the chronic inpatient multiples that I have met is the degree of relatedness and involvement that they engendered on the part of the ward staff. Not that their relationships with the staff were pleasant; on the contrary, in most cases the staff members were either angry at a patient or divided as a group in their feelings toward a patient. Yet they tended to interact with the patient vigorously as opposed to most other chronic patients on the same ward, who were simply cared for in a routine fashion. There is something about the relatedness of MPD patients that sets them apart from other psychiatric patients. Perhaps this is why so many therapists seem to become overinvolved with their first MPD patient or two.

Reviews of these patients' charts show that many of them had a pattern of erratic behavior, best reflected by significant ups and downs in their privilege status or other indicators of social functioning and ability to handle responsibility. Many came close to discharge on several occasions, only to have inexplicable regressions or other behavior that sabotaged their return to an outpatient setting. Often the staff saw them as manipulative and judged them not to be as "sick" as the other chronic patients on the unit.

They tended to create strong emotional responses on the part of the ward staff. These were expressed in the form of anger toward a patient and/or his or her doctor, while at the same time the staff might be working vigorously to help the patient in other ways. The patient's personality system would play into milieu splits by alternately placating and enraging the unit. For example, one patient being treated by a resident had an alter who periodically would emerge, put his clothes on backwards, and walk around the unit. This was that alter's way of declaring his difference from the host. The staff viewed this as purposeful, nonpsychotic behavior that was calculated to goad them, and would react by lowering his privilege status. At one point, this nonpsychotic, nonsuicidal patient had been restricted to his unit for over 6 months.

Patients with Posttraumatic and Pathological Grief Reaction

Another situation in which MPD seems to come to light occurs in patients who initially present with what appears to be either a posttraumatic stress disorder (e.g., rape trauma syndrome) or a pathological grief reaction. I have seen a number of cases where the MPD manifests itself in a woman in treatment at a rape counseling center for rape trauma syndrome. In most of these cases, the patient appeared to have been functioning well prior to the rape or attempted rape and had a significant deterioration in function following the trauma. Often the trauma reactivated nightmares and flashbacks of previous incest or sexual abuse, which were followed by increasingly frequent dissociative experiences such as time loss or minifugue episodes.

In some of these cases, the history given by the personalities suggests that the patient had achieved some level of integration or at least stability in the personality system, which was shattered by the sexual assault and the subsequent reactivation of dissociated memories and affects from prior sexual abuse. This presentation is likely to occur more often than one would expect by chance, since MPD patients seem unusually susceptible to rape (Coons & Milstein, 1984; Putnam *et al.*, 1986).

To date, I have seen four cases in which the presentation initially appeared to be a pathological grief reaction following the death of a parent. In each case, the patient was an established and successful adult, who had a precipitous decline in his or her level of functioning following the death of the parent. In one case, the multiplicity was not diagnosed for 3 years, during which time the patient had repeated hospitalizations for what was diagnosed as intractable temporal lobe epilepsy. The common link here seemed to be that in each case the parent who died was the primary abuser, and the death activated dissociated affects and memories.

Peers and Professionals

A fifth of the patients in the NIMH survey had graduate degrees (Putnam *et al.*, 1986). I know more than 20 multiples who are actively practicing professionals. They tend to be in the health professions, such as social work, psychology, and psychiatry, but my acquaintances include lawyers and judges. Having MPD does not preclude the ability to perform effectively in demanding occupations, but it is a handicap. The thought of a multiple being a peer or a professional is often greeted with horror or derisive humor by other professionals. In fact, many of the MPD professionals I know perform at above-average levels in their field. Unfortunately, many of these people are afraid to be in treatment, lest their multiplicity be revealed and cost them their jobs. We may hope that increasing professional and lay awareness of MPD will allow these people to be viewed for who they are—survivors of extreme childhood trauma.

SUMMARY

The major theme of this chapter on diagnosis has been that MPD is a chronic condition and that manifestations of dissociation will permeate a patient's past and present life. The key to diagnosis is learning how and where to look for this evidence. During the evaluation interview(s), one can often detect disruptions in the coherence and chronology of the patient's story; one must also be alert to defensive or compensatory maneuvers by the patient that seek to evade questions or divert the focus of inquiry. The interviewer seeks evidence of "time loss," as well as amnesias for complex behaviors or for the acquisition of knowledge or skills. Often there is amnesia for periods of childhood or important life events. Depersonalization, derealization, and out-of-body experiences are common. Such life experiences as being labeled a liar, flashbacks or intrusive recall of traumatic memories, and nightmares are often readily acknowledged, as well as experiences of "made" thoughts, feelings, and actions. The interviewer should seek specific examples of these experiences to examine in detail and should rule out their association with drugs or alcohol.

Within a given interview and across a series of interviews, one may see evidence of amnesia. Covert switching among alter personalities may be manifest by changes in affect, facial expression, and voice. The patient may occasionally make self-references in the third person or the first person plural. Common features of the mental status examination are summarized in Table 4-1. In some instances, special diagnostic procedures, such as the keeping of diaries, may be required. Although there are no definitive psychological or physiological diagnostic tests, the MMPI and Rorschach may provide suggestive evidence. And the often neglected physical examination is desirable to rule out certain organic conditions and look for evidence of self-mutilation.

The diagnosis is made by meeting alter personalities directly. They can often be elicited by direct or indirect questioning. The confirmation of the diagnosis is often in the patient's response to treatment. The patient can be expected to have an intense response to learning the diagnosis, and the therapist should approach this question gently but directly.

CHAPTER FIVE

The Alter Personalities

WHAT IS AN ALTER PERSONALITY?

The core feature of MPD is the existence of alter personalities who exchange control over an individual's behavior. It is important to state from the outset that whatever an alter personality is, it is *not* a separate person. It is a serious therapeutic error to relate to the alter personalities as if they were separate people. Although many alters will emphatically insist that they are separate people, the therapist must not buy into this delusion of separateness. The therapist can empathize with each alter's feelings of separation and each alter's unique perceptions of experiences and events. But the global message from the therapist should always be that *all* of the alters constitute a whole person. This is one of the first tests of the therapeutic alliance that occurs after the overt emergence of alter personalities. Certain alters may angrily contest this therapeutic stance and attempt to tie up the therapy with this issue. The therapist should not engage in protracted struggles or attempts at proof, but should simply impart and reinforce a message of implicit wholeness whenever the opportunity arises.

I do not think that anyone really knows what ultimately constitutes an alter personality. I conceptualize the alters as highly discrete states of consciousness organized around a prevailing affect, sense of self (including body image), with a limited repertoire of behaviors and a set of state-dependent memories. For our present purposes, however, the most useful clinical definition is the one developed by Braun and Kluft over the course of several American Psychiatric Association workshops on MPD. They define an alter personality as

> an entity with a firm, persistent, and well-founded sense of self and a characteristic and consistent pattern of behavior and feelings in re-

sponse to given stimuli. It must have a range of functions, a range of emotional reponses, and a significant life history (of its own existence). (Kluft, 1984c, p. 23)

Most MPD patients have some alter personalities who would meet this definition, as well as a number of "personality fragments" who are similar to full-fledged alter personalities except that they lack the depth and breadth of a personality and have only a very limited range of affects, behaviors, and life history (Kluft, 1984c). A personality fragment typically exhibits a single affect, such as anger or joy, or performs a single function, such as driving the car or protecting the body. Braun adds the further distinction of "a special-purpose fragment" that may only engage in a single, highly specified activity, such as cleaning the bathtub (Kluft, 1984c).

The distinction between a personality and a personality fragment can be difficult to make and is largely a matter of judgment. An alter's role in the personality system also changes over time, so that a given entity may be characterized as a fragment at one point and as a personality at another. In most instances, it is not necessary to establish firmly whether a given entity is a personality or a fragment, since the basic therapeutic interventions are similar for both.

Dimensions of Distinctness

An alter personality has a number of observable functions, attributes, and behaviors. The same personality will also have a number of "self-perceptions" that are important for its own sense of identity and overall role in the multiple's system. For the clinician, the observable phenomena are more impressive and lead to the acceptance of the diagnosis. For the multiple, the self-perceptions are more important in differentiating a given personality from others in the multiple's system. The clinician must develop a degree of empathy for a personality's self-perceptions, if he or she is going to establish a working alliance with that personality.

Observable Differences in the Patient

With repeated contact over time, an observer will notice that the alter personalities will differ from one another along a number of dimensions. Predominant affect is a major discriminator of alter personalities. Some alters will be continuously light-hearted and silly, whereas others will be unremittingly depressed and suicidal, and still others will always be

furious and hostile. A second dimension that discriminates alter personalities is observable behaviors. There will be differences in both spontaneous and elicited behaviors. Personalities may differ in posture, facial
appearance, body language, speech, and idiosyncratic mannerisms. They
may also react to the same stimulus in dramatically different ways. The
personalities will differ in their ability to recall memories of past events,
including previous interactions with the observer. Some alter personalities will manifest psychologically and often physiologically different somatic symptoms, such as headache or functional bowel disease.

Observable Differences in the Therapist

I would speculate that this disorder has come to be called "multiple
personality disorder" rather than something like "multiple psychophysiological states disorder" because the different alters elicit strongly individualized responses from people working with them. Repeatedly, I have
observed clinicians, other medical personnel, and various lay persons or
nonmedical professionals all react to the different personalities of a
multiple as though they were dealing with separate people. In watching
videotapes of myself working with multiples, I find that I also unconsciously change my demeanor when dealing with different alters. These
responses are expressed in all of the verbal and nonverbal forms of
communication that permeate our daily social interactions. In many
instances, the persons responding to different alter personalities are only
vaguely aware of the changes in their own outward behavior. I believe
that it is the evocation of these individualized responses to the alter
personalities of a multiple that many therapists find so compelling.

Differences Reported by the Alters

The alter personalities themselves will report having very different self-
concepts, body images, and values. They will see themselves as being of
different ages, and their behavior may vary along a developmental axis.
They may describe themselves as being of a different gender or race or as
having different sexual orientations. They will claim different relationships with significant others (e.g., some personalities may deny that they
are married or that their biological children are related to them). They
will also differ in their degree of awareness of the other alter personalities
and the past history of the individual as a whole. Some will recognize the
existence of the system of personalities and their function(s) within it;
others will vehemently deny that there are any other personalities.

Alter Personality Functions

Alter personalities can be thought of as performing specific functions or tasks required by the patient for overall functioning. Some of these tasks are related to the demands of the external world, such as performing a job, raising a family, or creating a work of art. Other functions have to do with the needs of the internal psychological world of the MPD patient. The external functions are the most obvious, but a therapist must be aware that many alters also perform important internal functions in addition to their external duties. Examples of internal functions include controlling which alter personalities are allowed "out" in specific situations, holding traumatic memories or intolerable affects, and transferring information across personalities. Often these internal functions are extrapolations of the external role. For example, an alter personality who functioned as a prostitute in the external world also functioned internally to titrate and buffer sexuality for the patient. This prostitute personality, initially thought to be of minor importance because of her infrequent overt appearances, turned out to be a prime mover in the personality system's internal politics.

Evolution of Alter Personalities over Time and Treatment

In most instances, alter personalities arise as a defensive response by the individual to what is experienced as an overwhelming traumatic experience (Kluft, 1984; Greaves, 1980; Bliss, 1980). Over time, alters may come to acquire a significant degree of autonomy and investment in their separateness (Kluft, 1984c). They may change from performing psychologically defensive tasks, such as screening out or absorbing unbearable experiences, to having their own independent objectives that are in conflict with those of the individual as a whole. Alter personalities change over time. They may acquire new functions or relinquish old ones. It is important to learn about both the external and internal functions of specific alter personalities and to recognize that these may change over the course of time and with treatment.

TYPES OF ALTER PERSONALITIES

Almost everyone hates to be stereotyped, and multiples are no exception. Therapists who have been exposed to a number of cases of MPD, however, quickly come to recognize that certain broad categories of alter personalities can be found in common across most patients. The overriding common denominators that allow characterization of alter personality types are the functions that the personalities serve and the affects and memories that they carry. Although each person with MPD is unique, some principles of organization are typical.

The Host Personality

All individuals with MPD have at least one alter who serves as the "host." The host has been defined as "the one who has executive control of the body the greatest percentage of time during a given time" (Kluft, 1984c, p. 23). Frequently this is the personality that presents for treatment and the one who becomes identified as the "patient" prior to the diagnosis of MPD.

The typical host personality is depressed, anxious, anhedonic, rigid, frigid, compulsively good, conscience-stricken, and masochistic, and suffers from a variety of somatic symptoms, particularly headaches (Kluft, 1984c). Host personalities are often overwhelmed by their life circumstances and present themselves as powerless and at the mercy of forces beyond their control or comprehension. In two-thirds of the cases in the NIMH survey, the host personality did not know about the existence of other alter personalities, and lost time when other alters emerged (Putnam et al., 1986). As Stern (1984) points out, it is more often the case that the host personality actively denies evidence of the existence of alter selves than that the alter personalities deliberately hide themselves from the host. When presented with evidence of alter personalities, the host may flee from treatment.

The host may not always be a single alter personality. In some cases, the host is a social facade created by a more or less cooperative effort of several alters agreeing to pass as one. These facade hosts may disintegrate early in the course of treatment, leaving the neophyte therapist wondering what has become of the "patient" who first entered therapy.

Child Personalities

Child and infant personalities are found in virtually every MPD patient's system of alter personalities (Putnam et al., 1986). Usually there will be a number of child personalities, and they often exceed the number of adult personalities. The child and infant personalities are usually frozen in time; they are locked into a given age until late in the course of therapy when, relieved of their psychological burden, they may "grow up" prior to integration. Child and infant alters frequently serve the function of holding memories and affects generated by earlier traumatic experiences. When these personalities come "out," they may repeatedly abreact the traumatic experiences in some fashion. Since many infant or small child personalities are nonverbal or only able to express themselves in an age-related manner, the abreactions often take the form of writhing on the floor, re-enacting the experience, throwing themselves into walls, or some equally disturbing and potentially dangerous behavior. They may also curl up into a fetal position or become unresponsive. It is not uncommon for them to perceive the therapist as if he or she were the original abuser.

Usually there will be other child or infant personalities who serve to counterbalance the frightened and abused ones. These child alters are often love seekers and may be very Pollyanna-like, seeing everything as wonderful and idealizing the abuser(s). They retain a childhood innocence that the other alters have lost. They can cause problems for a patient, however, because they lack the judgment or skills necessary to cope with situations into which they emerge.

Persecutor Personalities

At least half or more of MPD patients have alter personalities who see themselves in diametric conflict with the host personality (Putnam & Post, 1988; Putnam et al., 1986). This group of alter personalities, sometimes referred to as "internal persecutors," will sabotage the patient's life and may inflict serious injury upon the body in attempts to harm or kill the host or other personalities. They may be responsible for episodes of self-mutilation or for "suicide" attempts, which are actually "internal homicides" as persecutor personalities attempt to maim or kill the host. The perceived degree of separateness that allows one personality to believe that it can kill another personality without endangering itself has been labeled a "pseudodelusion" by Kluft (1984c) and a form of "trance logic" by Spiegel (1984).

Some persecutor personalities can be recognized as "introjects" of the original abuser(s); others have evolved from original helper personalities into current persecutors. Typically, they strike a contemptuous or condescending attitude toward the therapist and often actively seek to undermine treatment. In spite of their history of hostile behavior toward the patient as a whole and their negative reactions toward the therapy, they can be won over and enlisted in the patient's struggle to improve the quality of his or her life. In their anger, they contain much of the energy and strength that an MPD patient needs to survive and improve.

Suicidal Personalities

In addition to the persecutors who may attempt to kill the patient, there may be suicidal personalities who are driven to kill themselves. These alter personalities often have a single-minded dedication to their task of suicide and may have no awareness of the host or other personalities. They can be very difficult to reason with and may represent a signficant danger to the patient. The system of personalities, however, usually can be enlisted to hold in check the self-destructive impulses of these personalities.

Protector and Helper Personalities

Fortunately, most MPD patients also have an array of protector and helper personalities, who serve as a counterbalance to the persecutors and suicidal personalities. The degree of control that these protectors can exert on the more dangerous or self-compromising behaviors of the persecutors varies with each case and is also a function of the stage of treatment. In a patient who has not been actively treated as a multiple, the protectors may be too weak or only erratically available to aid the patient. As therapy progresses, and as more internal communication and cooperation is established within the system of alter personalities, the protectors will usually gain influence and control and will be able to intervene more effectively to suppress or redirect violence aimed at self and others.

Protector personalities come in a number of different forms, depending upon what the multiple requires protection from. There may be personalities who simply protect the body from any perceived external danger. In female multiples, these guardians are often male alters. Even in petite female patients, these protectors can be unexpectedly physically powerful. They will emerge if they believe that the body is in danger or threatened by circumstances reminiscent of previous trauma. They may be inadvertently triggered during therapy sessions. Since they are basically defensive in nature, it is important to assure and demonstrate to them that no harm is intended to the patient.

Protector personalities also serve as part of an internal system of checks and balances to counteract some of the self-destructive personalities. They may abort or sabotage self-destructive behavior or ensure that the patient gets help if a suicide attempt should occur. It is not uncommon for a suicidal or internally homicidal personality to take an overdose medication, and for a protector personality then to emerge and call the rescue squad.

The Internal Self-Helper

A special form of helper or protector personality is the "internal self-helper" (ISH), first described by Allison (1974a). Experienced therapists disagree about the nature of ISH personalities and whether they occur in all MPD patients. ISHs appear to occur in at least 50–80% of MPD cases where they have been sought. Typically, they are physically passive and relatively emotionless personalities, who provide information and insights into the inner workings of the system. Once they are identified, many therapists have found them to be invaluable guides, who can provide timely suggestions about problems and issues in therapy. Guidelines for eliciting, recognizing, and working with ISH personalities are described in Chapter Eight.

Memory Trace Personality

The memory trace, first recognized by Wilbur, is a personality who usually has a more or less complete memory of the individual's life history (Kluft, 1984c). This personality is commonly found in MPD patients and can provide historical information on past events and the activities of other personalities. The memory trace tends to be passive and usually must be sought out by the therapist.

Cross-Gender Personalities

At least half of all MPD patients have cross-gender alter personalities. In female MPD patients, child, adolescent, or adult male personalities are found in about half of cases. In male MPD patients, female alter personalities appear to be present in about two-thirds to three-quarters of all cases (Putnam et al., 1986; Loewenstein et al., 1986). These opposite-gender personalities often cross-dress and may be responsible for the unisex look adopted by many MPD patients. Female MPD patients frequently have short hair and wear clothing (blouse or shirt and pants) that allows their male alter personalities to emerge comfortably. As noted earlier, the male alters of female patients tend to serve in masculine roles, such as physical protection and operation of machinery. The male alter personalities of female MPD patients can be strikingly masculine in speech, mannerisms, and behavior.

In male MPD patients, the female personalities often are older, "good-mother" figures, who provide counsel and attempt to soften some of the angry and destructive behavior common in male MPD victims. The female personalities of male MPD patients are usually more active in the internal system's dynamics than in the outside world; consequently, they tend to emerge less frequently and as a rule are not as strikingly different. In both sexes, cross-gender alter personalities may be sexually active with either heterosexual or homosexual orientations, leading to much confusion.

Promiscuous Personalities

In most cases of MPD, there are personalities that express forbidden impulses. Often these impulses are sexual. Promiscuous alters may lead turbulent sexual lives, leaving the bewildered host wondering how he or she has once again gotten into a compromising situation. Promiscuous alters may also re-enact previous sexual abuse in and out of the therapy setting. A common scenario reported by female MPD patients is for a promiscuous alter to pick up a strange man, set up an intimate and often masochistic situation, and then vanish, leaving the frightened and usually sexually frigid host personality to contend with the stranger's advances. Not unexpectedly, the host interprets the outcome of this internal setup as rape. Prostitute personalities are common in female MPD patients. They may handle the sexuality for the personality system, as well as providing a source of income.

Administrators and Obsessive–Compulsive Personalities

Administrator and obsessive personalities are two types of alters who frequently emerge in the workplace and aid a multiple in earning a living. They may be quite competent professionally and often perform the additional internal function of organizing an otherwise fragmented individual. Coworkers typically see only these personalities, whom they "know" as the individual. Administrator personalities are often described as cold, distant, and authoritarian. Their aloofness discourages any familiarity that could disclose the existence of other personalities.

Substance Abusers

As previously discussed, substance abuse is not uncommon in MPD. Sedatives, hypnotics, and analgesics are the most commonly abused drugs, closely followed by stimulants and alcohol (Putnam *et al.*, 1986). The drug abuse in MPD is usually limited to specific alter personalities. There are many anecdotal reports suggesting that the alter personality who abuses a substance may be the only one within the multiple's system of personalities who experiences symptoms upon withdrawal. These reports have not been verified in a controlled setting, however.

Autistic and Handicapped Personalities

Personalities who appear autistic may be found within a multiple's system of personalities. Generally these are child or infant personalities. When active, they may sit and rock or self-stimulate in the manner of autistic children. They often are sent "out" when no other alter personalities are interested in being in control. They are particularly likely to emerge in situations where a multiple is being confined, controlled, or under intense scrutiny (e.g., in a seclusion room or wet-sheet pack in a hospital or under questioning by police).

Personalities with specific handicaps (e.g., blindness, deafness, loss of limb function) are relatively common in more complex MPD patients. The psychological meaning of the handicap may ultimately be understood in the therapy, but prior to recognition, these alters may create many difficult situations for the patient and therapist. I have seen four MPD patients who were in programs for the deaf because hearing-impaired alters were in control much of the time. None of these patients suffered from a physiological hearing impairment.

Personalities with Special Talents or Skills

Alter personalities who contain special abilities often exist within a multiple's system of personalities. These skills may be work-related, or they may be artistic or athletic. Typically, the alters who express these abilities tend to be personality fragments. They may be exceptionally skilled at what they do and exist purely for the expression of a specific ability or talent.

Anesthetic or Analgesic Personalities

Anesthetic or analgesic personalities are common in cases of MPD and often trace their origin to painful physical or sexual abuse (Kluft, 1984c; Putnam *et al.*, 1986). They deny feeling pain and are activated when the body is injured by self or others. They may be involved in self-mutilative behaviors.

Imitators and Imposters

Some multiples have within their system alters whose function is to mimic other personalities. When these imposters emerge, they appear and sound like the alter they are imitating. The intention will differ from case to case. In some instances they simply handle situations that the personality they are mimicking cannot; for example, one patient had an "imposter" who handled flirting and men for the asexual host. In other cases, the imposters may serve to confuse or sabotage the therapy and lead the therapist astray. Personalities who imitate the ISH personality have been reported.

Demons and Spirits

In some multiples, particularly those who come from rural areas or with fundamentalist religious beliefs, there will be alter personalities who identify themselves as spirits or demons. The spirits are often personalities who provide guidance along the lines of an ISH. The demons are usually malevolent, persecutor-type personalities and may identify themselves as Satan or one of his disciples.

Benevolent spirit personalities can be treated in the same manner as an ISH, described in Chapter Eight. Demons should be handled in the same fashion as other persecutor personalities. Attempts at exorcism or other religious practices to deal with these personalities are only transiently effective in suppressing them and are therapeutically contraindicated. Many therapists working with their first MPD cases will attempt to suppress the angry, hostile, and malevolent personalities. This does not work for any length of time and usually leads to problems in the therapeutic alliance, because the therapist is denying part of what the patient is experiencing. A more thorough discussion of working with persecutor personalities follows in Chapter Eight.

The Original Personality

Many multiples have a personality who is identified by the other personalities of the system as the "original" personality from whom all others are derived. Kluft has defined the original personality as "the identity which developed just after birth and split off the first new personality in order to help the body survive a severe stress" (Kluft, 1984c). Typically the original is not active and is often described as having been "put to sleep" or otherwise incapacitated at some much earlier point because he or she was not able to cope with the trauma. The original usually does not surface until late in the course of therapy, after much of the trauma has been metabolized by therapeutic abreaction. The host personality is not the original personality in most patients.

OTHER ASPECTS OF ALTER PERSONALITIES

Degrees of Interawareness among the Alter Personalities

The alter personalities of an MPD patient's personality system will possess varying levels of awareness of one another. The host personality, who usually presents for treatment, generally does *not* know about the existence of other personalities. Some types of personalities, such as ISH or memory trace alters, will claim knowledge of the entire system of alter personalities. Other alter personalities may know a subset of the other personalities, but not all of them. In many instances, personality A will know about the existence and behavior of personality B; personality B, however, may have no knowledge of personality A's existence. This property has been termed "directional awareness" and is typically exhibited by many of the personalities in a multiple's system.

In the older literature, various forms of directional awareness were used to classify cases of MPD into categories, such as "mutually amnesic," "one-way amnesic," and so on (Taylor & Martin, 1944; Ellenberger, 1970). These early classification schemes were based on generalizations from one or two cases and do not work when applied to a large number of patients. The NIMH survey found that three-quarters of

MPD patients had at least one personality who denied all knowledge of any other personalities, and that over 85% of cases also had a personality who claimed to know all of the other personalities (Putnam *et al.*, 1986). It is important for a therapist to recognize that knowledge about the system and other issues relevant to the life of the person are not shared equally across all alter personalities. One of the major tasks of therapy is to make available to the entire system of personalities the knowledge and secrets held by specific alter personalities. This generalization of knowledge gradually erodes the need for separateness and begins the movement toward resolution.

The dissociative barriers that separate the personalities are more permeable for some types of information than for other types. Ludwig *et al.* (1972) were the first to study this permeability systematically, although earlier researchers such as Morton Prince (Prince & Peterson, 1908) made use of this principle to investigate coconscious phenomena. The more emotionally charged or traumatically linked an idea or affect is, the more it will tend to be isolated within an alter and segregated from the larger domain of consciousness. Based on their paired-word and galvanic skin response (GSR) studies, Ludwig *et al.* (1972) observed, "The relative uniqueness of these personalities, however, as well as the boundaries separating them, tend to disappear for most emotionally neutral or non-affect-laden material" (p. 308). Hence, the alter personalities of a multiple will show extremely spotty compartmentalization, with a high degree of separation for some material and shared awareness of other material. Clever experiments have shown that one can subliminally feed information into one alter and demonstrate its existence to other alters, again indicating some leakage across dissociative barriers (Nissen *et al.*, 1988; Silberman *et al.*, 1985).

Attitudes of Alter Personalities toward the Body

Many of the alter personalities of an MPD patient show an amazingly cavalier attitude toward the safety and well-being of the body that they share. In addition to the "delusion of separateness" discussed above, even those alters who do recognize that they share the same body often do not seem very interested in the health of that body. I have told some personalities that they tend to treat their body the way employees of a firm often view a company car. It is seen as something to use, misuse, or abuse, but it is someone else's responsibility to keep it running. The personalities have in return provided their own explanations for their indifference to the well-being of the body they share. Common responses include the following: (1) Everyone else, particularly the original abuser, has mistreated the body, so the personalities do not feel that they should behave any differently. (2) The personalities exist outside of the body and only view it as a place to come for interaction with the physical world; they feel that it is unnecessary for their continued survival. (3) It is not their body, they do not like it very much, and they would change it (e.g., via a sex-change operation) if they could.

The other side of the coin is the fact that many of the alter personalities will see the body as being very different when they inhabit it. Some may see the hair as blond; others see it as brunette. Some see the body as short and fat; others see the body as tall and skinny. The ability of different personalities to "see" themselves as physically different is akin to the distortions of body image found in conditions such as anorexia nervosa. These perceived differences are part of each alter's internal representation and must be explored in order to understand the patient as a whole. In some cases, the personalities' perceived physical differences will concide with some of the external physical changes observed by the therapist. In many cases, they will not.

Names and Naming

Although identity is a complex concept, most of its attributes are collapsed into a single morpheme, a name (Seeman, 1980). Most personalities will have a name. Often they will have first and last and even middle names; in many cases, the names are some derivative of the legal name. So an MPD patient named Elizabeth Jane Doe might well have alter personalities with the first names of Elizabeth, Lizzy, Lizzie, Liz, Betsie, Beth, Bets, Jane, Janie, Lizzy-Jane, and so on. In addition, there may be different versions of a specific personality, so there may be Liz I and Liz II. These different editions usually vary along an age dimension, so Liz I may be a child and Liz II an adolescent.

Alter personalities may also be named by the external or internal function they perform (e.g., "the driver," "the maid," "the cook," "the gatekeeper" for a personality who performs the internal function of controlling which alter personalities in the system can emerge at a given time). Or they may be named for the affect that they manifest (e.g., "the angry one," "the sad one," "the scared one," etc.). Sometimes a function name may be disguised as a proper name; in one case, a memory trace personality was named "Stacy," which stood for "Stay and see." It is important to listen for double entendres in the names of the alter personalities; the therapist may thus avoid some confusion.

Many personality systems will have one or more "unnamed" personalities. Sometimes these "unnamed" alters use the same trick Ulysses pulled on the Cyclops: they go by the name of "No one." When the therapist inquires as to who in the system is responsible for some behavior, he or she will be told "No one." So the therapist should be prepared to inquire whether there is a personality known as "No one," "No name," or "Nobody." Most of the "unnamed" personalities will turn out to have names as the therapy progresses. Many alters are unwilling to reveal their names early in the course of therapy, because this knowledge allows the therapist to call them out. It is important to learn each personality's name and to use it in working with that personality as part of the patient's system. Chapter Six covers ways of learning about the names and functions of the alters in a patient's personality system.

SWITCHES AND SWITCHING

Switching is the process of changing from one alter personality to another and is a core behavioral phenomenon in MPD. Any therapist who hopes to make progress in treating a case of MPD must become adept at recognizing switches. Otherwise, the patient's behavior is not understandable, and the clinical leverage afforded by recognizing and confronting the alter personalities about their behavior is lost.

Degree of Control over the Process

Switching is a psychophysiological process that may occur in a controlled or uncontrolled fashion. A switch may be stimulated by the internal dynamics of the multiple's system, or it may be elicited by events in the immediate environment. In general, the alter personality present before the switch is replaced by another personality. In some cases, however, both personalities will be present simultaneously. In observing many multiples switch among their alter personalities, I have found a number of common switch elements (Putnam, 1988c).

As an MPD patient progresses through treatment, he or she gains control over the switching process. Early on, switches tend to be triggered by environmental cues or internal conflicts, and are experienced as being out of volitional control, particularly by the host personality. Many of the alter personalities will be unaware of one another and view life as a series of appearances and disappearances in which they often "wake up" in strange and unusual circumstances. There is a certain adaptive logic to the switching process, however, so that an appropriate alter personality is called out in most circumstances. The ability to switch and bring forth a personality appropriate to a given situation endows MPD patients with a chameleon-like capacity that they use in turn to mask the multiplicity. Hence, the existence of alter personalities may only be apparent to those people who observe the patient across a variety of different settings. In times of stress, however, alter personalities may emerge who are inappropriate to the situation, resulting in serious problems for the patient.

Manifestations of Switching

The manifestations of a switch can be divided into physical and psychological changes that may be observed when an exchange of alter personalities takes place. In many cases, the physical changes are the more observable, but the psychological changes are, in the long run, the more compelling. Switches of alter personalities can be overt or covert. The latter can be extremely difficult to detect, and it is only after one has observed a number of overt switches that covert switching is likely to be recognized.

    The degree of difference perceived in a switch between two alter personalities is influenced by several factors. The first factor is the degree of differentiation between the two personalities. A switch from a 10-year-old female personality to a 35-year-old male personality is more likely to produce a wide range of physical and psychological differences than is a switch between two adult male personalities who are similar along a number of dimensions. A second factor that seems to influence the observer's perception of difference is the observer's familiarity and past experience with the alter personalities. Many therapists report that initially they were only vaguely aware that a patient was changing in some fashion; they did not perceive this as a switch from one alter personality to another. As they came to know the alter personalities over time, they developed an ability to distinguish them more easily and to discern greater degrees of differences among them. Eventually, many therapists report that they can tell which personality is "out" from 50 paces.

Physical Changes

FACIAL CHANGES

    In some multiples, dramatic facial changes accompany the switching of personalities. These transformations are most apparent around the eyes and the mouth. Vertical wrinkles may be rearranged into horizontal creases, or the jaw may shift from an underbite to an overbite. In other cases, there may only be a subtle softening or hardening of expression. Most observers report that they notice a distinct change in the eyes. Usually this is not a quantifiable difference, only a qualitative one. I find that when I suspect that a patient may be covertly switching, it is important to carefully observe the direction and depth of the wrinkles, folds, and creases in the face, and then to watch for abrupt changes that erase or significantly rearrange these markers. The trick is to differentiate this process from the normal expressional changes that occur in all of us. Facial changes alone are insufficient evidence to confirm a switch, but together with other consistently observable changes, they can alert a clinician to possible covert switching.

POSTURAL AND MOTOR BEHAVIORAL CHANGES

Changes in body posture, body language, and motor activity frequently occur with the transition of alter personalities. The degree of difference observed between two personalities will be influenced by the factors described above. Many multiples have one or several alters who have distinctive body postures. This is especially pronounced with child personalities, personalities that contain memories for certain types of abuse experiences, and personalities that have specific psychosomatic conditions or deficits. Infant or small child personalities frequently curl up in fetal positions, crawl on the floor, or huddle in corners. Personalities that serve as reservoirs of memories and affect for traumatic experiences may re-enact those experiences in subtle or dramatic ways when they emerge. For instance, a 42-year-old female multiple had a 9-year-old child personality who continually rubbed her wrists and hands together when she was present. The subsequent history obtained from this alter indicated that she had been the one "out" when the patient was tied by the wrists, hung from a hook on a door, and beaten. She rubbed her wrists in response to the viscerally remembered pain and numbness from those experiences.

Alter personalities who suffer from psychogenic disabilities (e.g., blindness, deafness, mutism, or sensory anesthesias) will often have characteristic compensatory behaviors that are exhibited when they are present. Motor behavior across alter personalities may differ in other ways. The degree of motor coordination and manual skills for certain tasks can differ across alters. The level of available physical strength may also vary, so that certain alters are capable of feats of strength that other alters cannot duplicate. Tremors or unusual mannerisms may be present in certain personalities.

VOICE AND SPEECH CHANGES

Voice and speech changes have been repeatedly reported by clinical observers of MPD (e.g., Riggall, 1931; Morton & Thoma, 1964; Goddard, 1926; Mason, 1893; W. F. Prince, 1917; Cory, 1919; Peck, 1922; Congdon *et al.*, 1961; Thigpen & Cleckley, 1954; Burks, 1942; Lipton, 1943). Clinically, these changes are most apparent in pitch, volume, rate, articulation, accent, and language use. The male alters of a female MPD patient may drop their voices a full octave or more from the usual speaking voice. The child alters may raise their voices by an equal amount. In addition, the child personalities may speak "baby talk," babble, or use childlike grammar. Personalities who represent identifications with specific individuals may adopt their manner and style of speaking as well as imitating their voices. Voice spectral analysis studies of spontaneous and patterned speech of the alter personalities of subjects with MPD indicate that these changes often include format frequency changes that are not duplicated by actor controls (Ludlow & Putnam, 1988). In addition, speech defects, such as stuttering, may be present in some personalities and absent in others (M. Prince, 1906; Putnam *et al.*, 1984).

DRESS AND GROOMING

Changes in dressing style, grooming, and makeup are most apparent across several sessions. Several of the female MPD cases that I work with have male alter personalities who refuse to emerge if the person is wearing a dress. Consequently, as noted earlier, many of these people adopt a unisex look that permits male and female personalities to feel comfortable publicly. Changes in hairstyle can be very dramatic. In one case, a female MPD patient alternated between wearing her hair in an old-maid bun and a spikey, punk rock look. Neither personality was comfortable with the other's coiffure or social values. Some alternate personalities will have wigs that complete their identity. Changes in the use of makeup can be equally dramatic. Heavy use of makeup, false eyelashes, falsies, and so on is often seen in promiscuous or party personalities, whereas depressed and withdrawn personalities in the same individual may cultivate a nondescript appearance to help them escape notice.

BEHAVIOR DURING THE SWITCHING PROCESS

The actual moment of switching can last from fractions of a second to several minutes or even longer in a few cases (Putnam, 1988c). In most, but not all, instances where I have been able to videotape and study a switch, the initiation of the switch is signaled by a blink or upward roll of the eyes. There may be a rapid fluttering of the eyelids. Transient facial twitching or grimacing often accompanies a switch. In addition, there may be bodily twitches, shudders, or abrupt changes in posture. If the switch takes several minutes to complete, the individual may go into an unresponsive, trance-like state with blank, unseeing eyes. A few multiples have convulsion-like switches that have, on occasion, been mistaken for epileptic seizures.

In many cases, the patient has learned to disguise or cover up switching behavior. Women will frequently turn their faces away, momentarily shield their faces with their hands, or let their hair fall over their faces during the moment of switching. An alternate personality may time its emergence so that the therapist is looking away or is otherwise distracted. Alter personalities may also come and go very quickly so that they are only momentarily present. I have seen therapists who are unfamiliar with MPD often indicate their subliminal awareness that something has occurred in the patient by asking questions such as "Did you just hear a voice speaking to you?"

Immediately after a new alter has emerged, particularly an alter amnesic for the preceding interactions, a patient may exhibit a number of behaviors that MPD therapists refer to as "grounding." Typical grounding behaviors include touching the face, pressing the temples, touching the chair he or she is sitting in, looking around the room quickly, and shifting posture restlessly. Grounding behaviors are thought to be part of the orientation process for an alter who suddenly finds himself or herself in a new situation.

Psychological Changes

AFFECT

In many cases, the strongest indicator that a switch has occurred will be a sudden, otherwise inexplicable shift in the person's affect. Anger that comes "out of the blue," sudden laughter, or tears that are out of context are often manifestations that another alter has emerged with strong responses to the material being discussed. This apparently inappropriate and labile affect may contribute to the misdiagnoses of manic–depressive illness or schizophrenia in some MPD patients. It is important for the therapist to take note and follow up sudden and inexplicable shifts in affect. I often ask, "What are you feeling now?" The multiple may say something like "Angry" or "Sad." I then ask, "Does this feeling have a name?" Frequently a multiple will answer with a proper name (e.g., "Mary," "George W," etc.).

A multiple may show a sudden burst of an affect such as anger or laughter and then resume where he or she left off, without any recognition or acknowledgment that something unusual has just occurred. This is one example of intrainterview amnesia, discussed in Chapter Four. In fact, the alter that a therapist has been working with may have no awareness that he or she just said or did some inappropriate or outrageous thing. When the therapist inquires about what just happened, the patient may become panicked or tearful.

BEHAVIORAL AGE

Another manifestation of switching is an apparent change in the patient's level of maturity. Most alter personalities are younger than the chronological age of the patient. Consequently, when a patient switches, it is very likely that there will be some shift along the age dimension. Child personalities may be easily recognizable by their nervous fidgeting, movement overflow, and childlike gestures (e.g., rubbing the nose with the back of the hand).

THOUGHT PROCESSES

Alter personalities typically demonstrate a wide range in their cognitive abilities. Many of the child personalities will have difficulty communicating with the therapist because of an apparent difficulty in understanding ideas and language. Alters will differ in their ability to think abstractly, with some capable of adult-level reasoning and others being profoundly concrete (Putnam et al., 1984). If a therapist detects a sudden shift along this axis, it is likely that a switch has occurred.

The ability of personalities to remember past information or to learn new information will also vary considerably. Discrepancies between alters along this dimension may be greatest for cause-and-effect relationships. Some personalities will understand that a sequence of events will lead to a certain outcome, and others will arrive at a very different conclusion. If a patient is suddenly reinterpreting something that the therapist thought had already been clearly worked through, a different alter may well have emerged.

Psychophysiological Sensitivities

Both the clinical literature and the clinical lore on MPD are filled with accounts of psychophysiological differences to the same stimulus among alter personalities (Putnam, 1984a; Putnam *et al.*, 1986). The most commonly reported differences are in responsiveness to medications or alcohol. About a third of therapists will report that a given medication may have differential effects (e.g., ranging from sedation to activation, depending on which personality is "out"). Another common scenario is for one personality to get drunk and another to experience the hangover. Differential allergic responses have been reported and are the subject of current scientific investigation. The experience of somatic symptoms will vary across alter personalities. The therapist may observe that at one moment the patient appears incapacitated by a symptom (e.g., a migraine headache) and the next moment appears not to be experiencing any discomfort at all. This should suggest to the observer that a switch has occurred.

THE PERSONALITY SYSTEM

The alter personalities are fascinating, and the differences among them can be distinct and dramatic. It is important, however, always to remain aware of the patient as a whole person. The "personality" of an MPD patient is the sum and synergy of the system of alter personalities.

Numbers of Alter Personalities

The numbers of personalities in MPD patients range from two in the case of dual personalities, which are apparently rare compared to multiples, to reports of several hundred "personalities," most of whom are probably best conceptualized as personality fragments rather than alter personalities. Two recent studies, covering a total of 133 patients, both reported a mean of about 13 alter personalities per patient with a mode of about 8 alter personalities (Kluft, 1984a; Putnam *et al.*, 1986).

The number of personalities that an MPD patient has is probably determined by a number of factors. The NIMH study found a significant correlation between the number of different types of childhood trauma reported and the number of alter personalities a multiple had (Putnam *et al.*, 1986). This suggests that the more traumatized a patient was as a child, the more alter personalities the patient's system will contain. The age at which an alter personality is reported to first occur is also correlated with the number of personalities in the system (Putnam *et al.*, 1986). The younger the patient was when the first alter is retrospectively reported to have appeared, the more personalities he or she is likely to have. The clinical impressions of most experienced therapists support these findings.

The number of alter personalities in a multiple's system does have implications for treatment. Data published by Kluft (1984a) reveal a significant correlation between the number of personalities in a multiple's system and the length of time required from diagnosis to successful fusion, as defined by his stated criteria (Putnam *et al.*, 1986). The NIMH study found that MPD patients with large alter personality systems were more likely to engage in sociopathic behavior, externally directed violence, and suicide attempts than were patients with smaller personality systems (Putnam *et al.*, 1986). There were, however, no significant differences in the initial clinical presentations of multiples with large or small personality systems.

Personality System Structures

Since the earliest medical cases of MPD, therapists have used metaphors, maps, and diagrams to describe their sense of the internal world of the alter personalities. These metaphors can be useful or misleading, depending upon how literally they are interpreted. Each patient will have his or her own unique system metaphor or internal model that the therapist must come to understand and use in the course of treatment. Techniques for working with metaphors and system maps are discussed in Chapter Eight. There are, however, a number of common metaphors or structures that the therapist should bear in mind while working with an MPD patient.

Layering

"Layering" is a term introduced by Kluft (1984a) to describe a set of phenomena that many therapists find as they work through traumatic material with their patient. It is as if certain groups of personalities overlie each other or are buried beneath other personalities. Frequently one overtly recognizable personality will have been masking several covertly active personalities. In many cases, the alters involved are all related in some fashion to specific traumatic material or life issues. Therapists will frequently uncover layering when they begin to work with one personality and discover that new groups of personalities or personality fragments emerge who are connected to the issues being worked on with the first personality.

The existence of layering may only be deducible when the therapist begins to compare the accounts of several personalities about a specific experience. At some point, the therapist may discover that specific details or memories are missing. For example, personality A may be able to provide an account of events leading up to a specific traumatic experience such as a rape, and personality B may be able to recount what happened afterwards, but the actual memories of the rape itself are missing and contained within personalities C, D, and E, who may emerge for the first time in treatment at this point.

The failure to recognize and work through layering is an important cause of postfusion relapse (Kluft, 1984a). Therapists most often overlook layering when they fail to work through painful material completely. This means that much of the horrendous trauma suffered by MPD patients needs to be covered in graphic detail, and when gaps are found, layering should be suspected. Chapter Eight discusses ways of reassembling "memories" from the fragmentary recall of alter personalities.

Another variant of layering occurs as personalities within the multiple's system begin to fuse or integrate. The process of integration seems to open up certain niches within the system, which are filled by alter personalities who were previously dormant or inactive. For example, in one woman many of her child and adolescent personalities fused together into a single entity, which then "grew up." A short time thereafter, a number of "new" child and adolescent alters appeared, all of whom had by historical accounts been active personalities during high school, but had become dormant when the patient left her abusive home environment.

The experience of working with layering, with its levels within levels within levels of complexity, may leave the therapist feeling frustrated and wondering whether it will ever end. Layering phenomena are, however, just part of the defensive process of dissociation that binds pain and horror by dividing it into little parts and storing it in such a way that it is difficult to reassemble and to remember. Layering should be expected and should be looked for, particularly where there are unexplained behaviors or missing memories.

Families

As indicated previously, groups of related personalities often exist. The basis of their internal relationship can be a number of factors. Frequently personalities are related on the basis of sharing a common traumatic origin. Personalities may also be related because they trace their origin back to an earlier common alter from whom they were derived. Personalities may be grouped together by the functions they perform; for example, complex functions such as a job may be divided among a number of alters who perform subtasks required by the job. These personalities may see themselves as a group or a family.

These groupings or families are usually defined by the multiple's system and have implications for therapy. Personalities within a group or family are generally more aware of each other and have better access to shared pool of memories or skills than personalities across families. Often alters from one family will have no knowledge about the existence of another family within the individual. Complex MPD patients with large numbers of alter personalities may have several different families. Intrapsychic conflicts may also divide along family lines, with one family of alters engaged in an internal war with another family. Access to a family, or the transfer of information and memories from one family to another, is usually only possible through specific personalities in each family who serve as conduits into and out of that family. In many cases, one can only contact certain personalities by first eliciting the alters who serve as gatekeepers.

Tree Structure

Tree structures, such as those used to represent hierarchical relationships in an organization or family trees, can be useful models for the system of personalities. A typical tree structure representation of a multiple's system would have an original or core personality at the top or root vertex, with branching downward to other nodes (personalities), which in turn split and branch downward to more nodes (personalities). The bottom nodes of the tree structure, paradoxically called the leaves, represent the currently active alter personalities. This model is useful in charting the course of therapy, which often begins with the overtly active alter personalities (the leaves) and works backwards through this tree structure to the core personality or personalities (the roots).

One form of layering would correspond to uncovering several branches of personalities at a particular node. Families or personality groups would correspond to branching that has occurred near the root node or in the earliest stages of the tree structure generation. In this system, gatekeeper personalities would represent the nodes where branching, which divides the family groups, has occurred.

TYPES OF PATIENTS

Over the last century, a number of different classification schemes have been offered that seek to categorize MPD patients into subgroups. If anything, this process has accelerated with the dramatic renewal of interest in the disorder. At national meetings and other forums, one hears therapists characterizing their patient(s) with variously impressive sounding descriptive classifications. In most instances, the criteria for classification are ambiguous at best.

Allison and Schwarz (1980) have suggested that there are two major forms of MPD, based on the developmental period during which the first splitting off of alters occurred. Patients who undergo traumatically induced dissociative fragmentation early (from infancy to age 6 or so) have large personality systems with profound personality disorganization. Those who have their first splits after age 8 or so have fewer alters and better "egos." It is not clear whether this division has clinical implications, but the NIMH survey found a statistically significant relationship between more personalities and retrospective reports of earlier splitting off of alters (Putnam et al., 1986). There are other data suggesting that the developmental period during which a trauma occurs has a significant impact on later symptomatic expression in non-MPD patients (Browne & Finkelhor, 1986).

Bliss sees MPD as a "spectral" disorder with a wide range of forms and presentations (Bliss et al., 1983). O'Brien (1985) has suggested that there are three subtypes of MPD: a "coidentificatory" subtype, in which all of the alters identify physically with the same body; a "possessiform" subtype, in which alter "personifications" do not identify with the same body; and mixed forms, in which some alters are coidentificatory and others are possessiform. Classification schemes based on numbers of personalities, numbers of fragments, and internal dynamics have also been presented at meetings. The symptoms and phenomenology of the patients in the NIMH survey were grouped into 20 factors (e.g., depression, anxiety, somatic symptoms, etc.), and the data were analyzed using two separate cluster analysis algorithms. The results indicated that there were three rough subtypes of MPD patients, based on clinical phenomenology. The validity of this and of all other suggested classification schemes has yet to be demonstrated. One should be careful about accepting any treatment-related classification scheme for MPD until the reliability and validity of this typology have been documented.

On rare occasion, I think that I have seen MPD patients who were multiples in childhood and achieved a spontaneous fusion during late childhood or early adolescence (or at least the complete suppression of other alters), and who then experience the appearance of separate alters during adulthood in association with severe life stress. These "second-split" cases are rare, have a history of a limited and well-circumscribed childhood trauma, and generally function well in adulthood until overwhelmed by a major crisis. In two out of the three cases I have seen, when the crisis was successfully resolved, the alter personalities disappeared within days and could not be elicited even by hypnotic probing.

DIFFERENCES BETWEEN MALE AND FEMALE PATIENTS

Most of what we know about MPD comes from the study of female MPD patients. Male cases do occur, probably more frequently than is recognized. A review of the clinical literature shows that the percentage of male MPD cases is steadily rising as more cases are recorded (Putnam, 1985a). The major speculations on the disproportionate number of female patients have been reviewed in Chapter Three. Perhaps because of the relative rarity of male MPD patients, few investigators have addressed gender differences in the manifestations of MPD.

Bliss (1984b) found that female MPD patients tend to be more likely to present with symptoms referrable to anxiety, phobias, conversion reactions, and obsessional fears, whereas male MPD patients tend to have significantly more sociopathy and alcohol abuse. These data are congruent with the clinical impression that males tend to express their violence outwardly and often aggressively, whereas females tend to be more anxious and direct their violence toward themselves, either through somatic symptoms or through suicidal/self-destructive behavior (Putnam et al., 1984; Kluft, 1985a). Alcoholism appears to be a particularly common presentation for male MPD patients (Kluft, 1985a).

The NIMH survey data suggest that male MPD patients are somewhat more likely than females to have a cross-sex alter (Putnam et al., 1986). As previously stated, in males this alter is usually an older mother figure. Female MPD patients tend to have male alters who serve as protectors or mechanics. Females will also tend to have a number of boy alter personalities, whereas child cross-sex alters are somewhat rarer in males. A statistical comparison of symptoms and phenomenology between the male and female patients in the NIMH survey found essentially no differences between the sexes in most areas, however (Putnam et al., 1986).

Male MPD patients can be divided roughly into two clinical groups. The first group has host personalities who are outwardly effeminate and often homosexual in sexual orientation; the second group has host alters who are heterosexual, macho, and aggressive. The latter patients tend to be more dangerous to work with and, in my experience, rarely remain in treatment for any length of time. Patients in the former group, however, often have at least one alter personality who is a "Hell's Angel" type. It is my impression that, as a group, male MPD patients do not show the same dramatic degrees of difference across their alter personalities as do females. I find covert switching in males more difficult to detect. The male alters of female MPD patients are often quite masculine in appearance, speech, and behavior, but I find that the female alters of male MPD patients primarily exhibit only a softening of gesture and voice to manifest their presence. Kluft (1984a) has reported that his male MPD patients tended to have fewer alters and therefore briefer treatments, though his sample of eight males is too small to permit generalizations. A better characterization of the differences between male and female multiples awaits future investigation.

SUMMARY

This chapter has explored the range and roles of alter personalities in MPD. The basic premises are that alter personalities are not separate people and that the sum of the alters constitutes the individual. The alters differ along a number of dimensions, both observable and subjective. Differences in affect, behavior, cognition, appearance, and speech are more noticeable, but subjective differences in sense of self are more important to the patient. One must develop an empathetic understanding of these differences to conduct effective therapy.

The personalities perform different functions, both external and internal, for the patient and may evolve over time to some extent. The classic constellation of alters includes the following: a depressed and overwhelmed host, who is amnesic for the other alters; a series of frightened children, who hold traumatic memories; one or more malevolent persecutors, who often hold intolerable affects; and a series of protectors and helpers. Cross-gender alters, autistic alters, alters who express forbidden impulses, and substance-abusing alters are common. The alters will have differing levels of awareness of one another and typically exhibit a cavalier attitude toward the well-being of the body. Most alters will have names, though they may not reveal them for some time.

Transitions or switches among the personalities are a central feature of the disorder and may be covert, particularly early in treatment. Switches are triggered by external and internal stimuli and can be recognized by precipitous shifts in affect, cognition, appearance, speech, and behavior.

The personality system is the larger organizing structure on which the therapist should focus during treatment. This system is often composed of layers and/or families of alters that must be worked through. A number of different classification systems have been offered to type MPD patients, but to date, none have proved to have clinical utility. Male and female MPD patients probably differ in some respects, but we know very little about male MPD patients as a group.

CHAPTER SIX

Beginning Treatment

This chapter addresses the first steps to take in the treatment of MPD. It begins by discussing questions and concerns that many therapists raise when starting to work for the first time with a patient as a multiple. It then presents an outline of the overall "ideal" therapeutic course in MPD. The initial intervention process is described in detail, and the chapter concludes with some cautions about dynamics to be aware of early in the course of therapy.

THERAPISTS' CONCERNS ABOUT TREATMENT

Iatrogenic Creation or Exacerbation of MPD

It is to the credit of mental health professionals that the most common concern raised by a therapist beginning to work with an MPD patient is the question of possible iatrogenic induction of MPD or the exacerbation of the dissociative process by acknowledging and working directly with the alter personalities of the patient. This worry is usually expressed early after the first alter personalities have been overtly met, but before the therapist has become fully aware of the role that these alters play and have played in the patient's life. Often the therapist has already worked with the patient under another diagnostic label and has not "seen" any alter personalities. All of a sudden "new" personalities begin popping out all over the place. It is not uncommon to go from an initial meeting with one alter personality to discovering 6, 8, 10, or more alters in the next few sessions. Understandably, the therapist wonders where they are all coming from and what role the diagnosis of MPD and "suggestibility" of the patient play in the creation of these apparently "new" alter personalities.

A second phenomenon further intensifies concern about the iatrogenic induction of alters. While working with the patient under another diagnostic label, the clinician is often aware of precipitous shifts in mood, perceptions, and behavior occurring within the patient. These rapid changes are typically ascribed to "splitting" or other borderline dynamics, and no clearly recognizable alters are present. Following the diagnosis of MPD, however, the alters may suddenly become distinct and claim a differentiation from the host that was not previously present. Janet commented on this crystallization phenomenon a century ago: "Once baptised, the subconscious personage grows more definitely outlined and displays better her psychological characters" (quoted by Taylor, 1982, p. 86).

Two complementary processes seem to account for the sharpened differentiation of alter personalities immediately following diagnosis. The first is that the alters are "coming out of the closet" and no longer passing as the host personality. The diagnosis of MPD is often a liberating event for multiples, who have practiced deception and secrecy as a way of life. Alters are now overly eager to separate themselves from the host personality, who is usually perceived as pathetic and incompetent. The second process leading to an apparent increased differentiation among alters is actually a result of the therapist's evolving ability to "see" the distinctions among the alters. One of the effects of treating MPD is that it will change the way therapists see patients.

Not unexpectedly, the rapid appearance of "new" alters and the apparent crystallization of these alters into distinct entities often causes a therapist to raise the possibility that they are being iatrogenically induced. The most convincing evidence that the alters are not being iatrogenically created comes with time. Although new personalities may be created in therapy, the vast majority of alters in any given multiple's system will have a history of existence that predates the diagnosis and therapy by many years. This history, with sufficient documentation, will emerge as the therapist and patient reopen the past and fill in the gaps in time that previously were blank. In the long run, the question of iatrogenic creation becomes moot. Early in the course of therapy, however, most neophyte clinicians will be troubled by this possibility.

Fear of Eliciting a Violent Alter Personality

The second most frequent and appropriate concern raised early in therapy is that the therapist may elicit a dangerous or violent alter. This is a realistic possibility. The patient's past history with regard to violence is the best single indicator of whether there are dangerous alters within the system. In cases where the patient has a history of violence, appropriate precautions should be taken until it is clear that potential violence can be managed by contracts or other measures. Usually, this means that the therapist should see the patient with other people present or immediately available. Therapists have been assaulted by MPD patients, and this possibility should not be minimized or overlooked. In my experience, male multiples, while generally more dangerous to society, tend not to be so threatening in therapy, perhaps because they know what they can do. Female multiples may be more inclined to "play games" with violence and can be dangerous to a therapist.

Alters whose function is to fight, steal, or rape are more common in males. In females, the more dangerous alters are often protector personalities, whose function is to guard the patient from perceived danger (see Chapter Five). Protector or guardian personalities can be very concrete in their thinking and perceptions, and thereby misinterpret statements by the therapist as threats to the patient. For example, one therapist I know was collared by a body protector when he suggested that they "kick around" an idea. All he meant was that they should discuss it further. The body protector, who was monitoring the conversation between the therapist and another alter, perceived physical abuse as imminent.

The other side of the issue is that many multiples will exaggerate the dangerousness of some alters. Not uncommonly, a therapist will hear from other alters about the incredible earth-shattering rage of personality B, only to find that B, while appropriately enraged over some past event, is well controlled. This choice between taking what alters say at face value or with a grain of salt is a predicament that the therapist repeatedly faces during the course of therapy. In issues of dangerousness, it is best to err on the side of caution. The therapist should not, however, let such threats deter him or her from seeking out and meeting the alter personalities of the patient's system. Successful therapy depends on dealing with the personalities and the psychological material that they embody. Rumors of violence are often a form of resistance, augmented by the patient's own perception of the "dangerousness" of the information and affects held by that alter.

Concerns about Being Unqualified to Treat MPD

Another frequent experience for therapists new to the treatment of MPD is feeling "deskilled" by the diagnosis. Very few of us have had any formal training in the diagnosis and treatment of MPD. Although some therapists become "instant experts" upon seeing their first case, most feel that they do not have the skills necessary to treat these patients. Usually this is not true. The most important qualification for doing good work with MPD patients is the ability to do good psychotherapy. Most of the dynamics and resistances encountered in MPD patients are similar to those found in neurotic or borderline patients. The differences lie in the personification of these dynamics by the alter personalities. In many ways, this personification makes it easier to work directly with these dynamics.

In my experience, the feeling of being unqualified to treat MPD is expressed in two major ways. The first is an attempt to "give away" the patient. The dynamics of this are obviously complicated. Following the diagnosis of MPD in a patient previously thought to have another disorder, it is worthwhile to reconsider treatment options with the patient. In some cases, a transfer to another therapist may be best for one or both parties. In many cases, however, the therapeutic relationship has been formed and strengthened by, and in spite of, the chaos, suicide attempts, and hospitalizations that are common with undiagnosed multiples. In my opinion, the quality of the therapeutic relationship is an extremely important factor in the outcome of MPD. A therapist who has a good therapeutic alliance with a patient should seriously consider continuing to treat him or her rather than seeking a more "qualified" therapist. Working with the patient as a multiple, rather than as a schizophrenic, borderline, manic–depressive, or whatever, provides a tremendous clinical leverage that was previously missing.

Another manifestation of feeling "deskilled" and inexperienced in the treatment of MPD is the therapist's fear that he or she may do or say something wrong and inadvertently cause serious harm to the patient. Therapists who feel confident working with difficult and seriously disturbed patients may suddenly feel as if they are on thin ice with multiples, despite, in some cases, having seen the patients for years prior to the diagnosis. One should remember that MPD patients are survivors. They have survived incredible trauma and have perfected a defense that screens and protects them from trauma. A therapist cannot do anything to a patient that compares to what he or she has already lived through. If the therapist cares and follows the basic common-sense rules of doing sound therapy, no serious or permanent harm will ensue.

One situation that does warrant the serious consideration of transferring a patient to another therapist is an inability to make a commitment to treat the patient for at least a year or preferably longer. The treatment of MPD requires a year or more in adults and probably closer to 3–5 years on the average, although no systematic data exist to corroborate this impression. Students rotating through training placements or therapists working at facilities with mandated short-term interventions should refer MPD patients to treatment settings where they can have the continuity of therapy they need. Alas, this is often not possible. Nevertheless, the stability and continuity of the treatment situation is one of the most important factors in treating MPD patients. If an MPD patient believes, correctly or incorrectly, that the therapy is seriously limited or could terminate at any time, he or she will put up a corresponding resistance to engage in meaningful work; this is usually expressed by constant crises and acting out by alters.

Concerns about Treatment Setting

Immediately following the diagnosis of MPD, one may wonder about changing the treatment setting. At this point, neophyte therapists often mistakenly seek to hospitalize patients. Hospitalization has a definite role in the treatment of some MPD patients, but should be used only after careful consideration. In general, MPD patients do poorly on inpatient units, and the focus of therapy often becomes sidetracked by milieu issues. Outpatient individual psychotherapy settings are the preferred treatment setting for most MPD patients.

OVERVIEW OF THERAPY

The Tasks of Treatment

Establishing the Therapeutic Alliance

The tasks and stages of therapy with MPD patients are similar to those found in any intensive change-oriented therapy (Kluft, 1984a). These tasks include the development of a therapeutic relationship and the identification and replacement of maladaptive coping with more constructive behaviors. There is the additional issue of the replacement of internal division with some form of unity.

The development of trust is the key issue in establishing a therapeutic relationship with MPD patients (Horevitz, 1983; Wilbur, 1984b). This trust must be established across all of the alter personalities. The therapist should not expect this to happen quickly or completely for some time. A therapeutic alliance must be established with most alters separately. In some instances, this can be difficult and demanding; with other alters, simply meeting them and acknowledging their existence and needs are sufficient. It is important to listen attentively to each alter, including the child personalities. The therapist will be tested frequently to see whether he or she has heard, cares, and believes what the alters are saying. A common transference expectation is that the therapist is a cruel, harsh, and abusing parental figure (Kluft, 1984d; Wilbur, 1984b). Since many of the alter personalities lack the capacity to maintain a split between the observing ego and the experiencing ego, interpretation is not likely to change this perception, which is held separately by many of the alters (Kluft, 1984d). Instead, the therapist's behavior and attitude over time must serve to correct this misperception. The availability and empathy of the therapist in times of crisis will be critical to winning trust.

Consistency and continuity on the part of the therapist are also important parts of developing trust. These patients live in a discontinuous and inconsistent world. Their lifelong experience is that they drive other people away and dependable relationships are impossible. It is important to be on time and to keep appointments; when the therapist cannot avoid canceling a session, this must be done in a fashion that conveys this information to the personality system as a whole. Multiples are exquisitely sensitive to rejection and will perceive it where none is intended.

Caring for the patient is demonstrated by respect for each of the alters. All should be considered equally important, and the therapist should be careful not to develop favorites. Caring is also expressed by setting limits on dangerous or destructive behaviors. The therapist will be repeatedly tested for his or her willingness to stop inappropriate or dangerous actions on the part of one or more alters, as well as to stop inappropriate behavior directed at himself or herself. Part of showing caring for the patient is modeling self-respect.

A crucial issue in the development of a therapeutic alliance is the way in which the therapist handles traumatic material from the patient's past. Some of the abuses suffered by these patients are horrendous and will sicken the therapist when they are disclosed. The ability to listen to and work with this material is absolutely essential to the critical work in therapy. If the patient feels that the therapist cannot tolerate this material, then it will not be worked through in treatment. A related issue is the therapist's appreciation of the stress experienced by the patient during sessions when this material is worked with. Much of the past trauma will be relived in the office. The therapist's sensitivity to the effects of these abreactions on the patient and willingness to allow the personality system to recover and work through past trauma at its own rate will be critical in creating a therapeutic milieu.

Promoting Change in the Patient's Life

Therapeutic change comes through the identification of maladaptive behaviors and the substitution of more appropriate ways of coping. In MPD patients, there are two perspectives from which dissociative behavior should be viewed, the present and the past. The origin of the dissociative defenses is in past trauma. The manifestations of these defenses are in present behavior. Day-to-day events will trigger dissociative responses, but the root of this pathology lies hidden deep within the patient. At one time, usually in early childhood, dissociation was a highly adaptive response to overwhelming trauma. In adulthood, now that the patient is removed from the precipitating traumatic situations, frequent and easily activated dissociation becomes a seriously maladaptive response to the normal stresses of life.

Successful replacement of dissociative pathology with more appropriate forms of coping is, in large part, dependent on a recovery and reworking of the early traumatic events. Interpretations and insight will fail to achieve results in these patients until much of the precipitating trauma is exhumed, relived, and accepted by the patient. This is the major task in the therapy of MPD and represents the bulk of the therapy. This process, however, can only be successfully undertaken when a therapeutic alliance has been established and the patient's more overt self-destructive behaviors have been controlled. The patient must first be stabilized before the process of deeper change is attempted.

Replacement of Division with Unity

David Caul's often-cited remark, "It seems to me that after treatment you want to end up with a functional unit, be it a corporation, a partnership, or a one-owner business" (quoted by Hale, 1983, p. 106), is a statement that the final unity achieved by these patients need not be that of a single integrated personality. What is important is the achievement of a stable sense of unity in terms of purpose and motivation (Kluft, 1984d). Perpetuation of internal dividedness will lead to a perpetuation of chaos in the lives of these patients. Personalities can communicate and cooperate; it takes time for them to learn these skills, but once acquired they can be put to good use in the patient's daily life and in the recovery and metabolism of the past trauma. Some patients will choose to remain multiples; usually this means that all of the trauma has not been recovered and worked through. These patients may be satisfied by the improvement in their function, and/or may not be ready or willing to explore the deeper layers of trauma. In many instances, MPD patients leave therapy only to return for further work at a later date.

Many patients will wish to go on to complete integration. There are a number of ways to finalize this process, which are discussed in Chapter Eleven. Much of the real work of integration comes during the earlier stabilization of the patient and the painful slogging through of the precipitating trauma. Even when a final integration occurs, there remains a significant amount of postintegration therapeutic work. Few final integrations hold the first time or two, and even if they do, the patient has many new coping skills to learn and practice in order to fill the void left by giving up dissociative defenses. There is also much grief work to be done in finally coming to terms with the past and with the perceived loss of the distinct alters, who provided company and companionship during an otherwise lonely existence.

The Stages of Treatment

I have divided the treatment course of MPD into eight rough stages of tasks. In actuality, no treatment moves through this progression in a simple linear fashion. Many of these stages occur concurrently, but this division has heuristic value in that it permits a description of the treatment course as a series of discrete steps. Other authorities will no doubt divide up the course of treatment differently. What is important is that a therapist should have some general sense of the course and progression of treatment with MPD patients before becoming too deeply involved in the complexities of a specific case; that is, it helps to see the forest before plunging ahead among the trees.

Making the Diagnosis

Making the diagnosis is the first and most important step, for without a diagnosis, there can be no effective treatment. Chapter Three discusses the clinical phenomenology of these patients, and Chapter Four covers the process of making the diagnosis.

Initial Interventions

The subject of initial interventions is discussed in greater detail later in this chapter. The purpose of the initial interventions is to start the process of working with a patient as a multiple and to stabilize the patient so that the work of uncovering and abreacting the deep core of trauma can proceed. Until the patient and therapist can establish a working equilibrium, no major abreactive work can proceed without causing a serious disruption of the patient's life. The primary tasks of the initial interventions are to meet alter personalities, gather some history, and develop a working relationship with the personality system.

Initial Stabilizations

Techniques for stabilizing the patient and getting a handle on some of the apparent chaos are also discussed later in this chapter. Working with an MPD patient as a multiple provides the clinician with a variety of therapeutic interventions that were not possible when the patient was treated as having a single unified personality. The principal intervention is that of contracting with specific alter personalities and the personality system as a whole in order to control what were previously uncontrollable behaviors.

Acceptance of the Diagnosis

The acceptance by the patient of the diagnosis of MPD is an ongoing issue right down to the final integration. Most of these patients will have alters who refuse to believe that there are other alters. The host personality is usually foremost among the disbelievers, but is often aided and abetted by others. This is a major form of resistance to therapy. There is often, however, a period in the early stages of treatment when the patient struggles with and comes to some sort of acceptance of the existence of other parts. I include this process as a stage, although in many patients it is more of an ongoing issue than a discrete stage. I discuss some aspects of this process later in this chapter, and elaborate more on the denial of the diagnosis as an issue in therapy in Chapter Eight.

Development of Communication and Cooperation

The fostering of internal communication and cooperation is also an ongoing process right down to the final integration. Much of the groundwork, however, is laid early in the course of treatment. There are four primary aspects: (1) development of internal communication; (2) establishment of cooperation around common goals; (3) development of an internal decision-making process; and (4) the facilitation of switching. Once this process is under way, the patient will be able to function at a significantly higher level than was previously possible. Internal communication and cooperation can compensate for many of the amnesic gaps and thereby provide a sense of continuity that has previously been unattainable. The cooperation around common goals begins the task of replacing division with a form of unity. The development of an internal decision-making process within the patient continues the task of creating internal cohesion. Facilitation of switching relieves some of the internal tension and struggles among the personalities for "body time," which constitute a major source of internal conflict. It also further promotes cooperation as alters practice handing control over behavior back and forth to each other. I discuss these tasks at length in this chapter, with additions in the following chapters.

Metabolism of the Trauma

Metabolizing the trauma is a major treatment task in MPD. The therapist should not try to undertake it, however, until the patient has made some progress with the tasks outlined above. The recovery and abreaction of major trauma are exceedingly painful and will cause significant distress. Unless and until some stabilization has been achieved, the patient is likely to react to this stress with major dissociative pathology. Premature pursuit of early trauma can lead to serious consequences that may prevent further effective therapy. Once the groundwork is set, the therapist must then become more aggressive in discovering and uncovering the secrets of the past. A variety of techniques and issues associated with the recovery and integration of traumatic material are discussed in more detail in Chapters Seven, Eight, and Nine.

Resolution and Integration

Resolution and integration are not necessarily the same. Some multiples may elect to terminate therapy and remain multiples. This is the patient's right. In some cases it may be appropriate, and in other cases the patients would be better served by remaining in therapy and achieving a more complete unification. This topic is covered in greater detail in Chapter Eleven.

Development of Postresolution Coping Skills

The development of postresolution coping skills is a task that is often overlooked, particularly by therapists working with their first MPD patients. The world is not a bowl of cherries, and many multiples experience significant difficulties following a final integration. They must take on responsibilities that were previously split up among several alters or were not required of them because they were considered too ill. In many cases, it is only after integration that patients first fully realize what a tragic mess their lives have been and may still be, and feel the totality of the pain that was inflicted upon them. Integrated patients have been stripped of their primary psychological defense, dissociation, and have precious little to replace it as protection against the stresses of everyday life. Not surprisingly, a reactive depression often follows closely on the heels of the initial euphoria of becoming "one." No therapist should terminate an MPD patient's treatment immediately following a "final" integration. Complete treatment requires working with the patient through this trying and painful time. I discuss this topic further in Chapter Eleven.

INITIAL INTERVENTIONS

Working with a patient as a multiple means working directly with the alter personalities. Although there are experienced therapists who believe that one can do "good" therapy with multiples and not work directly with the alter personalities, in my experience this is not possible. In my opinion, it is necessary to meet and interact directly with alter personalities as part of the treatment of MPD. The process of meeting alter personalities has been covered in Chapter Four. In a case where the therapist is unable to elicit the overt appearance of an alter but continues to suspect the diagnosis of MPD, based on evidence of significant dissociative psychopathology in the patient (e.g., fugue episodes, amnesic spells, possible switches, etc.), then the use of hypnotic or drug-facilitated techniques covered in Chapter Nine may be indicated.

Once the initial introductions are over, the task becomes one of systematically meeting the alter personalities; determining their roles and functions; and assessing the levels of system psychopathology, system structure, and system strengths. The first step is to take a brief history from each alter personality who emerges. The first question often is "What is your name?" Names and naming principles have been discussed in Chapter Five. Most personalities will have names, but they may not share them with the therapist on the first request. An alter who avoids giving a name should be told that the therapist needs some way of asking for him or her, and should be asked how he or she would like to be addressed. If the alter still refuses to provide a handle, then the therapist should make one up, using some identifying characteristic that distinguishes this alter from the host and other alters. I will say something such as this: "Since you are not willing to share your name with me at this time, I am going to refer to you as 'the one who covers her mouth with a hand when she talks.'"

Names are useful in a number of ways. They help the therapist keep the different alters straight—a difficult task with complex multiples. They allow the therapist to call out specific personalities for questioning or contracting. One reason why alters are reluctant to share their identification is that it allows the therapist access to them more or less on demand. Names also help the therapist explain causal sequences to other amnesic alters, such as the host; for example, a patient can be told that the reason she found herself standing in the parking lot of her old apartment building was that the part of her called "Judy" still thought that she lived there. I keep a list of alters' names for each patient, with a brief biography and description of each alter's role in the personality system.

I will ask the personality what gender he or she is, if this is not obvious. I ask each alter how old he or she feels and what age the patient or the body was when the alter first came out. This is important information. The age of the personality is important in understanding his or her behavior, level of abstraction, and role in the system. The age of the patient or body at the time of the personality's first appearance will become relevant later when the therapist begins to explore for past trauma. Alter personalities are usually created during times of extreme stress for the patient. Knowing that a specific alter first appeared at the age of 6 years, for example, would suggest that there are specific traumas associated with that period of the patient's life.

I inquire about what the personality considers to be his or her function or role. It is worth asking several questions along this tack. What does the personality do? In what sorts of situations is he or she likely to become active or in control? Does he or she ever influence the patient's behavior without coming out? Does the host know of his or her existence? Does he or she have a special function or role to play in the patient's life? The therapist should make a note of the answers. They should not be taken to be the whole truth, but there usually is a kernel of fact in each. In the early stages of therapy, the therapist is likely to be misled or lied to on occasion.

The next important question to ask of each alter personality is about his or her awareness of other alters in the personality system. Whenever possible, the therapist should get proper names or good descriptions of the other alters. Again, the whole truth should not be expected. I call this process "chaining." In essence, it allows the therapist to acquire from the alters who emerge an overlapping list of names or descriptions of the alters who compose the personality system. Each time the therapist hears of a new personality who has not yet appeared, the therapist can ask to meet him or her. This technique will move the therapist around within the personality system and fill in some of the gaps. The therapist should not expect to meet them all on the first pass; chances are that new alters will continue to emerge up to the final fusion. Each time the therapist moves to a new layer or level of the system, it is important to go through this routine. In fact, each time the therapist hears of an alter personality who has not yet put in an appearance, it is usually necessary to meet this alter personality and go through the same list of questions. If the thera pist is consistent, it will become an expected routine.

If the list of alters is kept up to date, the therapist will acquire a great deal of valuable information about the size, composition, and structure of the overall personality system. The list will provide an idea about the minimum number of alters, though the system is likely to be several times larger than it appears on the first exploration. The list will also indicate something about the age range of personalities in the system. This is important, because personality systems composed largely of child and adolescent personalities seem to have different dynamics than do systems with more adult personalities. In addition, the list will indicate something about the perceived roles or functions of the alters. If the therapist compares the role descriptions that are obtained to the types of alter personalities described in Chapter Five, he or she can make an educated guess about who has not yet appeared. The therapist will also have some idea of which alters are likely to be responsible for specific pathological or dangerous behaviors; this information is important in the next stage of therapy. And finally, the list will give some idea of the awareness alters have of one another—information that is useful when the therapist begins to foster internal communication within the system.

As the therapist chains through the personality system, he or she will also get a general feeling for the level of psychopathology, as well as the internal cooperation and communication. A therapist seeing his or her first MPD patient will not have anything with which to compare the system; however, one seeing his or her fifth MPD patient will be able to make an educated guess about the length and difficulty of treatment. Chaining is useful not only in identifying the psychopathology of a multiple's personality system, but also in identifying the strengths. The therapist should keep in mind that the personality system arose as a coping mechanism, and that in its own fashion it still serves this function.

INITIAL STABILIZATIONS

Purposes of Contracts

The use of behavioral contracts between therapist and multiple to set limits on unhealthy behavior and to promote more adaptive behavior is a time-proven intervention in the treatment of MPD (Braun, 1986; Kluft, 1982; Wilbur, 1982). Behavioral contracting with multiples is, however, a fine art, and one in which even the most experienced therapist will be burned from time to time. Yet contracts are among the most useful and powerful clinical tools at the disposal of the therapist to set effective limits on what is otherwise out-of-control behavior. A number of general principles are worth keeping in mind when one enters into a contract with a multiple.

Thames (1984) points out that behavioral contracts serve two purposes in the treatment of multiple personality. The first purpose is to set safe and reasonable limits for the patient. These limits can cover a large number of areas, such as patient and therapist safety, treatment setting boundaries, and behaviors outside of the treatment setting (Sachs & Braun, 1986; Thames, 1984). The second purpose is to nurture a sense of cause and effect with regard to behavior for the patient. Multiples have a poor sense of cause and effect. In general, MPD patients come from highly abusive environments where parental behavior was erratic and inconsistent (Braun & Sachs, 1985). The child may have been punished for a given behavior on one occasion and praised on another. Some alter personalities have never seen the consequences of their actions; others may have been punished for behavior for which they were amnesic. Behavioral contracting with clearly delineated limits, obligations, rewards, and punishments helps to develop a sense of cause and effect that these patients need if they are to learn to deal with the world. I would add that the process of behavioral contracting also nurtures the development of internal communication and cooperation in direct and indirect ways.

Over time, the community of therapists treating MPD has learned the hard way that contracts with multiples need to be highly specific and very concrete. For example, the general contract to control dangerous behavior advocated by Kluft and Braun in the American Psychiatric Association course on MPD states, "I will not hurt myself or kill myself nor [hurt or kill] anyone else, external or internal, accidentally or on purpose, at any time" (Braun, 1984c, p. 36). Thames (1984) points out that specificity in contracting needs to cover at least five areas: (1) specificity as to what is required from the personalities; (2) specificity as to what is required from the therapist; (3) specificity as to the consequences of violating the contract; (4) specificity as to the length of the contract; and (5) agreement from the personalities that whoever breaks the contract is the personality who reaps the consequences.

I cannot overemphasize how important it is to be precise and careful in the wording of contracts with multiples. In every case, there will be alters who will seek out and exploit any loopholes that the therapist has neglected to cover. For these personalities it is a test, a game, and a challenge to sabotage the contract by exploiting an oversight on the part of the therapist. In one case, for example, a therapist with considerable experience in the treatment of difficult MPD patients made a contract with an anorexic multiple that she should eat a certain amount of food each day. The patient honored the letter of the contract by eating the specified quantity of food each day, but sabotaged the intent of the contract by eating only nonnutritious food, and continued to lose weight to a life-threatening level. Every therapist who has worked with MPD patients for any length of time will have a number of similar examples.

It is important to keep the wording of the contracts as simple and as concrete as possible. Contracts should be written down, at least during the early stages of therapy when the therapeutic alliance is fragile and the multiple is continually testing the therapist. An unwritten contract will result in the therapist's quibbling over wording with the multiple and being unable to enforce infractions of the contract with any authority. Also, the therapist should beware of making too many contracts. They may contradict or cancel one another, and an alter can be counted on to find and exploit any discrepancy. Multiples are paradoxical in that although they are fragmented and have amnesic gaps in memory, many can remember large amounts of material verbatim and keep track of many details that the therapist has forgotten. A second reason to avoid large numbers of contracts is that the quantity lowers the value invested in each.

Contracts can be negotiated in many areas. Thames (1984) provides a useful list. This list includes (1) the safety of the patient's body; (2) the safety of the therapist; (3) the privacy of the therapist; (4) the safety of the therapist's property; and (5) the safety of the property of other personalities. This last point is one that is often overlooked but is important for many reasons. Early in therapy, amnesic personalities such as the host will often find and destroy notes, letters, poems, artwork, and other personal property of other personalities as part of the denial of their existence. This naturally invites retaliation from those personalities whose property has been destroyed, and perpetuates the internal conflict. By contracting to prevent this from happening, the therapist is introducing the concept of respect for the rights of others within the personality system. This manifestation of concern for the rights of the other personalities will help win the trust of the system.

Contracts may cover the entire system of personalities, or they may be limited to specific personalities. This will depend on the specific circumstances. For example, contracts covering self-destructive behavior may be made with the entire system, whereas contracts covering the inappropriate emergence of child personalities at the patient's job need only be made with the offending alters. When I am making a blanket contract with the system, I spend time discussing the contract with as many alters as I can get to participate in the process. I invite them all "out," one at a time, to negotiate, comment on, or contribute to the contract's format and provisions. When we have arrived at a satisfactory draft, I again invite any holdouts to come out or be held to the spirit and the letter of the contract. It is clearly stated that any personality who does not emerge and negotiate is expected by me and by the personality system to honor the contract.

Determining the Consequences for Contract Violations

One of the most difficult issues in negotiating contracts is determining the appropriate consequences for a violation of a contract. Thames (1984) stresses that the consequences must be aversive but not abusive. This can be a fine distinction at times; the therapist can often get help from the personality system, however. I usually ask a number of personalities what they think the appropriate consequences for a violation of the contract should be. Not infrequently, I get reasonable suggestions that I would not have thought of myself. In cases where the consequences prohibit the offending personality from doing or having something for a length of time (e.g., being allowed to write or draw), it is important to specify that the length of time is time *in the body* (Thames, 1984). Otherwise, it may be meaningless for alters who do not have a sense of time when they are not "out."

The most difficult task is determining appropriate consequences for seriously self-destructive acts. Hospitalization or the termination of therapy may be necessary consequences. In cases where one or more alters present a serious danger to the therapist or the therapist's property, the consequence may be the termination of therapy. No therapist can effectively treat a patient he or she fears, and no therapist should try to do so. However, the temporary suspension of therapy sessions should not be used as a consequence for contract violations. An MPD patient needs to be seen on a regular basis, and the suspension of sessions will interfere with the ongoing work.

In cases where the contract is seeking to control self-abusive behavior (e.g., alcohol or drug abuse), the consequence can be that the alter who painted the town red must also endure the hangover. Multiples report that an alter can often avoid the consequences of such behavior by simply switching to another personality, who wakes up with a headache (Braun, 1983a). The same can be true for promiscuous behavior: One personality picks up a stranger, and another wakes up next to him or her in the morning.

Thames (1984) suggests that too much attention is paid to the consequence of contract violations and not enough to rewarding alters for honoring contracts. Rewards may be especially useful with child alters, and they can be awarded by the therapist or by adult alters who care for the internal children. The latter process is useful, as it nurtures self-parenting skills that help correct some of the deprivation of love and parenting suffered by many of these patients.

Length and Termination of Contracts

The duration of a contract will depend on the specific circumstances of that contract. Some contracts may run the length of the treatment and be terminated at the end of therapy; others may cover only the length of a single session. In many instances, one or more alters will only agree to a contract with a finite length. This is fine, but the therapist must never forget to renew the contract before the time limit is over. If, for example, a contract of a finite duration covers self-destructive behavior, the therapist must not forget to renegotiate before the contract expires; otherwise an unpleasant surprise may soon be waiting in the emergency room. Failure to renew a contract is viewed as not caring and as an invitation to act out. I make a bold note in my appointment calendar and on my progress notes when a given contract is set to expire. I try to renegotiate a contract at least one session prior to the expiration date. Such requirements are a pain for a busy therapist, but come with the territory. In general, it is best to assume a methodical and mildly obsessive stance when dealing with MPD patients, if only for one's own peace of mind.

Termination of contracts can occur in many ways. The most common situation is for the time limit to expire. If this is allowed to occur, then a clear statement to this effect should be made by both therapist and patient, and any rewards or consequences need to be enacted at that time. No contract should be left half finished, as this posture will undermine the therapeutic effectiveness of other contracts. In many cases, the contract has served its purpose and can be dispensed with. Again, if this is so, a clear statement should be made by all parties. If there is a possibility that the contract may be reactivated at a later date, then this should be discussed. All too often, a therapist will find that the contract has some loophole or provision permitting the continuation of the behavior that the contract was supposed to control. In these cases it is better to draw up a new contract than to patch an old one. When I have been outfoxed, I try to admit it, acknowledge my stupidity, and make use of the lesson just taught me. It may take several trial contracts before the wording can be made airtight.

My experience convinces me that multiples as a group generally honor the letter of contracts well. The difficulties occur when the wording is unclear or when the personality who is actually responsible for the behavior covered by the contract is somehow excluded from "signing" the contract. Although not all multiples are honest, as a group they seem to be at least as honest as the rest of us, if not more so. Most MPD patients can and will keep contracts as long as the therapist is careful to follow the principles described above.

Common Problems with Contracts

Some common pitfalls to be alert for in contracting with multiples include (1) the inadvertent reinforcement of pathological behavior; (2) failure to enforce a contract because of "mitigating circumstances"; (3) failure to determine whether certain child alters understand the contract; and (4) the use of inappropriate consequences, such as forbidding body time to specific personalities. The first situation is likely to occur when an alter actually receives gratification when a consequence is invoked. For example, an alter may repeatedly and deliberately violate a contract because he or she finds that the attention associated with the therapist's enforcement of the consequences is rewarding. In some instances, alters have used this as a tactic to monopolize therapy time. Obviously, a new set of contingencies needs to be negotiated.

"Mitigating circumstances" constitute one of the banes of contract enforcement. In general, a contract should be enforced as written. Not to do so sabotages the principle of contracting and invites the multiple to create situations in which the therapist is recurrently impaled on the horns of a dilemma. When I am backed into this corner, I usually enforce the letter of the contract and then invite the system to renegotiate the contract, based on what we have learned from the situation. Multiples will repeatedly seek to place therapists in positions of a "moral dilemma" or "double bind" (Braun, 1986). This is a way of testing the trustworthiness of the therapist. By definition, there is no acceptable solution. In such instances, the therapist should bite the bullet and enforce the concrete letter of the contract unless it is so obviously flawed that real harm may result if this is done, in which case the therapist should bite the bullet and admit fallibility!

Child alters often genuinely do not understand common abstract ideas (Putnam, 1984b). When a contract is drawn up that covers the behavior of child alters—and they should be included in any contracts concerning dangerous behaviors—the therapist should be sure to have them say in their own words what they think the contract means. Do they understand what the contract prohibits, what it encourages, what the time limitations are, and what the consequences are? The adult personalities can be asked to explain provisions of the contract to the children. Often the adult alters can do this much better than the therapist can and will know who should be covered in the contract. This technique also encourages a parental attitude on the part of the adult alters toward the child alters.

The therapist should be careful about dictating which personalities can have body time and how much. In most instances, this is not the therapist's business. I have discovered, much to my chagrin, that many of my patients are *very* different out in the world than they appear in my office. Preliminary experimental work by Loewenstein *et al.* (1987) reinforces this observation. The therapist may contract with the system to prevent the inappropriate emergence of specific personalities in situations where they may cause harm or embarrassment, but should not prohibit a personality from having body time. The personality system may instigate the restriction of body time for some alters, but the therapist should not become involved in the prohibition of certain alters without good reason. To do so is to become involved in the internal splits and conflicts, rather than taking an impartial, nonjudgmental attitude.

First Contracts

The first contracts should focus on (1) the type and duration of the therapy; (2) dangerous behavior; and (3) therapeutic boundaries. They should be made with the entire system of personalities, after the therapist has discussed the details and provisions with as many alters as possible. In the first stages of therapy, the therapist will probably know only a minority of the alters, so all contracts that concern general prohibitions such as suicide and assault need to be made with the personality system as a whole. The first contract I make with the system is the one developed for the American Psychiatric Association course on MPD. One version of this contract reads, "I will not hurt or kill myself or hurt or kill anyone else, internal or external, on purpose or accidentally, now or in the future." The therapist may want to spend some time arriving at a definition of "hurt" with the patient's system. At this stage in therapy I am primarily concerned with physical injury, which is easier to define.

Using a technique called "talking through," which is discussed in detail in Chapter Eight, I ask all of the alters to listen as I discuss the need for a contract covering violence toward the body and toward other people. I then invite the alters, one and all, to come forward and negotiate with me on the provisions and consequences. Usually a number of alters who act as representatives come forward, and we negotiate. I actively solicit suggestions, particularly with regard to consequences. Once a draft is agreed upon, the wording is set down, usually in the folder with the process notes, with specific start and stop dates. I clearly and explicitly say to the personality system that unless an alter comes forward to register his or her dissent to the provisions of the contract, all of the alters are bound by this contract. The amazing thing about this process is that it generally works. Using this type of behavioral contract, I have been able to discharge MPD patients from hospital situations where they had been under constant surveillance for suicidal behavior. In one instance, the patient was in four-way leather restraints and on continuous arms-length observation because she was so actively suicidal.

A second area where contracts are useful in the early stages of therapy is in setting limits regarding treatment. One must set limits on the length of sessions, the frequency of phone calls outside of sessions, and any inappropriate or intrusive behaviors. A single MPD patient can monopolize all of a therapist's time. Multiples push hard until they meet firm limits; it is one of the ways in which they interact with the world. For a variety of reasons, they tend to become special patients (see the section on countertransference issues in Chapter Seven) and use this status to extract extra time from the therapist. A therapist who allows this to happen will find that he or she is giving more and more to a patient who is making less and less progress.

ACCEPTANCE OF THE DIAGNOSIS

Multiples are not likely to completely accept the diagnosis of MPD until after their final fusion, if ever. In many cases, the host personality has been actively denying the existence of other alters for many years and is unwilling to accept the diagnosis of MPD easily. The host often destroys any evidence of other alters, and this denial, as much as any other reason, is responsible for the enmity that exists between the host and many of the other alters.

As discussed in Chapter Four, the patient may experience an exacerbation in dissociative symptoms following the discovery of one or more alters. Fugue episodes and suicide attempts (often internal homicides) are all-too-frequent responses to the initial diagnosis of MPD. On the other hand, a number of alters will be relieved at being able to interact directly with the therapist and/or family members. Their more frequent and overt appearances may increase the host's panic and sense of loss of control. The patient may appear to seesaw back and forth between the polar extremes of acceptance and rejection of the diagnosis. If the patient does not flee from therapy, usually by having a prolonged fugue episode, he or she may appear to come to some acceptance of the diagnosis. Usually the host will try to avoid the subject, or may acknowledge the existence of others in an abstract way but continue to act as if there were no other alters. In addition to the host, there will probably be some other alters within the multiple's system who do not accept the diagnosis.

I do not think that it is necessary to convince the host or any of the other disbelievers in the multiple's system that the patient is a multiple. Many therapists attempt to prove the diagnosis to their patients at some point. In my experience, this does not work and usually becomes a resistance that deflects the focus of the therapy. Instead, I chip away at this issue in a number of ways. First, I always try to make sure that the host is filled in on any events that occur during a therapy session for which he or she is amnesic. And when I do, I mention the names of any personalities with whom I have been interacting, or I may suggest that the host ask a specific alter for additional information. I try to do this in a matter-of-fact manner. I also point out the obvious. If the host was sitting in a chair when another personality took over, and returns to find himself or herself sitting on the floor (as often happens when child alters emerge), I will bring this change to his or her attention. Pressing the issue too hard may precipitate a panic or dissociative response from the host or another alter. Over time, the weight of such examples as the one above has a cumulative effect on the denial.

Multiples will attempt to find out everything that there is to know about MPD and then use it to prove to the therapist that they are not multiples. Prolonged "logical" discussions of whether or not a patient is a multiple should be avoided; the patient will usually win! This search for knowledge about the disorder should be interpreted as part of a wish to get better. I do not believe that such discussions are countertherapeutic in the long run, but it may make the therapist uncomfortable to find that a patient knows the clinical literature better than he or she does. It is better to concede to patients whatever expertise they wish to claim, and just practice sound psychotherapy. It should be kept in mind that if they were able to treat themselves effectively, they would not be in therapy at all.

At some point in the treatment, the converse situation is also likely to occur: The patient will "accept" his or her multiplicity and often seek to affirm it in some public fashion. The therapist should not fall into this trap, either, and should be wary if and when the patient decides to go public with his or her diagnosis. It is one thing for a patient to confide the diagnosis to family, friends, and coworkers, and a different situation when the patient calls the local newspaper with his or her life story. This latter situation usually results in some serious problems, and all too often I am aware of the therapist's active participation in this "educational" project. The aggressive acceptance and sudden desire for public acknowledgment of the multiplicity constitute a resistance to treatment and should be worked with as such.

Another form of denial of multiplicity occurs when the patient makes a "flight into health" and admits to having been a multiple but denies that this is a current problem. Many patients will seek to leave therapy at this point. In some cases, all overt evidence of their multiplicity may vanish. I have never seen it last, but I have seen several patients drop out of treatment as "cured." Again, the overriding dynamic appears to be an expectable reluctance to confront traumatic memories. In many cases an alter or two reappears after a few sessions. In some instances, however, this apparent disappearance of personalities will continue for several months. Spontaneous integrations are possible, but probably occur far less often than they are claimed. Other aspects of the "flight into health" are discussed in Chapter Eight.

COMMUNICATION AND COOPERATION

Principles

Interpersonality communication is probably going on in every multiple most of the time. The therapeutic concern is more with the direction, quantity, and quality of this communication. Most host personalities hear voices, usually critical and disparaging comments. This is a form of unidirectional communication between one or more hostile alters and the host. Other alters may report being able to see and talk with one another while they are not "out." The host may experience this communication as conversations within his or her head. The host may find notes, letters, poems, drawings, or other evidence left by alters, which comprise yet another channel of communication. Retrospective reports by adult MPD patients and work with child multiples suggest that the level of bidirectional communication between hosts and other alters is higher in children and declines during adolescence. By adulthood the host is often not on speaking terms with any of the alters and is terrified and tormented by the voices. The task of the therapist is to reopen the channels of communication and re-establish dialogue in the personality system.

If the therapist has chained through the personality system and kept some record of what personalities have appeared and who else they are aware of, he or she will have a rough idea of the channels of communication that exist within the patient's personality system. The therapist should also have some idea of who is aware of, and therefore in a position to communicate with, whom. Now, in most cases, this will be an incomplete picture of the system, but this is the place to begin. I try to reinforce the idea of communication at every opportunity. Typically, I subsequently hear that there was actually much more communication going on in the system than I was initially led to believe.

Internal communication is one of the major therapeutic processes that produces change in MPD patients. This communication leads to a breaking down of the amnesic dissociative barriers that divide the patient into personalities, and leads to internal cooperation that displaces the previous competition among alters. Internal communication also allows the multiple to perform an internal "reparenting process," which helps promote healing.

Techniques for Promoting Internal Communication

The Therapist as a Go-Between

The first technique is simply for the therapist to act as a "go-between." This entails listening to one alter and then relating what that alter said to whoever else in the system needs to hear it. Often this is the only way to initiate a dialogue between the host and other alters early in the therapy. There are a lot of problems with this process, however. It is frequently difficult for a therapist to maintain a neutral stance while relaying hostile and vindictive comments back and forth. The net result is that the therapist falls into the internal splits and may feel forced to support one side against the other. This, of course, is one of the dynamics of MPD to which every therapist should be alert. A multiple will attempt to back the therapist into a corner where he or she feels compelled to support some personalities against others. However, things are not usually what they seem, and siding with one party against another will blow up in the therapist's face at a later point.

In the beginning, however, acting as a go-between may be the only way to initiate a dialogue within the system. The therapist should try to be neutral and to convey information as accurately as possible. It is useful to remember that one is involved in another person's internal conversations, and not Henry Kissinger engaged in Middle Eastern shuttle diplomacy. The therapist should watch out for efforts to enlist his or her support on behalf of one side or another. It should be continually suggested that the personalities have the capacity to talk directly with one another if they wish. The host is usually the most resistant to this idea and will claim not to be able to talk with the others. This is part of the host's denial process and will decline with time. I urge the host to "say things internally," or to just think what he or she wishes to say to the others and to listen internally for an answer. Eventually most host personalities will begin this process, which marks an important transition in opening up internal communications. The therapist should not become a fixed part of the internal communication process, or the patient will be unable to maintain an internal dialogue in the therapist's absence.

The Bulletin Board

The next level of communication technique that I introduce to a system is what I call the "bulletin board." The principle is simply that the patient has a place where personalities can "post" messages for each other or the system as a whole. The actual medium is up to the patient. In most instances, I suggest that the patient buy a small notebook that he or she can carry easily. Personalities are then instructed to write messages in the notebook to one another. The messages should have a heading (e.g., "To Jim and George," "To everyone," etc.), and should be dated and signed. The dates and sequential order of the messages allow the patient to track the dialogues chronologically, which provides a form of continuity.

The host may be resistant to this technique because he or she does not like finding mysteriously written messages that provide tangible evidence of the alters' existence. The host may also be disturbed by the content of these messages and protest that he or she does not believe or feel what the messages say. I urge the host to persist in this experiment and not to assume responsibility for the content of the messages. The host should be encouraged to post notices about his or her needs and schedules and to check the notebook several times a day, even if he or she is sure that nothing has been written in it. Host resistance is the major obstacle, and this process may need to be restarted several times before it takes hold and becomes a useful tool for promoting internal communication.

I prefer a notebook as the communication medium because it is cheap, can be carried around privately, is easily accessible, keeps all of the messages in one place, and provides a sequential record of the communication. Some multiples will prefer another medium. I know a multiple, for example, who uses her telephone answering machine to relay messages back and forth among the alters. She prefers this because the illiterate child personalities have more access to the bulletin board through an oral medium. Multiples will also use tape recorders for the same purposes. The access of illiterate alters to a written bulletin board can be facilitated by identifying adult personalities who will help the child alters write and post messages. Again, this task fosters the reparenting process within the multiple's system. Occasionally one of the alters will destroy part or all of a notebook.

Internal Conversations

The internal conversation is the preferable form of internal communication, but one that usually does not become widespread until later in the treatment process. Two or more alters simply carry on an internal dialogue, as opposed to the unidirectional monologues previously present. The capacity for such communication is probably present in every multiple's system; the difficulty lies in promoting it. I encourage alters to communicate in this fashion from the beginning, and use the go-between and bulletin board techniques only as intermediate and temporary steps in promoting dialogue. In many cases, the patient finds the idea of alter selves so frightening that communication only succeeds when it is first distanced and filtered through the therapist or a bulletin board. The "face-to-face" quality of an internal dialogue can only be tolerated after some measure of familiarity and trust has been gained through the other channels.

The process of developing internal conversations changes the hearing of voices from a frightening or distracting experience to a useful and rewarding activity. Initially, the derisive comments heard by the host are considered evidence of being "crazy" and are experiences to be denied or blocked out. Internal conversations now become a doorway into the other rooms of the self previously denied to the host. Eventually the patient may experience group discussions among many of the alters. Like members of any group, they must learn some rules of order, such as yielding the floor appropriately. The ability to carry on internal conversations allows the patient to simulate the more continuous existence of a unified personality and to fill in gaps in continuity caused by alter switching. Again, host resistance is the primary hurdle to be overcome in the development of this ability.

Topics for Conversations: Working toward Common Goals

Eventually, and ideally, anything and everything may be accepted as an appropriate topic for internal communication, regardless of the medium. At first, however, it is best to begin with needs. The person as a whole has many needs and many obligations that must be fulfilled. Often the host, with the help of administrator and helper alters, is struggling to meet these needs. Apparently simple tasks (e.g., getting the oil changed in the car, picking up laundry, etc.) become overwhelmingly difficult when there is no good internal communication. It is this type of task that I first ask the host to "post" on the bulletin board as an announcement, with all the particulars about the specific task or obligation that must be fulfilled. Other alters can use the bulletin board to post their own needs, requests, or comments. If a notice is unclear, the host or other alter can post a request for more information or clarification. It often takes a while for the system to make full use of this process. As it begins to smooth out difficulties and make possible things that were previously exceedingly difficult to accomplish, however, the host and system will become more adept in communication. Increasingly effective internal communication shows the personality system that there are direct and immediate benefits from working together.

A second appropriate topic for early internal communication is the filling in or replay of information that the host is missing because of amnesic gaps from switches. One of the reasons why the host seeks to suppress or deny the other alters is the anxiety that he or she feels about what actually happens during the blank periods associated with switches. Many hosts fear that they engage in inappropriate or even criminal behavior during their amnesic episodes. Not knowing what happened, however, is usually much worse than the facts. Alters should be encouraged to communicate to the host a summary of what occurred during any extensive period when they were "out." The host should be urged to ask what occurred whenever he or she loses a significant amount of time.

Internal Decision Making

Initial Expectations

Among the major stressors on the personality system are the conflict of interests and values and the competition for body time among alters. For various reasons, this seems to increase in intensity when a therapist first begins to work with a patient as a multiple. Against this background of increased competition, for therapy time as much as anything, the therapist must begin to lay the groundwork for an internal decision-making process. Some sort of decision-making process has always been in effect, but usually one or several dominant alters have imposed their will on the system, with other alters seizing control at various times to impulsively act out forbidden wishes. The results speak for themselves!

In the beginning, the most that can be expected is limited cooperation around general tasks in which most of the alters have a common interest. This may include being discharged from the hospital, should the therapist have made the diagnosis during an acute hospitalization. In one patient, for example, the initial therapeutic work on cooperation and decision making was focused around who was going to be "out" during a dental appointment. The patient had had several bad experiences in which all of the alters refused to be present while a tooth was being extracted. As a result, a child alter was shoved "out" and behaved in an embarrassing way. There was a common interest in correcting some serious dental problems, but no alter who had the ability to arrange dental treatment was willing to experience it. After lengthy debate, a compromise plan to divide the experience among several alters was worked out. For the most part, the alters were able to stick to the plan and did succeed in obtaining the necessary dental care.

If some degree of internal cooperation is to be achieved, an effective means of internal communication must be in place. There also must be a sense of fairness or justice within the system. Usually this is present. In fact, many multiples are exceedingly moral individuals with a strong sense of fair play. The therapist can ask the alters to begin working on some of the practical problems in the patient's everyday life. Who is to be responsible for certain tasks in the patient's life? Who pays the bills? Who makes sure that the patient gets to work each day? Having to formally make such decisions highlights the need for a decision-making mechanism and demonstrates to the multiple and therapist the nature of the processes already in place. The therapist should work through and examine some initial decisions with the patient's system. In many cases, the groundwork for a cooperative decision-making process exists and needs only to be modified to achieve a greater degree of internal consensus.

The basic nature of the decision-making process should be along democratic lines, with as large a representation of alters as is feasible. To exclude an alter is to invite trouble. Some alters will remain unknown to the therapist and system until a later point in the therapy. Every time a major decision is made, all "unknown" alters can be invited to step forward and register their comments and opinions. This will smoke out some holdouts from time to time. Whether the actual decision-making process is explicitly a one-alter, one-vote system or a representative system with decision-making councils who act after hearing the various arguments will depend on each MPD patient's system. The latter situation may function better, as it is less cumbersome.

Long-Term Expectations

The long-term expectation is that the patient's personality system will put in place a smoothly functioning mechanism to match the allocation of resources with the person's overall needs. This decision-making process will include all of the alters in some manner, and will be perceived as fair and impartial, with the overall system's best interests as its mandate. When such a system is in place, it has tremendous power and will represent a major stabilizing factor in the patient's life. Patients without such a system are at the mercy of an internal law of the jungle, which results in erratic and often self-destructive behavior. Once an internal governing system has a consensus mandate from most of the other alters, it can enforce its will on the personality system with a consistency and power that no single helper or administrator alter personality can.

Control over Switching

As multiples progress through treatment, they seem to acquire an increased ability to control the switching process. Untreated multiples generally appear to be at the mercy of environmentally triggered switches that produce chaos in their lives. With time and practice in treatment, switching into and out of specific alters becomes easier and more under the multiples' control. In the physiological research studies conducted at the NIMH program in Bethesda, we have learned to use multiples who have been in treatment for 2 or more years, as they have acquired more control over who is "out" and how long they can remain there (Putnam,

1984b). As control over the switch process improves, many of the "impulsive" pathological behaviors decrease correspondingly. I do not believe that any unintegrated multiple has complete control over environmentally evoked personality switches, but observation suggests that many can gain a substantial degree of voluntary control over the switch mechanism.

Host Fears

Among the early impediments to increased control over switching are the host's frequent attempts to suppress all other alters. In many cases, the host is at some level unwilling to allow other alters "out," either in therapy or in other settings. This suppression is almost always incomplete and provokes acting out by other alters, who struggle with the host and one another for body time. The host's suppression of the other alters is usually motivated by fears that he or she will lose control completely if he or she allows any alters to emerge. The host may also fear that he or she will never come back if another alter emerges. Many hosts describe a "death-like" experience of fading into nothingness when another alter takes over. This void can be terrifying and is an experience that they dread with phobic intensity.

The host may also be concerned about inappropriate behavior by another alter. Based on past experience, this is probably a realistic fear. In therapy, the host may be concerned about possible rejection if the therapist meets an inappropriate or aggressive alter. The host may experience the switch process as embarrassing and resent the loss of time that occurs. Time loss is an aversive experience and leaves the host worrying about what he or she might have said or done during the blank space. The host may also be concerned that the therapist will come to like some of the other alters more and consequently will spend more time with the others. The host and other alters are all capable of an intense sibling-like rivalry for the affections of the therapist.

Facilitation of the Switching Process

Increased control over switching is desirable; it gives the patient more control over his or her life and enables the therapist to plumb the system more effectively for past traumas and current psychopathology. Control is achieved in a gradual fashion over time and is probably the result of several factors. The first is the host's acceptance of the diagnosis and willingness to meet the other alters. The second is improved internal communication within the system that allows for smoother and more appropriate switching. The third factor is the increasing internal trust that develops among alters as a result of better communication. As they come to know one another better, there is a greater willingness to share the body. As each alter's needs become known to the system and a centralized decision-making process begins to acknowledge and meet these needs, the alters are correspondingly more willing to wait their fair turn and are less likely to seize the body opportunistically to fulfill their own wishes. The fourth factor is that improved communication also fills in the gaps in time, and fears about what might have happened during amnesic spaces are alleviated. There are undoubtedly other factors that also result in improved control over switches.

The therapist can set the stage for acquisition of improved control over switching in several ways. The first is to allow the host to have some benign experiences with switches to help offset prior aversive experiences. Hypnotic techniques, such as those described in Chapter Nine, are particularly useful in relaxing the host and allowing other alters to step forward while the host watches from a comfortable position. These techniques are helpful in working with a host who is frightened by "death-like" experiences associated with previous switching.

A second important intervention is to ensure that the host returns after a switch to one or more alters occurs during therapy. Hosts find it especially disconcerting to "wake up" outside of the treatment setting and not know what has occurred. They may fear that they have harmed the therapist or something bad has happened. It is also important to make certain that the host is informed of what occurred during any portion of therapy for which he or she is amnesic. As internal communication improves, the therapist can delegate this responsibility to the personality system, but in the beginning it is important to tell the host what personalities emerged and what was said, so that he or she understands that therapeutic work is going on during these amnesic episodes.

COMMON PITFALLS IN THE EARLY
STAGES OF THERAPY

Overreaction to Pathological Behavior

Multiples seem to teeter continuously on the brink of total disaster. Every improvement is followed by a relapse. Hostile alters threaten suicide, internal or external homicide, and assorted other catastrophes.

The therapist must learn to live through these and perform useful therapy, despite apparent calamity at every turn. The ability to tolerate a high level of background noise is an essential attribute for therapists working with MPD patients. Some therapists find that they just cannot adjust to this continuous cataclysm and opt to transfer these patients. If a clinician wishes to work with MPD patients—and the rewards are great—it is important to remain calm and unruffled by much of this chaos. Often it is simply a resistance to getting on with the hard work of abreacting earlier trauma. R. P. Kluft (personal communication, 1985) describes his demeanor in therapy as an attempt to "bore my patients into health." I would similarly advocate a "laid-back" approach to much of the noise generated by these patients. Suicide and homicide threats must, of course, be evaluated, but most do not warrant hospitalization of the patient. Control can often be better imposed from within rather than from without.

A therapist can expect a range of quasi-psychotic phenomena, conversion symptoms, and psychosomatic manifestations in an MPD patient (Kluft, 1984d). This is part and parcel of a major dissociative disorder. It is important not to overreact to these symptoms, but rather to explore who and what is responsible. The power of working with MPD patients as multiples is that the therapist can often sidestep the pathology by engaging the personality system to find out who is responsible for these symptoms. Then the therapist meets with the appropriate alters and works out a contract or other measure to limit the symptoms to an acceptable level. Attempts to impose control from the outside play into a resistance that seeks to divert the therapist away from painful areas.

Overinvestment in Multiplicity as a Phenomenon

Overemphasis on multiplicity per se is a common mistake made by therapists new to the disorder. MPD is a fascinating phenomenon that makes one question most of what one has learned about the human mind. A reading of the case report literature from the earliest cases to the present shows that one of the common impulses on the part of therapists is an attempt to document the differences among the alter personalities of their patients. The lay media are also primarily interested in emphasizing these differences. This fascination with the differences of the alters sends a clear message to patients that these are what make them interesting to therapists and others.

I do not think that one can be both an investigator and a therapist of the same patient. I never involve any patient that I directly treat in research, and vice versa. The transference–countertransference issues, which are overly complex in MPD anyway, become overwhelming. The message of investigation is that the researcher is primarily interested in the differences among the alters. The message of treatment should be that, taken together, the alters are ultimately one person, and the goal of treatment is a resolution of the perceived differences and the development of internal unity. For a therapist to send both messages to the patient is to create a significant level of confusion that will ultimately spill back into the therapeutic process.

Development of Favorites

A common mistake made by therapists new to MPD is the development of favoritism among the alter personalities. Over time the therapist comes to know a range of personalities, some of whom are more functional and socially desirable than others. The therapist may actively dislike some of the internal persecutors and may be uncomfortable in relating to child or seductive personalities. Consequently, he or she may attempt to encourage and promote specific alters over others who are viewed as pathological. The therapist may seek to prohibit some personalities from having time in the body, and, in extreme cases, may attempt to hypnotically "lock" personalities in a closet or bury them as a way of suppressing them. As one therapist said to me while describing his attempts to promote the attractive work personality and suppress the hideous self-mutilator, "If only I could keep her [the work personality] out all of the time, everything would be all right." This is not true. The therapist should not make the error of believing that the patient has "good" and "bad" personalities and that the task of therapy is simply to promote the good and suppress the bad.

Every alter must be treated as an equal. Every personality was created for a reason and with a purpose. To selectively encourage some and ignore or suppress others is to ask for trouble. Favoritism is easy to slip into. Some personalities are more appealing and pleasant to be with; they demand less and threaten less. It is an understandable reaction on the therapist's part to encourage the presence of personalities with whom he or she is more comfortable. Unfortunately, very little work will get done in the treatment setting, and a great deal of acting out will occur outside of therapy. The therapist has to work with them all. Doing so will show many of the "bad" personalities to be "good" in the long run. Their "badness" is often due to the fact that they are the keepers of pain and rage, which frees up the "good" personalities to function.

Going after Past Traumas Too Soon

A major focus of the treatment of MPD is the recovery and therapeutic abreaction of earlier traumas. This represents a core task of the therapy and is necessary to achieve a stable resolution or integration. I think, however, that it is a mistake to jump into this part of the treatment process before the patient has been adequately stabilized and is prepared to begin the hard and painful work involved. Premature exploration of early trauma is likely to produce marked dissociative symptoms, including prolonged fugue episodes, suicidal or internal homicidal behavior, and other crises that will effectively disrupt the therapy. The initial interventions and stabilizations discussed in this chapter should be in place before the therapist makes a serious attempt to work with the trauma.

A patient may allude to past events suggestive of earlier trauma in the beginning stages of therapy. It is important to follow up on any such references, if only to let the patient know that the therapist has heard what has been said and understands what is in store for the future. I would, however, refrain from an aggressive and/or abreactive exploration until a measure of trust, together with a degree of internal communication and cooperation, has been established.

Fear of Losing One's First Case

Multiples are special patients. They make sure that they are in many ways. In fact, many are quite extraordinary and talented people. Their relatedness (which is usually more intense than that of most other psychiatric patients) and a multitude of transference and countertransference feelings generated by the various alters tend to break down many of the usual patient–therapist boundaries. Therapists experienced in treating other disorders often find themselves relating and behaving toward their MPD patients in ways that they would never consider doing with any other type of patient. Transference and countertransference issues are discussed more fully in Chapter Seven.

One of the early countertransference issues that occurs in a therapist working with his or her first MPD patient is the fear of losing the case. The fear seems to be that the patient will quit therapy or perhaps transfer to another therapist. This may happen. Some multiples wander the country, sporadically initiating treatment with whoever is available and then abandoning ship as soon as the going starts to get rough. I think that some percentage of multiples—R. P. Kluft (personal communication,

1985) has suggested roughly a third—cannot sustain or are not yet ready to sustain meaningful treatment. They may show up for some crisis intervention work and then bail out before one can get close to the real issues. These patients cannot be held in treatment. It is best to let them know what is available and what is is required on their part. If and when they are ready for treatment, they will find a way to make it happen.

Belief–Disbelief Cycle

"When I am with her I believe it—and then when I go home at night, I think that I must be being taken; it can't be real. And yet when I see her again, I think it really is real." The therapist who shared those thoughts with me was going through what I call the "belief–disbelief cycle." There is a great deal about MPD that stretches one's sense of credulity. In the early stages of treatment, many therapists working with their first multiples will find that they swing between belief in the reality of MPD and fear that they are being duped by clever actors. This experience may in part be responsible for the strong wish of therapists to document the differences across the alters of their patients. The real test of the authenticity of MPD is the test of time. Therapists will find that with the exception of flights into health, real multiples behave in a consistent manner session after session. In using actors as a control group in our physiological studies, we have repeatedly observed that actors go out of character when stressed, fatigued, or distracted. They do not have the day-in, day-out consistency of the multiples. With time, a therapist is likely to come to accept the reality of a patient's psychological organization as a series of alter identities.

Overdependence on Medication

In many cases, the diagnosis of MPD is made after the patient has received treatment under another diagnostic label. Frequently the patient is already on one or more psychotropic medications. The interactions and effects of medication on MPD are very complex and are covered in detail in Chapter Ten. The primary treatment modality in MPD is psychotherapy/hypnotherapy, and medication is useful primarily as an adjunct or supportive measure (Barkin *et al.*, 1986; Kluft, 1984d). It is a mistake to attempt to use medications to suppress the symptoms and manifestations of MPD. Transient symptom suppression may be possible with high doses of neuroleptics, but this inevitably causes an unacceptable deterioration in the patient's level of functioning.

In most instances, it is preferable to wean the patient off all medications after a diagnosis of MPD has been established. Medication can be reinitiated, if appropriate, once the therapist has gained some familiarity with the personality system and is in a better position to evaluate the differential effects of the medication across the various alter personalities. In many patients, reinstitution of medication will not be necessary because the symptoms and behaviors can be managed by contracts and other psychotherapeutic interventions.

SUMMARY

This chapter has begun with an exploration of concerns commonly voiced by therapists new to the treatment of MPD. These include the fear of creating or exacerbating MPD by working with the alter personalities; fears of violent alters; concerns about being unqualified to treat MPD; and concerns about the appropriate treatment setting. I have sought to provide reassurance that one cannot iatrogenically induce MPD; that dangerous alters can be safely managed; and that rumors of dangerous alters are often dynamic exaggerations. The ability to be a good psychotherapist is the primary prerequisite to working with MPD patients, and an outpatient setting is generally best.

Next I have outlined the tasks and steps in a "typical" treatment. The important overall tasks include (1) establishing a therapeutic alliance; (2) promoting appropriate changes; and (3) replacing internal division and conflict with some form of functional unity. The course of treatment is divided for heuristic purposes into eight stages or steps. The first step, making the diagnosis, has been covered earlier in Chapter Four.

The second and third steps of initial interventions and stabilizations have been discussed here in some detail. Techniques for meeting alters and gathering information on the personality system are presented, and the principles and benefits of contracting are detailed, stressing the need for highly specific and very concrete wording of written contracts. I have noted the difficulties inherent in determining and enforcing the consequences for contract violations. Useful areas for first contracts include (1) the type and duration of therapy; (2) control of dangerous or self-destructive behavior; and (3) appropriate therapeutic boundaries.

The fourth stage, acceptance of the diagnosis, is usually more of an ongoing theme in therapy. Typically the patient attempts to force the therapist to "prove" the diagnosis or distracts the therapist with heated arguments over the diagnosis. At other times, the patient may seek to exploit the diagnosis by going public, too often drawing the therapist into this destructive resistance. Flights into health and other forms of denial of the diagnosis may occur at various points in treatment.

The fifth step, the development of cooperation and communication within the personality system, also represents an ongoing task. Although more communication and cooperation are present than may be immediately apparent, the therapist must identify and build on what is already there. Specific techniques for fostering communication are discussed, as well as the principles of internal group decision making. With most of these techniques, it is best to begin with the mundane chores of daily life. I have also discussed ways to help the patient gain control over personality switching.

The last steps in the course of treatment—metabolism of the trauma, resolution or integration, and postresolution coping—are discussed in subsequent chapters. This chapter has concluded with a few common mistakes made by therapists early in the course of treatment. These include overreaction to pathological behavior; an overinvestment in the weirdness of MPD; favoritism of some alters over others; beginning to explore the trauma too early; a waxing and waning of belief in MPD; and an overdependence on medication to control the patient's symptoms.

CHAPTER SEVEN

Issues in Psychotherapy

The treatment of MPD is, in essence, the psychotherapy of a traumatic neurosis. Chapter Six has described the initial sequence of interventions necessary to stabilize a newly diagnosed patient and create a therapeutic milieu in which treatment can take place. Every patient–therapist dyad is unique and will necessarily have its own special treatment issues and problems; it is impossible to anticipate what these may be. I have found, however, that a number of common themes and issues regularly occur in treatment with MPD patients. This chapter is devoted to an elaboration of these issues and themes as they affect the psychotherapy of MPD.

BOUNDARY MANAGEMENT

Frequency of Sessions

In many instances following the diagnosis of MPD, there is an opportunity for a re-evaluation of all aspects of the therapy. One of the most frequently asked questions at this time is "How often should an MPD patient be seen?" Obviously no single answer will suffice for all patients, or even a single patient under a variety of different circumstances. In general, I find that for outpatients a frequency of two or three times a week seems to work well. Less frequent sessions tend to lead to stalemated therapies, whereas more frequent sessions often result in highly enmeshed and chaotic treatments. I will see a patient as often as I think may be necessary in a crisis situation. As a matter of policy, however, I do not think that seeing a patient more often results in more rapid improvement. Certain aspects of the treatment—for instance, the acceptance of the diagnosis, the development of trust, and the metabolism of trauma—have intrinsic rates of their own that cannot be significantly increased by more frequent sessions. The therapist should pace the treatment accordingly. The average patient is likely to take several years of treatment to reach a satisfactory resolution, whether he or she is seen twice a day or twice a week. Therapist burnout will not be helpful to either the therapist or the patient.

Length of Sessions

Most of the points made above also apply to the length of sessions. MPD patients tend to overstay their allotted time and run into the next patient's hour. They may prolong a session in several ways. Commonly, some alter makes a grand appearance just as the therapist thinks that he or she is wrapping the session up for the day. I have learned to say, "Well, our time is up. I'll be glad to talk with you at our next session." Alters will learn that if they really wish to speak with the therapist, they are going to have to emerge earlier in the session.

I generally work with a session length of an hour and a half for MPD patients. A 50-minute hour is too short for much of the work that needs to be accomplished in a session. This is particularly true for abreactive work, which requires time to be initiated, run its course, be processed, and achieve closure. A patient is naturally reluctant to plunge into the throes of a painful abreaction and tends to delay the start of such reactions until well into the session. Once initiated, an abreaction should be allowed to run its course. Time must be taken afterward to reorient the patient, start the processing of recovered memories, and provide a degree of closure on the experience. Failure to help the patient stabilize afterwards can result in postsession dissociative behaviors that disrupt future therapy and increase the patient's reluctance to undertake further abreactive work.

It is unfortunate that this type of work does not fit neatly into the traditional 50-minute psychotherapy hour. One solution is to schedule a multiple as the last patient of the day, so that the therapist can accommodate a longer session length. Whatever session length is chosen, the therapist should stick to it. It is important to maintain this boundary; otherwise the MPD patient will consume ever-increasing amounts of time with diminishing returns. The therapist should not expect the patient to be the one to end the session on time!

Availability of the Therapist outside of Sessions

An MPD patient is going to have periodic crises. Kluft (1983) notes that crises requiring a therapist's intervention occur in up to 80% of multiples.

Being available for emergency work or consultation with other therapists working with a patient comes with the territory. The crucial point is ensuring that the therapist's availability is not abused by the patient. In the early stages of therapy, the therapist may receive a large number of phone calls at the office and/or home from various alters. It is important to negotiate a contract with the whole personality system regarding the number of calls and the conditions under which calls are appropriate. If this is not done, the therapist will receive 10 calls in a night as each personality calls up to give his or her opinion of what another alter just said in the preceding call.

The therapist should not be surprised if an MPD patient shows up at the office at times other than the regular sessions, or is found in the parking lot or sitting on the front steps at home. This can be disconcerting and even frightening at times. It is important to control this behavior by contract immediately. If this behavior persists, and the therapist feels threatened or intimidated, he or she should perhaps seriously consider terminating the treatment. When a multiple begins to intrude into the therapist's private life, it is a danger sign that should not be ignored or condoned.

Special Sessions

Special sessions are likely to constitute an important part of most successful treatments. They may include extended sessions for prolonged abreactive work, sessions to view videotapes, or sessions in which child personalities are rewarded by special treats. In one case, I met with a patient at the zoo for several sessions, as this facilitated access to certain child alters who would not come out in the clinic setting where I was seeing her. Obviously, therapy boundaries must be watched carefully in such settings. Special sessions or sessions in special settings need to be thought through clearly. What does the therapist expect to accomplish with the session, and why is a special session or a special setting needed? There often are valid reasons for such sessions, but they should not become the rule.

COMMON THEMES AND ISSUES IN THERAPY

This section discusses a number of themes that recurrently emerge during the course of therapy with multiples. The roots of these themes lie in two major domains: trauma from the past and trauma in the present. The first involves experiences from the past, primarily the experience of being abused by parents or other caretakers. Trauma in the present involves the myriad of difficulties that arise for a multiple in trying to fit into a society that stresses the continuity of time and self. In many instances, the first expression of these themes occurs in the context of everyday experience, but in fact they are driven by earlier, deeply buried experiences. Lindy (1985) has described a similar process, which he labels "the special configuration of the traumatic event," in victims of natural and human-caused disasters.

One of the factors, however, that differentiates the themes and dynamics of multiples from those of other victims of traumatic experience is the sheer volume of trauma endured by most MPD victims. The victims of a flood, an airplane crash, a nightclub fire, or the like are contending with a single, relatively brief, simply explained traumatic incident. Multiples are usually facing years of terror and trauma at the hands of people who are supposed to have loved and cared for them. Thus, although many of the themes and concepts developed from work with disaster victims are applicable to MPD, they are uniquely reconfigured by the chronicity of the trauma and the fragmentation of the self found in MPD victims.

Control

The issue of control can become a major dynamic in the treatment process, and if not properly addressed it may lead to a therapeutic impasse (Caul, 1985a). The theme of control in MPD patients usually manifests itself in two arenas: control of self and control of others (primarily the therapist). The host personality usually experiences himself or herself as being out of control. This experience, in part, contributes to the depression and sense of being overwhelmed and helpless that many host personalities describe. The frightening amnesic voids, repeated experiences of being confronted with evidence that they have said or done something that goes against their judgment and values, experiences of watching themselves as if they were detached observers, and passive influence experiences all contribute to host personalities' perception of nearly complete loss of control over themselves and their surroundings.

What sense of self-control a host personality does possess is the result of an exhausting internal struggle of self-repression. The fragility of this sense of self-control and the fear that once lost it can never be regained are part of the host's resistance to allowing any of the other alter personalities out. The host often seeks to reinforce internal control by external means. Some hosts are rigidly obsessive and attempt to suppress other alters by ritualized behaviors. Other hosts are controlling of the therapist and stifle inquiry or exploration into areas that might provoke the emergence of alter personalities, all the while apparently remaining oblivious to the existence of alters. A host may control the therapist by indicating that the therapist's more or less continuous presence is necessary to prevent switching. In a number of my cases, the hosts joined the military in hopes that the highly structured routine of service life would provide a mechanism of control that they could not.

Host personalities often express fears about loss of control with statements of impending doom. Usually these statements imply that some unspecified catastrophe is going to occur in the near future. A patient may express a deep sense of dread and inevitability about an ultimately disastrous outcome. Yet, at the same time, the patient is extremely vague about the details.

The desperate quality of the host's struggle to maintain control and the apparent frailty of this control are often mirrored in the therapist's feelings of loss of control over the treatment process. It is easy for a therapist to become co-opted into the unquestioned assumption that the host must maintain control at all costs. Embedded within this supposition may be the therapist's own fears of multiplicity and of frightening alters who might emerge, wishes that the patient would stabilize and stop ceaselessly changing, confusion as to "who" is the real patient, and reluctance to compound the patient's suffering by uncovering hideous memories. The host must learn to relinquish control if the multiplicity is to be treated. The therapist should be careful of an overidentification with the host's fears of loss of control.

The other side of the coin is expressed by alters, usually with apparently malevolent intentions, who claim complete control over the fate of the individual. These alters may emerge and sneeringly tell the therapist that nothing that he or she can do can prevent their ultimate triumph. Like the fears of total destruction expressed by the host, these claims of total power are greatly exaggerated. The gambit here is to engage the therapist in a struggle for control over the patient. In any such struggle, the therapist will lose. Thus, struggles with persecutor alters for control of the patient should be consistently avoided. I pre-emptively concede all control over the ultimate fate of the patient to the patient, *as a whole*, in the early stages of therapy. Struggles for control serve to divert the therapist away from dealing with real-life issues and exploration of past trauma. The malevolent alters are often simply performing in their larger role of protecting the patient.

Caul (1985a) notes that one form of control over the therapy commonly involves the patient's changing subjects or untracking the focus of the session. He states that it is all right to allow this to continue for a moment, but the therapist should soon regain control and bring the session back on track. Another tactic is for an alter to prevent the therapist from talking with other alters. Caul (1985a) suggests, "While the therapist should understand the reason that this is taking place, the patient should be told that the other personalities have rights and that the therapist has a responsibility for treating them all" (p. 4).

The therapist will undoubtedly be drawn into many struggles for control with, and over, the patient. In the short run, the therapist may, in emergency situations, have to take control from the patient through hospitalization or other measures. In the day-to-day therapy, the therapist must also be responsible for maintaining the treatment boundaries and focus of the sessions. In the long run, however, the real control over the person's life must be returned completely to the patient. Struggles for control in therapy should be understood as mirroring internal struggles among the alters for control of the patient's behavior; struggles for control of the dissociated material the patient is permitted to experience consciously; and the need of a victim to be in control so that "it" never happens again.

Rejection

Multiples are exquisitely sensitive to any form of rejection and will often perceive it where none is intended. Responses to this perceived rejection may include self-mutilation, suicide attempts, fugue episodes, and missed sessions. The flip side of this dynamic is that many multiples will repeatedly force the therapist into acceptance–rejection situations as part of the testing that goes on in therapy.

The basis for this sensitivity lies in an MPD patient's past history. To be an abused child is to be profoundly rejected by the people who are supposed to love and care for the child. Many multiples report creating personalities whose function was to be pleasing to their abusers in an effort to reduce the rejection and abandonment to which they were subjected. No matter who was created or what they did, however, the rejection continued. I think that it would be difficult to overestimate the feelings of rejection and abandonment that these patients have experienced in childhood. Rejection by an important person may also have been a prelude to an abusive episode. In some cases, one parent's rejection would signal the other parent that that parent could now do what he or she wished.

This sensitivity to rejection is often compounded by later experiences in adult life. Many multiples have experienced important relationships' ending painfully and unexpectedly because of something that they "did" but were not aware of. A common scenario is for one alter to sabotage the relationships of the host or another alter. Rejection may also have taken the form of denial of multiplicity by prior therapists.

It would be nice if a therapist never had to reject a patient, but experiences of rejection, intended or otherwise, will undoubtedly occur more than once during the course of treatment. In fact, the patient will see that it happens. The important thing is to care, to make it manifestly clear that the therapist is not abandoning the patient, and to continue to pursue the goals of the treatment. In time, the patient will come to see the larger acceptance of who and what he or she is that the therapist's commitment to the treatment represents. A therapist who believes that he or she is being set up to reject a patient should call it, lay out what he or she thinks is happening, and look at the consequences of both sides of the issue with the patient. The therapist does not pass a multiple's test by blindly accepting the side of a forced choice that he or she thinks will please the patient. If the patient is a multiple, there will be alters on both sides of an issue, and to accept one side of the proposition is to reject the other. The only way out of most of these no-win setups is to call them for what they are.

Secrets

The theme of secrets permeates all therapeutic work with MPD patients. Secrets exist on many levels. Alters keep secrets from the host, from the therapist, and from one another. The secrets involve past experiences and present behavior. Much of the treatment involves the slow unwrapping of secrets and the processing of their contents.

The secrets usually begin with the abuse. Abusers (particularly sexual abusers) often threaten children, and/or people and pets important to them, with injury or death if the children should ever tell anyone about the abuse. For the child personalities of an MPD patient, with their timeless unmetabolized trauma, these threats still retain all of their gruesome power.

> In every case, as these memories are shared for the first time, patients experience genuine terror. It is as though that same feeling of vulnerability—intact and alive from the time of original trauma—is reexperienced. In none of the cases with which I am familiar could this terror be understood solely as a dyadic transference phenomenon. The terror is as though patient and therapist convene in the presence of yet another person. The third image is the victimizer, who long ago de-

manded silence and whose command is now being broken. The numbing intensity of these occasions, when patients feel as though they are risking their lives to tell their stories, suggests that as long as there has been any desire to unburden, confess, or heal, there has also been the shadow of this third person. Psychologically, the relationship with this person has continued since the time of the threat. (Lister, 1982, p. 875)

Other dynamic bonds between victim and abuser may still be operative in maintaining these secrets. Lister (1982) has pointed out that trauma may occur at an age in which a degree of psychic fusion with an abuser is a developmentally normal process. To reveal a secret, and break this bond, may produce a separation that is experienced as a loss of a primary object tie. This dynamic is clearly active with some child alters. A related dynamic, identification with the aggressor, may also contribute to the keeping of secrets. Lister describes a further dynamic in which the child, by originally tolerating the abuse and now by continuing to remain in psychological bondage, may be attempting—by "love, manipulation, or magic—to 'cure' the parent" (p. 874).

There are several dynamics between patient and therapist that may be involved in further preventing the patient from revealing secrets (Lister, 1982). The first is the shame and guilt so often felt by victims of trauma. The second is the defense of magical thinking—"if I don't speak of it, perhaps it never was." The third is the fear that the therapist's response to hearing about the abuse will be disappointing and will further compound the feelings of abuse or associated shame and guilt. The fourth is that the therapist may question the truth of the patient's report and force the patient either to leave the therapist or to abandon his or her understanding of what happened. And, finally, the therapist may not be able to tolerate hearing the details of the abusive experiences. All of these dynamics, together with the sequestering of memories within alters and amnesic barriers across alters, serve to keep traumatic secrets deeply locked within the patient.

The secrets of the past are not the only secrets kept by multiples. In the vast majority of cases, they have continued to live a life of secrets. They have kept their true nature, multiplicity, hidden from others and often from themselves. They have learned to compensate and cover for time loss and its associated inconsistencies in their behavior. Many multiples lead double and triple lives. The coexistence of widely discrepant social roles, such as librarian by day and streetwalker by night, is not uncommon in MPD patients.

Secrets can only be shared, and therefore ultimately revealed, when trust has developed between patient and therapist. In general, the patient will gradually lead the therapist through the hierarchy of secrets, starting with those that are least traumatic and only moving on to the more highly charged secrets if the therapist passes the first tests. Lister (1982) has vividly described the process of abreaction associated with the first revelation of secrets that are linked with past threats to the individual.

Secrets have a power of their own that pressures the patient both to conceal and to reveal them. The therapist's efforts are best spent in creating a therapeutic climate in which the revelation of these secrets and all of their attendant trauma can safely occur. The first hints are usually casually dropped and immediately glossed over; the therapist cannot be expected always to recognize these first clues. The patient will, however, provide a pattern of information that over time will point to a secret. The therapist should facilitate this process through careful listening and support, but should not "drag" the secret out of the patient.

Setups and Tests

Every interaction with an MPD patient is at some level a test. Multiples test a therapist repeatedly in subtle and not-so-subtle ways. The tests are directed at determining "trustworthiness." The issues, circumstances, and goals of these tests will vary, but the overriding concern on the part of a multiple is whether the therapist can be trusted.

A core concern of most multiples in treatment is a primitive fear that the therapist will turn on them and abuse them, as their parents or other caretakers did in so many cases. So, paradoxically, they will often maneuver a therapist into situations where he or she may symbolically recapitulate an original abusive situation. Trust does not come easily for MPD patients, and too many therapists are lulled into believing that their patients have complete faith in them. Such hubris can lead to serious problems. Personalities will constantly attempt to lead the therapist astray by suggesting actions or situations that are symbolically abusive. If the therapist shows no ability to recognize these traps, to set limits, or to extricate himself or herself from these setups, then how can he or she be trusted?

Setups and tests frequently occur around contracts and boundary management issues. Will the therapist leave some loophole that permits self-destructive behavior? Will the therapist allow the multiple to transgress a therapy boundary? Will the therapist enforce a contract, or can he or she be "bought off" in some way? This is part of the testing that accompanies all contractual interactions with multiples and is one reason why contracts need to be explicitly stated and consistently enforced. The therapist will gain more points with an MPD patient by being scrupulous in contract making and enforcement than by attempts to win goodwill by letting the patient "off the hook" when infractions occur. The willingness to overlook a contract violation is for the patient comparable to the willingness of important figures in his or her past to overlook the abuse and suffering. The therapist cannot be trusted to make a deal and keep it.

Another area ripe for testing is the therapist's ability to hear, recognize, and deal with traumatic material. In the beginning of treatment, references to abuse and trauma are often symbolic, mentioned vaguely in passing, or embedded in current life-situational material. Is the therapist tuned in and listening? Does the therapist believe in the reality of the abuse? Can the therapist tolerate the explicit details? Will the therapist find the patient to be the degraded and worthless human being—or, even worse, the monster—that abuse and trauma have convinced the patient he or she is? Will the therapist be contaminated by the abuse? One must remember that the patient's ideas, feelings, and attitudes about the abuse were, by and large, formed during early childhood and have remained unaltered since that time. A great deal of magical thinking and primitive symbolism will be embodied in all issues related to past abuse and trauma.

A therapist cannot pass these tests by being clever or by wanting to do the right thing. He or she must be sensitive and honest, listening on many levels for references to past trauma. The therapist must let the patient know when he or she does not understand something, and must follow up obscure comments and passing asides. The therapist should also be impeccable in all of his or her interactions with the patient. This does not require being distant and aloof, but it does mean being strictly honest. The therapist should not make a promise that he or she cannot keep. Promises are special tests, and failing them can have serious repercussions for the therapeutic alliance. The therapist cannot pass all of the tests; in fact, many of the tests are deliberately constructed to be no-win situations, and the therapist should beware of forced choices.

What Really Happened?

"I don't know if this really happened, or if I dreamed it—or even made it up." Multiples and other victims of severe trauma often have difficulty in determining the origin of the dreamlike images that flood their inner awareness at times. These images may be vividly intense and accompanied by powerful emotions, and yet at the same time seem unreal and alien. Often the images are fragments of an action scene in which figures perform or other events occur. There may be elements in the scene that seem clearly impossible; for instance, one patient kept seeing a ball of blazing fire roll around a room. These images will have an intrusive flashback quality, yet the patient may not be able to relate them to anything remembered as having actually occurred. The patient may feel trapped between the compelling affects generated by the images and an inability to make any sense of the content.

Multiples, like Billy Pilgrim in *Slaughterhouse-Five*, Vonnegut's (1970) semiautobiographical account of the Dresden holocaust, are "unstuck in time." The past and the present intermingle and follow each other in chronological confusion. Flashbacks, with their accompanying distortions of age and body image, send a patient hurtling backwards to relive trauma that seems more vivid now than when it actually occurred. As one husky man told me, "When I go back I look at my arms, and they are the skinny arms of a 12-year-old boy." Time is discontinuous for multiples. The breaks are more than the simple lapses in continuity produced by the personality switches; inversions and reversals in a patient's sense of time are produced by flashbacks to past events. Reality testing is impaired by the lack of a firm "now" against which to measure what is past and what is present.

The questions of what really happened and when it happened are usually sources of painful confusion for MPD patients. Confusion of past and present; of real and unreal; and of dream, fantasy and memory may overwhelm them at times. Not uncommonly, patients will retreat into a phase during which they announce that they "made it all up." Closer questioning will reveal that they do not know how or why they made it all up, and this assertion will quickly crumble under scrutiny. Understandably, both patients and therapists will wish for some tangible truth as to what really did happen. Sometimes this is forthcoming. Dr. Wilbur was able to meet with Sybil's father and hear him confirm the truth of what she had been told (Schreiber, 1974). Unfortunately, in the majority of cases, no hard incontrovertible evidence remains beyond the physical and psychological scarring of the patients.

Anger at or Idealization of the Abusers

Severe and chronic child abuse can produce a strange bonding between abused and abuser. This seems to be particularly true with incest. One patient described how incredibly angry she became at me when I suggested that her incestuous father had abused her. How dare I accuse her father of being a child abuser! Child abusers were the scum of the earth. I was talking about *her* father. She disappeared and did not return for several months, at which time she was willing to accept the possibility that she might have been an abused child. Virtually every multiple will have a group of alters who idealize the abuser(s) and who have no memory or knowledge of the abuse. Such alters were, and may remain, adaptive for a child living continually with his or her abuser. They served as a respite from continual terror and allowed the child to make use of whatever nurturing and love the abuser was able to provide.

In the same personality system there will be alters who harbor murderous rage toward the abusers. They frequently will not acknowledge them as "their" parents and will refer to the abusers by their proper names or some epithet. They may threaten to kill the abusers if they get a chance, thus putting the therapist in a difficult legal situation, given the current *Tarasoff* guidelines for notification of intended victims. I do not know of any case in which these threats were actually carried through, but each instance deserves careful evaluation. Unfortunately, much of the anger these personalities feel toward the abusers will be scapegoated onto the therapist. In the early stages of therapy, interpretation usually has little impact on this process. The therapist must set limits and not allow a patient to abuse him or her in any fashion. Modeling this behavior has the secondary effect of demonstrating that there are other ways of dealing with potential abuse besides killing the abusers.

Recapitulation of the Abuse

Recapitulation of the abuse usually occurs on at least two levels: within the personality system and within the therapy. Typically, it also occurs in relationships outside of the treatment. The need of victims to re-enact their previous trauma has been repeatedly described in the literature on the psychological consequences of disasters (Horowitz, 1985). Children may relive the events through repetitive play; adults may do so by flashbacks and retelling. Multiples seem to need to recreate abuse equivalents within the therapy. In most instances these abuse equivalents will be symbolic, but in some cases of therapist psychopathology, they may lead to seduction of the therapist or sexual acting out.

The most pathetic examples of abuse equivalents in a therapy setting occur in situations where the therapist feels forced into some "abusive" behavior in order to "save" the patient. In one case, as a child the patient had been repeatedly tied up and forced to perform fellatio on her father. During her last hospitalization, she became severely suicidal and anorexic. The staff members tried to feed her through a naso-gastric tube, but she kept pulling it out. Consequently, they felt compelled to place her in four-way restraints. The patient was now tied to her bed and having a tube forced down her throat in an ironic re-enactment of her earlier trauma, all in the name of saving her life. Once the similarity of these "therapeutic" interventions to her earlier abuse was pointed out to all parties, it became possible to discontinue the forced feedings. The patient was able to leave the hospital shortly afterwards and maintain herself independently. A therapist who feels forced to do something aversive to the patient for the "sake" of the patient should think again.

Re-enactment of prior abuse within the personality system usually takes the form of internal persecution. Specific alter personalities will inflict abuse on the body, and nominally upon other alters, that is either the same or symbolically the same as the abuse suffered during childhood. The multiple's personality system contains both victimizer and victim. The victimizer personality may be a more or less direct introject of the patient's original abuser. These internal persecutors are activated by a number of factors. They may be stimulated by events in the patient's daily life that were cues for abuse during childhood. More often, they are activated when the patient begins to relate details of past abuse to the therapist; when this occurs, they will "punish" the patient for telling about past trauma. Naturally, this increases the patient's resistance to further disclosure. Not only is the abuse painful to recall and relive in an abreactive fashion, but to do so may bring on further abuse from these abuser introjects.

The patient may create re-enactments of abuse through external relationships. For example, most sexually abused multiples will have promiscuous alter personalities who set the patients up for traumatic sexual experiences. A common scenario involves a promiscuous personality's picking up an abusive sexual partner and then turning the body over to the frightened and often frigid host at the height of sexual degradation. When asked why she did such a thing, one such alter told me, "I had to take it for her [the host] when she was little—now I want her to feel what it was like."

The dynamics of re-enactment are complex, but probably include several driving forces. The traditional view is that re-enactment is an attempt at achieving a belated mastery of the trauma and overcoming the feelings of helplessness the patient originally felt (Fenichel, 1945). I believe, however, that a second dynamic is more important in MPD patients; this is the attempt to transfer remembered pain across the amnesic boundaries of the alter personalities. Part of the therapeutic effect of abreaction is the wider sharing of past traumatic experiences that were previously sequestered within a single or small group of alters.

This process of larger group sharing of painful memories acts to dilute the intensity of the remembered experience and aids in its ultimate metabolism. Many of the acts of internal persecution that appear to be senselessly brutal to an outside observer may actually be misguided attempts to share, and therefore to dilute, unprocessed pain.

Guilt and Shame

Guilt and shame are responses to trauma that multiples share with victims of natural disasters and with victims of physical and sexual abuse who do not have MPD. A number of sources usually contribute to this sense of guilt. Most multiples have low self-esteem, also seen in non-MPD victims of child abuse (Putnam, 1988a), and feel that they have no right to be alive. In some cases, the patient has witnessed the death of pets or siblings; this may lead to a sense of "survivor" guilt, in which they question why they survived while others died. Some alters may feel that they deserved what was done to them because they are bad and ugly. Other alters may believe that they were responsible for provoking or eliciting the abuse, just as non-MPD abused children may assume an unrealistic sense of responsibility for the behavior of their parents.

There may well be reality-based guilt feelings. Many multiples have done things to themselves or other people of which they are ashamed. The therapist must determine which feelings are reality-based and which are "neurotic," and work with them accordingly. This can be a difficult distinction to make, because many of the current behaviors, such as promiscuity, for which there may be a sense of guilt or shame have their roots in prior trauma and unrealistic assumptions of responsibility.

Competition for the Body

Early in the therapy, competition for time in the body will be a hot issue among the alters. The problem of who is in the body is a perennial issue with multiples, but it may be that competition for time in the body increases as a patient begins to accept his or her multiplicity. Prior to diagnosis, at least some of the alters now clamoring for equal time will have actively tried to avoid being "out" or recognized. The process of chaining through the system may also stir things up and activate alters who previously emerged infrequently.

Manifestations of this competition include direct demands by alters for time; threats by alters that they will seize the body and do something destructive or self-destructive; and actual escapades by alters that are experienced as fugue episodes by the host. Some alters will be demanding more time in therapy, and some will be demanding more time "out" outside of therapy. I think that the responsibility of the therapist is to address issues of appropriate and inappropriate behavior, communication and cooperation, and social responsibility, rather than becoming involved in determining exactly which personality has how much time when to do what. The personality system should determine and enforce the allocation of time "out."

Body Image Issues

Multiples frequently experience dramatic distortions of their body image. Many child personalities will experience themselves as small and weak; consequently, they may not attempt tasks that are well within the physical capabilities of the body. Some alters will experience themselves as attractive or physically powerful, whereas others will perceive themselves as hideously ugly or contaminated by the abuse and even contagious toward others. Cross-gender alters may see the body as having a different gender. In cases where a cross-gender alter perceives the body's actual sex, there may be attempts to change it. These may run from crude mutilation of the genitals or breasts to seeking sex-change operations. One female multiple complained to me about the fact that she was getting arm muscles "like a man." The culprit turned out to be "Billy," a 17-year-old male alter who liked to lift weights. He kept telling me, "I got to get this body back in shape, man!"

Not surprisingly, the lack of a unified sense of the physical body can lead to a cavalier attitude on the part of some alters toward the safety and well-being of their mortal flesh. The therapist should not overlook opportunities to help develop and reinforce among the alter personalities an awareness of the vulnerability and ultimate common mortality that they all share. When the personality system comes to realize that if one dies, they all die, there is usually a significant improvement in internal cooperation.

The Wish to Meet Another Multiple

A multiple often demonstrates an approach–avoidance conflict when faced with the possibility of meeting another multiple. On one side is the wish to meet a fellow traveler, to prove that one is not alone, and to discover that other people exist who are more of an "us" than an "I." The flip side of this ambivalence is that meeting another multiple would confirm the reality of MPD.

When multiples do get together, they interact as well as anyone else. Despite the incredible number of possible personality interactions between two multiples, the dynamics of their systems usually serve to bring out the most appropriate pairs of alters. Administrators will deal with their counterparts, and child alters will play together. There is often an intense initial bonding that later gives way to a more realistic relationship as the two multiples come to know each other better. One of the more difficult aspects of these relationships occurs when one multiple attempts to relate to another multiple as he or she might relate to someone without MPD. This may include covert switching or other deceptions that multiples use to conceal their multiplicity. Such behavior can produce a strong negative reaction from another multiple, who is more perceptive on this score and recognizes that the first multiple is not being "honest" with him or her.

Distribution of Energy in the Personality System

Working with multiples may make a therapist believe that these patients have higher levels of energy than the average person. Many report that they only sleep a few hours each night, and when one alter becomes tired another comes "out" and takes off at full tilt. The energy within the personality system is, however, finite. At times therapists will see some previously robust alters appear to weaken and fade away; they may report that they are "dying." Novice therapists are often panicked by this apparent crisis and attempt to save the dying alters. In most cases, these dying alters will reappear after a period of dormancy. Personalities rarely, if ever, permanently disappear unless they become integrated into a larger whole. Alters may, however, become inactive for periods of time. Most multiples will have layers of inactive alters who represent past functions that are not currently needed by the system.

The process of redistribution of energy and activity within the personality system represents one of the mechanisms by which this psychological structure evolves to meet changing needs. A therapist's allegiance must be to the personality system as a whole and not to specific alters. The redistribution of energy among alters represents ongoing change within the personality system and usually is something to be welcomed rather than feared. The therapist should not become involved in struggles to preserve and protect specific alters who are fading away, but instead should talk about this process as a personality system decision in which the alters as a group share control.

Ambivalence

Ambivalence is a property of the larger personality system. Individual alters rarely show any degree of ambivalence. In fact, individual alters typically demonstrate a single-minded sense of purpose or mission that is unmatched by most non-MPD individuals. The suicidal alter is committed to suicide; the depressed alter is incurably depressed; and the internal persecutor is unremittingly hostile toward the host. This will remain the case until some degree of communication and cooperation has begun to produce a larger sense of system as "self." When one sees ambivalence manifest in an MPD patient, it is usually in the form of doing and undoing, as one alter performs an action and another undoes it. It is important not to mistake such behavior for the actions of a single "ambivalent" alter. A therapist must identify and work with all of the alters who are responsible for this vacillating behavior.

Insight

Experience with MPD patients suggests that there is a great deal of truth to the old therapeutic saw about the difference between intellectual and emotional insight. Many multiples will have alters, particularly internal self-helpers (ISHs), who can explain the patients' psychological dynamics with penetrating intellectual insight. Yet the patients as a whole are rarely able to make use of this understanding. It is noteworthy that the alters containing these insights are generally characterized by a neutral or flattened affect and may relate both past traumatic memories and frightening future possibilities in a mechanical, affectless manner. Effective insight comes only much later, when most of the dissociated affect has been brought into a larger, shared, conscious awareness.

TRANSFERENCE ISSUES

Transference in Multiples

Although the treatment of this patient was along psychoanalytically oriented lines, I found some formidable obstacles for the patient in this type of therapy. Most significant, I believe, is the fact that it simply is not possible to know what is going on in the transference at any given moment as accurately as one would like because (a) the transference changes, sometimes quite abruptly, often slowly and subtly, and (b) it is not just one transference that confronts the therapist but a whole group of them, one for each personality or ego state. (Jeans, 1976b, p. 250)

Within a short period of time, it will become evident to most therapists working with their first multiples that these patients are capable of generating highly complex transference and countertransference responses (Wilbur, 1984b). "Transference" may be defined as "responses to a therapist that are primarily based on, and displaced from, significant childhood figures, especially parents and siblings" (Langs, 1974b, p. 151). Transference reactions are often overdetermined, condensed, archaic, infantile, and primary-process responses. Transference involves a displacement, usually from an important person ("object") in the patient's past, onto the therapist. This displacement may involve a single traumatic incident or repeated traumatic episodes. One should not forget, however, that every patient's reactions to a therapist exist somewhere on a continuum ranging from appropriate responses to reality-based stimuli to grossly inappropriate or psychotic responses that are not reality-bound.

Most classical discussions of transference are defined in terms of a patient–therapist dyad. The alter personalities of a multiple, however, may have semi-independent transference reactions to a therapist, leading to an additional level of complexity. Classical dyadic transference reactions can be conceptualized as layered, in that any given response may draw upon several earlier experiences with a number of important persons from several different periods of the patient's life. There may also be a number of different transference fantasy systems within a unified personality patient that form a hierarchy, with some reactions serving to mask or repress other reactions (Langs, 1974b).

In a multiple, the transference reactions of any given alter will usually be based on discrete events from a specific period in the patient's life and will not reflect the type of layering seen in patients who do not have MPD. The layering seen in an MPD patient occurs because many of the alters will have different, semiautonomous reactions to the same stimulus. For example, if a therapist physically touches a multiple, some alters may have a transference experience of the therapist as an important childhood figure who was nurturing and comforting. Simultaneously, other alters may experience the therapist as an abuser or rapist and the touch as extremely aversive. These conflicting transference reactions may be expressed simultaneously, sequentially, or in some combination thereof.

Working with Transference in Multiples

When working with multiples, in most instances the therapist will be faced with discrete transference reactions rather than with an organized transference neurosis such as occurs in classical psychoanalysis. In the case of a formal transference neurosis, defined as "an emotional illness that evolves from, and is an elaboration of, transference responses and fantasies" (Langs, 1974b, p. 195), the goal of the treatment is a resolution of this neurosis; this is conceived of as a recapitulation of past experiences currently experienced in the present with the therapist. Transference reactions, however, are not as well organized and usually need to be worked with in a more piecemeal fashion. In many instances, the transference aspects of the material should be ignored altogether, and the therapeutic focus should be on the reality content of the material and its impact on the patient. Generally, in the treatment of MPD, the therapist should not search out, emphasize, or refer to passing transference phenomena unless they represent major obstacles to therapeutic progress.

The principles enumerated by Langs (1974b) for working with transference reactions in psychotherapy are generally applicable to the treatment of multiples. These include (1) tracing out the transference reaction's intrapsychic roots and determining the person or persons to whom the patient related in the past and on whom the patient's behavior toward the therapist is based; and (2) identifying the period from the patient's life during which the past experiences generating the transference reaction occurred. This second point is important in establishing the level of functioning present at that time, which may be embodied in an alter personality's reactions. The material transferred usually will contain a mixture of memories, fantasies, and past perceptions (both realistic and unrealistic).

Precipitants of Transference Reactions

Transference reactions in multiples may be precipitated by a variety of stimuli. Reality-based experiences, both in and out of therapy, constitute a major source of precipitants. The highly sensitized, extraordinarily vigilant perceptual system of a multiple will pick up and react and/or abreact to many apparently innocuous experiences. In many instances, the host may initially embody the transference reaction and yet may have absolutely no idea as to the stimulus or the source of the experience.

Many transference reactions are therapist-evoked. Sources of these reactions include the following:

1. Aspects of or items in the therapeutic setting. For example, one patient had a major abreactive episode in which I was perceived as her incestuous father, when I wore a blazer similar to one her father owned.
2. The therapist's theoretical or therapeutic stance.
3. Therapeutic interventions, if they are sufficiently reminiscent of disciplinary or other experiences from childhood.
4. The inevitable nonintervention aspects of therapy, such as billing, canceled sessions, vacations or other separations, or unexpected interruptions during sessions.
5. Misdirected or poorly executed therapeutic interventions. MPD patients are extraordinarily sensitive to a therapist's errors.

In multiples, a major source of transference reactions is simply the uncovering and eliciting during the course of therapy of alter personalities who embody past trauma. The therapist's gender or mere presence is often all that is required for his or her inclusion into a highly emotional transference reaction. In these cases, there is often such a profound perceptual distortion that the patient will hallucinate the therapist as the transference object. This can be dangerous for the therapist.

Forms of Transference Reactions

The precipitant of a transference reaction will inevitably influence its form. The primary determinant of form, however, is the makeup of the multiple's personality sytem. The nature of the alter personalities present, and their hierarchical access to overt or covert control over the patient's behavior, will largely determine the form that a transference reaction takes. Wilbur (1984b) states, "[I]t must be understood that the transference feelings which are experienced by each alter depend on that alter's role in the complex of personalities in relation to the conflicts and affects with which that alter is concerned, and the defenses it has evoked" (p. 31).

If, for example, a multiple's system is composed largely of highly traumatized and fearful infantile and child alters, transference reactions in which the therapist is perceived as the past sexual abuser may be manifested by regressed behavior, such as whimpering or hiding under furniture. On the other hand, if the system contains adolescent alters who handled sexual abuse, there may be manipulative or seductive responses to a therapist perceived as the sexual abuser. In many multiples, a range of alters, representing responses from different periods within the patient's life, will participate in a transference reaction. This often produces complex, shifting behaviors that confuse a therapist.

Transference reactions can be directly focused on the therapist within the therapy setting. As such, these reactions are often distorted and dominated by primary process. Transference reactions may also be manifested by acting out beyond the treatment setting; such reactions will result in direct or indirect sabotage of the treatment. They may take the form of the patient's acting out promiscuously or violently outside of treatment, or, more insidiously, seeking to bring other parties (often well-meaning therapists) into the treatment process. An all-too-common scenario involves an alter's showing up in an emergency room with an overdose or other self-destructive act because of something that occurred in a recent therapy session. The alter may then seek to involve other parties in the treatment by relating incomplete, distorted, or confabulated information about the therapist. Unfortunately, many professionals do not attempt to uncover the whole story before trying to "rescue" the patient from the evil therapist. A little skepticism and a little charity are in order when one hears a multiple relate the injustices that he or she has suffered at the hands of a therapist. With a multiple, there are usually more than two sides to a story.

COUNTERTRANSFERENCE ISSUES

MPD patients often evoke unique and complex countertransference reactions from therapists (Davis & Osherson, 1977; Kluft, 1984d; Saltman & Solomon, 1982). "Countertransference" in this context is defined as those responses on the part of the therapist toward the patient that, although evoked by some event within the therapy, are primarily directed at gratifying the therapist's needs rather than advancing the patient's treatment. In this section, I describe a number of situations and responses that I have repeatedly encountered in treatment and supervision of the treatment of MPD. This list is by no means complete, but does cover some of the more common countertransference reactions that thwart progress in treatment.

Many of the alters of a multiple patient are likely to engender distinct and separate countertransference responses within the therapist. Thus a therapist working with a multiple may simultaneously be aware of hostility toward one alter, sexual feelings toward another, and a wish to hold and nurture a third alter. A therapist may feel pulled one way and then another throughout a session with a multiple, struggling to identify what is going on in the patient as well as within himself or herself. The disorder itself also evokes a variety of responses within a therapist, ranging from fascination to fear.

Who Is the Patient?

I have seen a number of therapists struggling implicitly or explicitly with the question "Who is the patient?" while working with their first MPD cases. In such an instance, the "patient" in the therapist's mind is originally the host personality, who presents for treatment. Following the diagnosis of MPD and the overt emergence of other alters, the therapist becomes confused as to who really is "the patient." This confusion occurs in situations where the host is complaining of significant distress caused by other personalities. The therapist may experience a strong sense of loyalty to the host as the patient and feel that the other alters have less claim on him or her as a therapist. This sense of confusion is further heightened in cases where the host personality is actually a facade created by the covert cooperation of several alters colluding to pass as a unified host. With the diagnosis of MPD and permission to be openly multiple, such a facade host often dissolves before a therapist's eyes, leaving the therapist wondering what has happened to the person he or she knows as "the patient."

A therapist facing the apparent loss of "the patient" and the replacement of this patient with a collection of different entities, some of whom express hostility toward the therapist, often feels deceived, betrayed, and abandoned. The very nature of the therapeutic contract appears to have been violated. Sometimes a therapist's impulse is to try to resurrect the host, which usually leads to an impasse with the patient as a whole. The therapist must come to recognize that the patient really is a multiple and that the therapeutic work involves the whole personality system. Initially, this may produce feelings of loss or failure in a therapist who sees "the patient" disappear to be replaced by an alien entity. The overt emergence of alters, however, should be understood as an expression of trust and not misunderstood as deception.

Keeping the Patient Straight

Keeping two essentially different histories, sets of feelings and perceptions clear and apart while doing therapy was another difficulty. Both personalities had very definite and opposite reactions to people and situations. Obvious differences between them, such as their sexual preferences, were easy to remember correctly, but there were more subtle areas, such as their reactions to family members, which were dynamically important but more difficult to recall. (Davis & Osherson, 1977, p. 512)

Many therapists feel overwhelmed by the sheer volume of information that they must continually track and process while engaging in therapy with MPD patients. Some alter personalities compound this difficulty by being insulted and angered when a therapist incorrectly attributes some fact or feeling to them that actually belongs to another alter. Repeated experiences of anger and contempt from alters toward the therapist for his or her failures to keep information straight will eventually take their toll in the form of countertransference feelings of anger and resentment toward the patient.

There is no simple way to eliminate this problem. In general, a therapist can deal with it by keeping a card file or other record of the alters and their attributes and by updating this information as part of the process record or progress notes. Still, the therapist will make mistakes or forget who said what, where, and when. Multiples seem to have an uncanny ability to remember this sort of information. Many MPD patients have explained their obsession with tracking the minute details of patient–therapist interactions as part of their compensation for time loss and amnesia. When the therapist makes a mistake and receives a harsh correction, it is better to admit fallibility and ask for clarification than to get into a dispute over the details.

Being "Real" with the Patient

"I find myself having to be much more 'real' with her than I am with my other patients," a dyed-in-the-wool psychoanalyst commented to me after working with his first multiple for several weeks. Multiples push against every traditional therapy boundary and can cause discomfort in therapists wedded to a particular theoretical orientation or therapeutic stance. Such therapists often find themselves caught between their pragmatic observations of what works with an MPD patient and the dictates of their professional training.

Most multiples cannot tolerate the traditional unresponsive, "neutral" therapeutic stance advocated by psychoanalytic theory. They will force the therapist to relate to them in other ways, or there will be a rupture of the therapeutic alliance. This pressure on the therapist to abandon his or her usual manner of relating to a patient can produce feelings of being manipulated and having one's therapeutic authority undermined by the patient. Every therapist must come to some equilibrium between the reality-based need of the multiple to be responded to in an active, direct, and real manner and the therapist's need to maintain a therapeutic stance toward the patient in which he or she is both comfortable and effective. One must be flexible in order to be effective with multiples, and yet one must be rigid with regard to certain treatment boundaries or the therapy degenerates into chaos. Such paradoxes permeate the treatment of MPD.

Ceaseless Change in the Patient

"Is it possible that this is never going to end? That new personalities are just going to keep on coming? That it's a bottomless pit?" These questions were addressed to me by a clergyman working with an MPD patient in pastoral counseling. He was working with a difficult and highly fragmented MPD patient, who nonetheless was functioning and showing demonstrable improvement. He was, however, worn out and overwhelmed by the hordes of "new" personalities and fragments that continued to emerge and create new crises. Therapists working with complex MPD patients often despair that there will ever be an end, fearing that the personalities will continue to multiply in a Malthusian fashion and outstrip their ability to meet and work through the issues that each personality contains.

A related feeling experienced by therapists working with MPD patients is a sense of frustration because a patient's personality system never holds still long enough for a therapist to become comfortable with a set of active personalities. Alters will come and go, and the relationships among them and the energy and abilities that they embody will continually change, so that the therapist cannot always be sure from session to session who the principals are.

It is normal for therapists to wish that the patients would stop ceaselessly changing, but transformation is a cardinal feature of a dissociative disorder. It is important to keep in mind that change is often desirable and part of the therapeutic process. The appearance of new alters and the shifting balance among the alters represent new accommodations within the personality system, probably in response to the therapy. Alters can be created by the therapy, but most of these entities will be special purpose fragments with a finite role and life span. In pathological therapies, more permanent alters may be created by an abusive therapist–patient relationship, but this is the exception. The mercurial quality of the patient can be lessened by focusing on the personality system as a whole rather than on specific alters.

Difficulties in Hearing Details of Past Trauma

Working with an MPD patient will ultimately bring the therapist into contact with graphic details of past traumatic experiences. Since a multiple may undergo the transformation from victim to victimizer, there may be material related to the patient's infliction of violence upon others. The details of these events may activate within the therapist countertransference feelings of anxiety, rage, revulsion, and an existential fear of death. There may be accompanying strong feelings of concern, sympathy, and a sense of helplessness. Empathic reactions elicited in the therapist by the details of childhood physical and sexual abuse can be powerful. The therapist may find that the explicit details of the abuse activate sadistic, punitive, or voyeuristic impulses within him or her that may be disturbing to acknowledge.

A second, related countertransference phenomenon involves the effect of the recall of traumatic material upon a patient, much of which takes the form of painful abreaction or revivification. The disorganizing effects of an abreaction can be profound and may reverberate for days. Many patients will blame the therapist or accuse him or her of compounding their suffering when therapeutic exploration triggers an abreaction. Patients often overtly or covertly accuse the therapist of making them "worse, not better" following such an experience.

Consequently, therapists are often doubly sensitized to traumatic material and may be reluctant to follow up hints or clues left by patients about the existence of undisclosed trauma. A core therapeutic task is the recovery of dissociated traumatic material and the integration of this material into a patient's larger memory and sense of identity. A therapist must be aware of his or her countertransference feelings about listening to such material. Kluft (1984d) notes that empathizing with an MPD patient's experience of traumatization can be a grueling experience for the therapist: "One is tempted to withdraw, intellectualize, or defensively ruminate about whether the events are 'real'" (p. 53). A patient will know if the therapist is unable to tolerate hearing what has happened to him or her, and therapeutic progress will come to a standstill. In such cases, it is better to acknowledge the problem and, if necessary, transfer the patient to a therapist who can face the trauma with the patient.

Seduction

Seduction is a real possibility with MPD patients. There are no hard data, but I have heard a sufficient number of anecdotes from both multiples and therapists to believe that MPD patients become sexually involved with their therapists much more frequently than do other patients. Sexuality in MPD patients is usually compartmentalized within a few alters. A female patient not uncommonly has one or more alters who have been involved in prostitution. The host personality is usually asexual or obviously frightened by sexuality. Child personalities are usually asexual, but may ask to be held or hugged or to receive other forms of affection from the therapist. Sexualized adolescent or adult alters can come "out" during these displays of affection without the therapist's being immediately aware of the switch or its consequences.

Seductive behavior by sexual alters is both a form of testing the therapist to see whether he or she will behave like past abusers and an attempt to gain control over the therapist (Saltman & Solomon, 1982). Seduction was often the only control that the patient had over his or her abuser in the past. More than one patient has told me of learning to seduce an abuser because it gave the patient control over the timing and circumstances of the inevitable sexual abuse. In some cases, the seductive behavior was also a protective attempt to draw the abuser's attention away from younger siblings and represented a significant self-sacrifice on the part of the patient.

At some point in the treatment course, most multiples will have an alter who will try to seduce the therapist; in fact, the therapist can virtually count on this. I think that therapists who get into trouble at this point do so because they have already violated many other treatment boundaries and believe that the rules do not apply to them. This is particularly true for therapists working with their first multiples.

A related issue is the "sexual abuse" of the therapist by some MPD patients. I have had the experience of being sexually harassed by specific alters of a few MPD patients. This harassment has on occasion involved attempts at grabbing or fondling me. More commonly, an alter may start to strip in the office or leave sexually explicit suggestions or comments on the telephone answering machine. This behavior, which I view as a form of aggression directed at the therapist, needs to be quickly brought under control by contracts with the personality system and, if possible, with the specific alter personality involved. If this is not possible, the therapist should terminate the treatment. I consider such behavior equivalent to violence or the threat of violence toward the therapist, and as such it cannot be tolerated. I handle overtly sexualized behavior in much the same fashion as I handle potentially violent behavior, including seeing the patient with other staff members present.

Reparenting

Multiples evoke the desire and fantasy of reparenting in many therapists. The child alters especially seem to beg for good parents to hold and nurture them. Their painful history and current torment may elicit strong parental feelings. Some reparenting is inevitable with most patients, whether or not they are multiples, and is part of the transference dynamics. As with so many other issues, however, multiples will push this process to an extreme. In some cases, therapists have taken multiples into their homes and tried to raise them anew. This does not work and will ultimately cause serious problems.

Instead, I believe that the reparenting process must occur from within the multiple. The adult personalities must come to first acknowledge and then ultimately protect, care for, and raise the child alters. In my experience, this works well. The adult alters learn to let the child alters "out" at appropriate times in appropriate contexts and to provide the child alters with nurturant experiences. They also learn to help the child alters share the dissociated traumatic experiences that so many of them hold. It is useful to have one or more adult alters "hold" a child alter while the child recounts or abreacts a traumatic memory. With appropriate internal reparenting, the patient can correct many of the harmful developmental experiences, at the same time gaining a greater respect for the personality system and the role it has played in his or her physical and emotional survival.

The Fantasy of Being the Greatest MPD Therapist in the World

Multiples have a way of pumping up one's vanity—and then pricking it with a pin. Their past experiences have left them suspicious and cynical about human nature. A therapist should remember that when he or she begins hearing (explicitly or implicitly) from an MPD patient, "You are the most special therapist who ever treated MPD." Part of the patient wants to believe that this is true, and so does part of the therapist. Another part of the patient wants to set the therapist up for failure, and thus to demonstrate once again that all important figures in the patient's life are really frauds and are not to be trusted. I think that the experience of being told by MPD patients just how special and great they are is behind much of the instant "expertise" acquired by new MPD therapists. Such therapeutic grandiosity will be laid low in the not-too-distant future. Therapists' tendencies toward feelings of omnipotence and grandiosity are actively fostered by MPD patients as part of testing and set-ups. A therapist should thus be careful and humble.

Being "Bad-Mouthed" by an MPD Patient

The other side of the coin is being publicly degraded by a patient. Usually this is not done to the therapist's face, but occurs in ways that get back indirectly. Multiples talk and compare therapists constantly. They will drag other therapists or interested parties into their treatments whenever possible. I have heard multiples say terrible things about therapists I believe to be impeccable in their conduct, and I have heard some of the terrible things that they say about me. It hurts and it makes one angry, particularly when a therapist believes that he or she has worked hard to help the patient. Since many of the things said are reported out of context and often have a significant degree of distortion, a defamed therapist may feel deceived, betrayed, and abused by the patient.

I believe that one should understand this demeaning of the therapist as one of the inevitable dynamics of multiplicity. Whenever there are strong positive feelings on the part of one or more personalities, there will be a counterweight of negative feeling. Most multiples want to believe that their therapists are good, caring, all-knowing, and all-powerful. They also believe that all important figures are bad, unreliable, and abusive. They are afraid to become too close or too dependent, and yet within a short time most multiples become highly dependent on their therapists. The "bad-mouthing" that goes on over the course of therapy is an expression of the polarization of feeling that multiples experience in regard to important transference objects. If it becomes a problem between therapist and patient and serves as a resistance to progress, it should be interpreted as part of the transference. In the meantime, a therapist should be charitable toward fellow therapists and take what is said about them with a grain or two of salt, because it is likely that somewhere out there similar things are being said about himself or herself.

Concern about Colleagues' Reactions

While serving as a *de facto* national resource center for therapists treating MPD over the past 8 years, I have observed that many clinicians treating these patients have kept their work secret from colleagues out of concern that they would be ridiculed or discredited. The inclusion of MPD in the DSM-III and DSM-III-R, and the increasing body of clinical literature, have allayed these fears to some extent. Yet many therapists remain reluctant to admit to working with MPD patients. This is particularly true for psychologists, psychiatric nurses, and social workers who depend on medical backup from psychiatrists.

It is difficult to convince another professional who has never "seen" an MPD patient of the existence of the disorder. Even eminent therapists such as Cornelia Wilbur have been publicly accused by ignorant professionals of perpetuating a *folie à deux* with their patients (e.g., see Victor, 1975). I have learned to stop arguing with those who, either out of ignorance or malice, attempt to deny the existence of MPD. At the present time, it is sufficient to point them gently toward the DSM-III-R and a list of references (Boor & Coons, 1983; Damgaard *et al.*, 1985) and let the sheer volume of evidence argue on its own behalf. Gratifyingly, in a number of instances, these skeptics have discovered MPD in their own patients. I find that nothing makes a skeptic a more dedicated believer in the existence of MPD than making the diagnosis for himself or herself.

SUMMARY

This chapter has been devoted to a discussion of the themes and issues that commonly arise during the course of psychotherapy with MPD patients. It begins by exploring the problems of boundary management, stressing the cardinal principle that although MPD patients often demand (and may require) special arrangements, the therapist must remain clear about boundaries and availability, or the treatment will quickly degenerate into chaos.

Control is a central issue in the lives of these people and will surface in a variety of forms during treatment. Struggles for control and fears about loss of control act as resistances to uncovering work. In emergencies, the therapist may need to assume temporary control through hospitalization or other measures. In most instances, however, it is best to concede all control to the personality system as a whole and focus on the work of therapy.

Secrets and their powerful dynamics permeate the psychotherapy of MPD. A variety of psychological mechanisms perpetuate the primitive power of these secrets. The patient will be torn between revealing and concealing this material. It is the task of the therapist to create a therapeutic climate in which the traumas can be disclosed, processed, and accepted. Secrets should be helped to emerge instead of being extracted.

A major dynamic is testing the trustworthiness of the therapist. The patient may attempt to seduce the therapist or to maneuver the therapist into recapitulating past abuse experiences. One should expect repeated testing, and one should beware especially of force choices or bids to back one side of the personality system against the other.

Multiples generate complicated transferences and countertransferences. Although these patients do not usually develop a formal transference neurosis, they typically exhibit a range of transference reactions and responses. The therapist as abuser is a common manifestation. Often there are multiple, simultaneous, conflicting transference reactions experienced by different alters, adding to the confusion of therapy.

Therapists will also have multiple countertransference reactions to the range of alters that compose the patient. Confusion as to who constitutes the patient, resentment over ceaseless change, difficulties in hearing about past traumas, and strong parental feelings are often described by therapists. Yet most therapists I know report learning a great deal about the art of psychotherapy from working with MPD patients.

CHAPTER EIGHT

Psychotherapeutic Techniques

This chapter details specific techniques and approaches that have been found to be useful in working with MPD patients. Some of these techniques are directed toward the personality system as a whole, and others are focused on specific types of alter personalities commonly encountered in MPD patients. Much of what constitutes psychotherapeutic technique is ineffable, however. What may work well for one therapist–patient dyad may fail miserably in another.

TALKING THROUGH

"Talking through," or talking to the personality system as a whole, is an effective and useful technique in working with an MPD patient (Braun, 1984c; Kluft, 1982). It is useful in making contracts, in establishing general principles or boundaries, in informing the patient about events affecting the therapy (e.g., vacations), and in working with the patient in times of crisis. Although one should always assume that all of the personalities are listening all of the time during therapy, this is often not true. This assumption is useful because it forces the therapist never to make interventions or remarks that he or she would not wish all of the personalities to be aware of. Talking through is a technique to ensure that as many alters as possible actually are listening.

When talking through, I usually begin by saying something like this: "I want everyone in there to give me their full and undivided attention. I want everybody to be listening." I will usually repeat this several times. There is no way to know whether all of the alters are listening, but usually enough are tuned in that the effect is achieved. I may also specify that if any alters are unable to listen, then someone else in the system must take responsibility for informing them of what they may need to know. After getting the personality system's attention, I tell the patient whatever it is that I wish to communicate. I usually repeat the message several times at different levels of abstraction. I may also ask some of the adult alters to help the child alters understand whatever it is that they need to know. I then invite all of the alters who have questions or comments to come "out" and speak with me directly. It is usually clear pretty quickly whether I have gotten my message across.

The advantages to talking to the personality system as a whole are for the most part obvious. It saves time and energy. It addresses the patient as a whole. It fosters internal cooperation and coconsciousness, and it reaches alters that the therapist may not even suspect exist. The major problem that I have had is when the personality who is "out" during the talking-through process is an amnesic host personality who may not accept the diagnosis of MPD. Talking through an unaware host to the rest of the personality system may produce strong feelings of depersonalization or passive-influence phenomena (Kluft, 1982). On a number of occasions, an amnesic host has become upset and told me to stop it because I was causing discomfort. I respond by asking the host to relax and listen quietly. Often the host will go into a trance-like state during the process of talking through and will be amnesic for much of the content. It is usually worthwhile to make sure that the host has also heard the message directed to the larger system.

An example of how I use talking through involved a newly diagnosed MPD patient whose personality system I did not know well at all. The host kept finding herself in the parking lot of her old employer, miles away from where she was supposed to be at that hour. Her current employer had threatened to fire her if she continued to be late for work. I was unable to elicit an alter who took responsibility for these actions. I then talked through the amnesic host to the personality system as a whole, explaining that I did not know many of them yet, but that collectively I would require them all to make sure that they made it to work each day on time. I explained that it was necessary to keep a job if they as a group were going to be able to remain financially independent and continue in treatment. The minifugues ceased. At a later point, I met the alter who was responsible for these episodes; "he" had been dealing drugs in the parking lot.

ASSEMBLING WHOLE MEMORIES
FROM FRAGMENTS

Even in non-MPD patients, traumatic experiences often produce fragmentary recall of an event. In a multiple, the memory of a traumatic experience may be contained within a single alter, or it may be spread across several alters. When a memory is divided among several alters, each alter may contain a fragment of the event, or one alter may contain the memory for the details of the event while others hold the affects generated by the event. It is the therapist's job to help the patient reassemble the whole memory, both content and affects, and to integrate this structure into the person as a whole.

This is slow, methodical work. In the beginning, little is going to make sense. The therapist will meet some alters who exhibit powerful affects for which there is little content; other alters have bits and pieces of vivid memory detail, but are unable to place this content into a larger context. This is a large, multidimensional puzzle that the therapist and patient have to assemble one piece at a time. The patient will continually provide clues, but he or she does not know the answer either, and powerful psychic processes are at work that attempt to suppress, distort, or otherwise impair recall of traumas. Time, patience, trust, and working through alter by alter, level by level, will slowly assemble a coherent and chronological picture of the trauma that precipitated and perpetuated the patient's fragmentation into a multiple personality.

The puzzle metaphor is a useful one to keep in mind. With a puzzle, one usually begins by assembling pieces with a common background into small units, fitting the units roughly together, and then filling in the gaps that separate these units from each other. A similar process often occurs in assembling the life history of an MPD patient. Affects are often a useful place to start. Braun (1984c) has described his work with a modified form of the "affect bridge" technique originated by Watkins (1971). This involves identifying a strong, but often contentless, affect and tracing it through alter personalities. Braun's modification involves allowing the affect to change (e.g., from anger to fear) and to trace this new affect to its roots. The use of affect bridge techniques is discussed in greater detail in Chapter Nine.

Memories may also be traced in a similar fashion. Braun (1984c) suggests starting with the last piece of memory and working backwards in time, eliciting alters who have the next piece in a sequential fashion. Often one traces memory and affect in a parallel fashion, slowly assembling a coherent whole from the bits and pieces of abreactive fragments. In one patient, for example, the work began with a feeling of overwhelming sick dread that was evoked by the sound of a train. The patient was unable to associate any memories to this stimulus, but the sounds of a passing locomotive or train whistle would result in rapid switching of alters who exhibited affects of fear, horror, grief, and anger, respectively. The angry alter threatened to kill the patient's father because he was a bastard, but provided no other details. The grief-stricken alter mourned the death of a dog who was her only companion on an isolated Midwestern farm. The horrified alter reported watching her father tie her dog to the railroad tracks that passed behind the family farm, and the fearful alter was still bound by the threat that this would happen to her someday. The memory that emerged was of her father taking her pet, tying it to the railroad tracks, and making her watch the yelping dog ground to pieces by a freight train. He threatened that the same would happen to her if she ever revealed his incestuous activities to anyone.

The memories (often recalled as intensely vivid images), together with the affects generated by this experience, were divided among several alters. There were several additional alters connected with this episode who were not discussed above, but all were connected to memories or affects associated with this event. Once the general outline of the event was determined, it was possible to deduce some of the missing pieces and search for alters who contained these elements. Unfortunately, this was just one of many traumatic experiences endured by this woman.

CROSS-INVENTORYING

"Cross-inventorying" is a technique developed by David Caul (1983) that I have found to be of great use in the treatment of MPD. Like many such techniques, its effect is probably dependent to a large extent on the way in which it is implemented. The basic process is simply to have each alter personality state in detail his or her opinions about the strengths and weaknesses of the other alters. The therapist listens carefully, sorting out the negative and positive aspects, and comments on instances of complementarity between pairs or across groups of alters. The comments need to be subtle and directed to both the alter who is "out" and the personality system in general. The therapist should not favor the presence or absence of one trait or ability over another, but rather should convey the sense that the combination of traits (e.g., anger in one alter and passivitiy in another) provides the personality system with a wider range of responses to the world. Caul (1985b) stresses that the therapist should constantly focus on the positive aspects of the personalities and attempt to identify the negative influences within the personalities without making them feel guilty or ashamed.

The point of cross-inventorying is to help the alters recognize that (1) even though they may hold antithetical values and ways of responding to events, the responses of other alters to the same stimuli may be appropriate in some circumstances; (2) the personality system as a whole gains from having the flexibility inherent in a wider range of complementary strengths; and (3) the weaknesses of one alter are compensated for by the strengths of another. It is a way of showing the alters that they do, in fact, fit together to make a larger whole that is more powerful and effective than any one of them is individually. The technique is most effective when used in a background manner (i.e., continuously and subtly), so that over time the personality system repeatedly receives input about the nature of the larger whole. After a while, the alters will begin telling the therapist about how they compensate for one another's strengths and weaknesses.

DREAM WORK WITH MULTIPLES

Although nightmares, night terrors, hypnagogic and hypnopompic phenomena, and other evidence of traumatic sleep disturbances are common in multiples and other victims of trauma, little has been written about the role of dreams in the dissociative disorders. Marmer's (1980a) chapter on the dream in dissociative states is the principal reference to date. Dreams can play an important role in uncovering buried trauma and identifying secretive alters (Jeans, 1976a; Marmer, 1980b; Salley, 1988). Not infrequently, an MPD patient will bring to therapy dream material containing information about past trauma that is unavailable in the waking state. Ferenczi (1934) and Levitan (1980) have observed a similar phenomenon in the traumatic neuroses.

Marmer (1980a) describes analyzing dream material as expressions of split ego functions. He states,

> By focusing interpretations in the way in which I did, the personalities saw that they all had to deal with the same material, that they had all experienced the same traumatic events, that they each had their unique defensive styles, and that these became recognized as reactive instead of being regarded as primarily destructive as had previously been the case. (p. 174)

He believes that a great deal of the work of building a common ground among the alters can be done by using dream material to demonstrate to the personality system that dissociated and disowned experiences are expressed in dreams that are the alters' own creations. Marmer (1980a), as well as many other therapists working with MPD patients, suggests that individual alter personalities may shape or create dreams separately from other alters.

My experience with dream material from MPD patients suggests that it can provide access to deeply hidden trauma that is difficult to elicit even with hypnotic techniques such as age regression or the affect bridge. Dreams containing traumatic material are usually repetitive and leave the patient with sustained strong affects or profound feelings of depersonalization upon awakening. The patient may be afraid to go to sleep for fear that the dream will recur. In some cases, patients will request sleeping medications or use alcohol to suppress dreams and nightmares. The dysphoria associated with these dreams is so intense that few patients seem to be able to record the details upon awakening. Fragmentary recall usually persists, however, so that it is possible to glean details at a later date.

When listening to this material, I treat it as a dissociative experience similar to, for example, an out-of-body experience. The details and setting of these repetitive traumatic nightmares seem to be more clearly based on actual settings than are most dreamscapes and can often be used to determine what age the person was and where he or she was when the trauma occurred. One can search the personality system for alters who were created during this time period in the patient's life. The postdream residual affects are also important and can be used as a starting point for affect bridge work. MPD patients seem to be more willing to share and work with dream material than with other forms of memory for trauma.

THE INTERNAL SELF-HELPER

Definitions

The internal self-helper, known as the ISH, was first described by Allison (1974a). The importance placed on identifying and working with the ISH varies with different therapists. Allison (1978b), for example, emphasizes the importance of incorporating the ISH into the therapy. Kluft (1984c), on the other hand, defines ISH personalities in passing as "serene, rational, and objective commentators and advisors" (p. 23), but nowhere discusses the use of the ISH in any of his otherwise important and thorough discussions of treatment. Braun (1984c) and Caul (1984) make passing references to the use of the ISH with varying degrees of emphasis. It is not clear whether an ISH is a universally present alter or only occurs in some MPD patients. There may be more than one ISH present within a given multiple.

Working with an ISH

The literature has few examples of the uses of an ISH, although a number of therapists privately report significant success in incorporating an ISH into the therapy. Allison (1978a) describes the ISH and the therapist as carrying on a dialogue about the patient as a third party. He states that "there is no human to human relationship with which to compare this partnership. It is so unique a relationship it has to be experienced to be believed" (p. 12). The ISH will discuss the patient's strengths and weaknesses and tell the therapist what needs to be done to help the patient. Braun (1984c) describes substituting the ISH for the therapist in a technique he calls the "switchboard," which is used to foster inner dialogue in a manner similar to the model of the therapist as go-between, described in Chapter Six.

Caul (1978a) believes that in the course of therapy the ISH should be identified as soon as possible. He states:

> The therapist must not be afraid to "horse trade" with the ISH, who will always be protective of the personalities and will see to it that therapy is provided and that the personalities will get the best deal possible. If the therapist becomes stymied, it is recommended that the therapist inform the ISH that special help is needed from that source in order to proceed with the therapy. The ISH will almost never play all of his cards at once. The therapist must learn and understand that for the most part the ISH can do more and exert more influence than the therapist realizes. (pp. 2–3)

Caul (1984) provides a number of examples of the stabilizing influences of ISHs in his paper on group and videotape techniques. In one notable example, he describes the ISHs of two multiples commiserating with each other about their similarly angry alters.

My own experience with ISHs has been limited. I have met several, and find that in some cases they are invaluable sources of information and guidance in working with multiples. I certainly have not found an ISH in every multiple, although I usually do find at least one alter who is primarily focused on seeing that the patient gets appropriate treatment. I usually seek an ISH in the same way I seek other alters, by directly asking. I ask whether there is one who sees itself as a guide, helper, or healer, and who can assist me in working with the patient. The first personality to step forward after this request is often not the ISH, so the therapist should not accept an alter's statement that it is an ISH at face value. A true ISH will prove itself in the long run. The other alters can also help in deciding whether or not the therapist is working with a true ISH.

I see the ISH as a guide or a source of information about the personality system and the direction that the therapy needs to take. As Caul has indicated in the passage quoted above, the ISH will rarely reveal more than a small amount of information at a given time, and that information may be incomplete or contain unstated assumptions that the therapist does not understand. ISHs are enigmatic, leaving the therapist with the problem of deciphering their Delphic statements. The therapist can ask for clarification, but will not always get it. In general, if I believe that I am talking to an ISH, I will try to incorporate his or her advice into my interventions, but I take it with a grain of salt. There are ISH imposters who can give misleading or destructive advice, so the therapist should be wary.

There will often be a number of ISHs within a patient, each having authority over a group or family of alters, but none having access to the whole system. Therapists new to MPD often become upset when, as they move to a new level in the personality system, their former ISH fades out or abandons them. The ISH has simply reached the limit of its knowledge or authority, but a new helper can usually be found as the therapy progresses. It should also be noted that ISH personalities often lack staying power and cannot remain "out" for lengthy periods (Caul, 1984).

The principle embodied in the ISH is that at some level the patient has an observing ego function that can comment accurately on the ongoing processes and provide advice and suggestions as to how to aid the rest of the patient in achieving some insight and control over his or her pathology. One can often find this type of function in non-MPD patients as well as within one's own self. It is important to listen to these voices of inner wisdom, but it is a mistake to view them as all-knowledge-able or all-powerful. When one is struggling with a difficult patient, one often wishes for some miraculous intervention, and I think that this wish is what leads some therapists to ascribe omniscience to ISHs. One should of course listen to the patient, particularly if an ISH appears to be available, but in the long run one must use one's own therapeutic judgment.

THE USE OF JOURNALS AND DIARIES

Many therapists and MPD patients report that the keeping of a diary and/or the writing of a life history is a valuable therapeutic task that aids in learning more about the personality system, recovering amnesic material, and, in the patient, gaining a sense of his or her continuity across time. Kluft (1984c) advocates the use of a daily writing exercise as a form of sequential task useful in the diagnosis of MPD. He suggests that the patient write whatever goes through his or her mind each day and bring the written thoughts to the session. He reports that many alters first announce themselves through this medium. Caul (1978a) suggests that patients write a "chronologue" of their past history.

In addition to the bulletin board technique described in Chapter Six, I have found that keeping a diary (and/or writing an autobiography or other form of life history) is a very powerful technique for uncovering information about how the personality system fits together with the patient's life history. Initially the patient, particularly the host personality, may balk at a suggestion that he or she consider doing this. This reluctance is usually caused by the experience of losing time or becoming profoundly depersonalized during these writing sessions, and sometimes finding strange, obscene, threatening, or frightening messages in the journal.

In later stages of therapy, when there is some acceptance of the diagnosis, MPD patients often become hypergraphic and bury the therapist with lengthy excerpts of autobiographical writings. In some cases, these autobiographies become important projects that unite the alters around a common theme and serve as a focus of internal collaboration and self-revelation. Each alter can add his or her piece to the puzzle, and each can come to know the others through their contributions. The patient first assembles himself or herself on paper as preparation for fusion and integration. Abreactions may accompany the recording of some past experiences, but many patients learn to take this in stride and use it as a technique to continue the work outside of the treatment setting. Because of the extensive trauma suffered by most multiples, it is useful if the patients can do some of this abreactive work on their own time.

WORKING WITH INTERNAL
PERSECUTOR PERSONALITIES

Internal persecutor personalities are found in the majority of MPD patients (Putnam *et al.*, 1986). The persecutor personalities usually direct their acts of hostility toward the host personality. The various forms of harassment and the patient's reactions to them constitute a major source of torment for an MPD patient. In personality systems that contain persecutor alters, the therapist must engage and work with these personalities. They will not go away spontaneously, and they cannot be exorcised. On first meeting, they will be fearsome, loathsome, demon-like entities totally committed to the malicious harassment and abuse of the patient. In the long run, they often prove to be one of the therapist's strongest allies and can play a major role in the healing of the patient.

Forms of Internal Persecution

Among the most common manifestations of internal persecution are critical and condemning voices usually heard by the host personality. These voices will berate and belittle the patient, threaten or urge suicide, and sarcastically and gleefully taunt the patient about their *total* control over him or her. Hosts who are unaware of or unwilling to acknowledge other alters will react to these voices with terror and/or despairing resignation at their apparent imminent destruction. The voices can also distract and disturb a host at times when he or she is attempting to concentrate on a difficult task. Some multiples refer to this experience as "jamming." The patients are often reluctant to admit the existence of voices, lest they be thought to be "crazy."

Direct injury to a patient's body is usually the form of internal persecution that disturbs therapists most, although many patients regard this as less troublesome than some other forms of persecution. Suicide is an ever-present issue with multiples. The internal persecutors may be threatening to commit suicide themselves, threatening to kill the host (internal homicide), or urging or commanding the host to kill himself or herself. The host may also be considering suicide as the only way of ending the ceaseless torment. What few data there are suggest that the overall lethality in comparison to the number of attempts and gestures may be relatively low. That does not mean that a therapist can ignore the possibility of suicide; however, the therapist must come to terms with a high background level of suicidal ideation within the personality system. Suicidal gestures are frequent, and serious attempts are not uncommon. Frequently these are aborted by other alters. But most multiples seem to teeter continually on the knife's edge of destruction through the early stages of therapy.

Self-mutilation by persecutors to punish the host or other alters is common (Bliss, 1980; Putnam *et al.*, 1986). The host may "wake up" to find that he or she is covered with blood or injured in some fashion. These experiences are terrifying for the patient. The host may also find threatening notes or even more graphic warnings of future mutilation; for example, one patient found a threatening message written in her own blood on her bedroom wall. Episodes of self-mutilation are frequently triggered by disclosures in therapy of past trauma, and the warnings or messages left by the persecutors often explicitly specify that any further revelations will be met with more injury or death. Needless to say, such experiences often stifle the patient's attempts to remember or reveal the past. This is, of course, one of the primary functions of the persecutor personalities.

Persecutor personalities may harass the patient in other ways. Disruptions of the patient's family, social, and occupational life are common. Many multiples become socially isolated because the persecutors deliberately alienate their friends. Persecutors can make a patient's family life difficult, resulting in divorce and in rejection by their children. Other forms of social sabotage may involve huge debts for the patient or legal problems resulting from the behavior of the persecutor alters; the latter may be more common in male MPD patients. A particularly virulent form of sabotage involves the persecutor personality's setting the patient up for rape or physical abuse. Disruption of therapy is another form of harassment undertaken by the internal persecutors. They may prevent the patient from attending sessions in a number of ways. They may threaten to harm the patient if significant information is revealed to the therapist, and in some cases they may threaten to harm the therapist unless the host withdraws from treatment.

Origin and Functions of Internal Persecutors

Therapists working with their first cases of MPD are often baffled by the apparent hatred of the persecutors for the host or the patient as a whole. There seems to be no justification for the intensity of their malevolence or for the unremitting hostility and violence wreaked upon the poor, defenseless host. "What did she ever do to you to deserve this?" one therapist demanded of a persecutor after his patient was hospitalized for esophageal ulcerations caused by the persecutor's swallowing a corrosive drain cleaner. The persecutor, who was in no apparent discomfort (although the host was in significant pain), replied, "She is a total loser and deserves to die." This is typical of the rationale given by internal persecutors to justify their harassment and self-mutilation. They usually express extreme contempt toward the host. Beahrs (1982) points out that, paradoxically, the dominant emotion of the persecutor toward the host may really be love.

Beahrs (1982) makes the observation that many of these "demons" are angry children. My experience supports his observation that persecutors tend overwhelmingly to be child or adolescent personalities. Bliss (1980) states that "all of the personalities begin as friends and allies, or, if you will, invited guests" (p. 1390). Kluft (1985b) concurs that in child MPD patients there is a "notable" absence of persecutors as well as of pure ISH alters. He speculates that the persecutors develop both from a masochistic turning inward of hostile affect and from early helper personalities who were initially created to suffer abuses and over time have come to identify with the aggressor and to resent suffering for the others. The clinical impression at this time is that the majority of the persecutor personalities initially began as helper or abuse-absorbing personalities and have been transformed over time into the hostile, punitive alters found in most adult MPD patients. It is worth keeping this origin in mind while dealing with some incredibly vituperative persecutor alter who is gleefully threatening the total destruction of a patient.

I think that the persecutors serve a number of important functions within the personality system, and that acknowledging and understanding these functions help the therapist and the personality system to develop an alliance with them. In many instances, persecutors contain the energy and affects that the depressed and apathetic host cannot sustain. Often, this is why they are so contemptuous of the "weak" and "wimpy" host. Beahrs (1982) points out that if one ignores the content and focuses on the energy and affects, these "demons" contain much of the patient's life force.

The persecutors also function to maintain the silence and secrecy that have surrounded the past abuse. Initially, this may also have been a life-protecting role. They protect the past by threatening the patient and/ or the therapist with disastrous consequences if it is revealed, and by creating such an uproar in therapy that the therapist never has a chance to focus on the past. Lindy (1985) has described the concept of a "trauma membrane," in which a survivor of a catastrophe is protected from intrusive or inquisitive inquiry by relatives or close friends. The trauma membrane serves to keep noxious reminders of the experience at a distance. The persecutor alters often serve as an MPD patient's "trauma membrane." These alters and the personality system as a whole must be convinced that the therapist is a healing agent and that it is safe to allow him or her behind the shield.

Relating to Persecutors

The therapist must remember that ultimately all of the personalities, persecutors included, have a role and a place in the patient as a whole. The therapist should relate to all of the personalities with honesty and respect, though Caul (1983) cautions that this does not mean indulgence. It is important to be nonjudgmental when dealing with persecutors. They are not bad per se; it is the things that they are doing to the host, the others, and the body that are bad. The therapist should try not to get into struggles with the persecutors over control of their behavior or the patient as a whole; since they are part of the patient as a whole, they have more power to influence the outcome, for better or for worse, than the therapist does. Instead, the therapist should talk with them, bargain with them, contract with them, and try to make friends with them. It often seems surprisingly easy, until one remembers that most of them are really like frightened children filled with rage and an infantile sense of omnipotence. They welcome the attention and relief that a therapist can bring to them. Obviously, one does not reinforce their destructive behavior, but rather their cooperation.

Many therapists initially avoid their patients' persecutor personalities. They are afraid to have them come out in sessions and often seek ways to banish, exorcise, or suppress them. I usually try to get them to appear and stay "out" for at least 15 minutes during a session. They may emerge roaring, but often leave meekly. Simply keeping them "out" for a period of time seems to deplete their energies. Repeatedly, I have had the experience of having a ferocious persecutor tell me that he or she is getting tired and has to go now. When a persecutor comes out, I try to find out all I can about his or her origin and present role in the personality system. When did he or she first come? When did he or she first start to come out? What was his or her original purpose? What is his or her role now? I try to get him or her to tell me all about his or her relationship with the host and with other alters, and I empathize with this alter as with any other.

It is important to validate the existence and importance of persecutor alters—to recognize that they represent needs, feelings, hopes, and fears. One of the common fears is that the therapist may attempt to do away with them. They should be reassured that this is not so; that the therapist has neither the power nor the wish to kill them off; and that the therapist recognizes that in some way, at some level, they must be doing what they are doing because they believe that it is necessary to help the patient. They should be reminded of their past and of the fact that they originally came to help the patient deal with what he or she could not face.

In cases where a persecutor seems to be functioning as a trauma membrane to protect the host from the recovery of painful memories, the persecutor should be assured that the therapist will work with him or her to allow the host to "remember" the material in a way that is tolerable for the personality system as a whole. The therapist should ask the persecutor's advice about how this may be accomplished. One of the dynamics of the internal persecution process is the persecutor's attempt to transfer back to the host and other alters some of the trauma and affects that he or she originally absorbed to protect the patient. It is often done in a childish attempt at recapitulation of abusive experiences ("I took that for her and now she's going to feel what it was like"). The therapist needs to help the persecutor understand that there are other ways for the patient as a whole to reown painful memories and affects.

In many instances, the host is actually abusing the persecutors. Usually this is through an unknowing suppression or a dimly aware rejection of the persecutor. Helping the host acknowledge the persecutor's existence, and the fact that the persecutor part represents needs and feelings, often helps to lower the intensity of the internal conflict. Ultimately, the patient as a whole needs to reown and reabsorb all of the persecutors. Fortunately, the persecutors, despite their apparent attempts at annihilating the patient, are often willing to give up the pain they contain and work with the others. Many of these destroyers become healers at a later stage in the therapy.

Levels of Persecutors

Like ISH personalities, internal persecutors often exist at a number of levels in the personality system. As a given persecutor begins to mellow and becomes cooperative, he or she will tell the therapist about another persecutor lurking in the background, who is "10 times worse." The therapist should question these estimates of malignancy, as they are usually derived from the persecutor's infantile omnipotence and rage. The increasing "anger" of the deeper levels of persecutors stems from the fact that they are usually the guardians of more traumatic layers of dissociated memories and affects. If the patient is layered (and many MPD patients are), then the therapist must work through each layer, dealing with the alters at each level. This can be a monumental task. On the other hand, after working through a number of layers, the therapist will have a good idea of who and what to expect in subsequent layers.

MAPPING THE PERSONALITY SYSTEM

The idea of mapping the personality system of MPD patients is not new; both Morton Prince (1909a) and Walter Franklin Prince (1917) published diagrams of their understanding of how the alter personalities of their patients fit together. Bennett Braun (1986) has expanded the idea of mapping into a useful therapeutic technique.

In essence, the personality system is asked to produce a map, diagram, or schema of the alters' best understanding of how they fit together or their sense of their inner world. The exact form of the map should be left up to the discretion of the personality system. I have received Mercator projection maps, pie charts, architectural blueprints, organizational personnel charts, target-like arrangements of concentric circles, clock faces, lists, and some totally unclassifiable documents. What is important is that all of the personalities be represented on the map in some fashion. The results are quite variable, and a substantial percentage of MPD patients are not able to produce any form of map at all. In some cases, however, the patient creates a useful document that can tell the therapist (and patient) a great deal about the dynamics of the personality system and indicate areas of further therapeutic work.

Some of the most useful pieces of information contained in the map are the blank areas where the patient feels that something or somebody should exist. This should alert the therapist to the existence of hidden alters who must be met. The juxtapositions of alters on the map are also potentially useful data and can help identify which alters are likely to be able to fuse easily during the series of partial fusions that build toward the final fusion. The form of the map also provides information about the personality system's internal metaphor, which can be used in working with the system. Some MPD patients, for example, liken their bodies to houses in which the alters live in separate rooms. A map of such a system may resemble a blueprint with the alters' rooms opening into a central hall or room. A therapist can use this structure to locate the alters, set up lines of communication, arrange meetings, and so on. The therapist should use the map as a source of metaphors for generating images or explaining concepts to the personalities. Complex MPD patients often represent separate families of personalities on their maps. This enables the therapist to see which alters group together and which alters serve as connection points between separate families.

Once a map is generated, copies should be kept by both the patient and therapist. The map should be updated periodically, at which times newly identified blank areas can be added, partial integrations incorporated, and newly recognized alters added. Before any "final" integrations, the patient and therapist should go over the map looking for loose threads or ambiguous areas that signal undiscovered alters or incomplete work.

RESISTANCES TO TREATMENT

Definition

Langs (1974a) defines resistances as "all of the devices (e.g., defenses) used by the patient to interfere with the progress of his treatment and to prevent the affective expression of the potentially disturbing derivatives of unconscious, conflict-related fantasies in the sessions" (p. 464). In the case of multiple personality patients, one might replace "fantasies" in this definition with "dissociated memories and affects." Resistances occur in all psychotherapies, and the therapies of multiples are no exception. Not every defense, however, is manifested as a resistance. In MPD patients, resistances are most frequently expressed around uncovering work. As with all other patients, resistances in multiples are overdetermined, unconsciously driven processes that take place largely out of the patients' awareness.

Resistances are also important manifestations and indices of therapist error. Incorrect or inadequate therapeutic interventions may heighten current manifestations of resistance or elicit new forms. A therapist must always bear in mind his or her possible contribution to a patient's suddenly increased resistance following a "therapeutic" intervention. Not all expressions of resistance threaten the therapeutic alliance, but all disruptions of the therapeutic alliance are major expressions of resistance (Langs, 1974a).

Manifestations of Resistance

The form of resistance is determined by a number of factors, including the relationship between the patient and therapist, the point in the course of the therapy (e.g., early or late in treatment), the traumatic material that the resistance is concealing, the patient's personality system, and the circumstances of the treatment (e.g., inpatient vs. outpatient), to name only a few important influences. Langs (1974a) has described a number of typical resistances seen early in treatment with many types of patients. These include blaming others, mistrusting or having paranoid feelings, acting out, using a significant other to oppose treatment, denying emotional problems, having financial or time problems, and fearing treatment and the therapist. Multiples may exhibit all of these classical forms. In addition, however, multiples often have a number of unique forms or unique expressions of the more classical forms of resistance.

Fugues, Trances, and Depersonalizations

Dissociation is a multiple's primary defense against trauma. Not too surprisingly, it also becomes a major form of resistance to treatment. In the treatment setting, resistance is often manifested in trance-like states or profound depersonalization. During trance-like states, the patient may become minimally or completely unresponsive and stare off into space. The therapist will have great difficulty making contact or communicating with the patient. Things often reach a crisis point when the hour has ended and the therapist has another patient waiting. Alternatively, the patient may experience profound depersonalization and respond with a floating detachment to all interactions.

Outside of the treatment setting, minifugue episodes are a frequent manifestation of resistance. The patient will leave the treatment session and then wander in a dissociated state for several hours until he or she finally "comes to" in an unfamiliar place and calls the therapist in a panic. In a session, the patient may bolt for the door in a panicked or dissociated state. These experiences, which usually produce significant discomfort for both the patient and therapist, will often dampen the active uncovering of traumatic material.

Acting Out

As a resistance, acting out takes a myriad of forms, but the manifestations that are most troubling to the therapist are suicide gestures, externally directed violence, and self-mutilation. The suicide gestures or self-mutilation may directly follow sessions in which attempts have been made at uncovering traumatic material. Persecutor personalities, with their mandate of guarding secrecy, are often responsible for these actions.

Internal Uproar and Acute Regressions

Multiples, with their child and infant personalities, are capable of acute and profound behavioral regression. During moments of extreme anxiety, they may collapse into a thumb-sucking, preverbal state as an infant personality emerges. Tyrannical 2-year-olds or other child alters with disturbed reality testing may emerge, keeping the therapist preoccupied with "babysitting" rather than psychotherapeutic work. In many instances, these infant or child personalities are sent out by the system to thwart uncovering work. If a personality cannot talk, he or she also cannot disclose highly charged material. Such a regressed state can be disturbing to the neophyte therapist, who perceives this as a deterioration in the patient's condition. A common mistake is to respond to these regressions with "supportive" interventions or medication.

Internal uproars, in which the personality system degenerates into a screaming mob within the patient's (usually the host's) head, often prevent further work by overwhelming the patient with internal stimuli. They may also produce conversion or "hysterical" symptoms, which in turn become the focus of the therapy rather than the traumatic material. Conversion symptoms in MPD are usually highly symbolic of the material they conceal.

Involvement of Others in the Therapy

As mentioned earlier in this chapter, MPD patients frequently involve others in their treatment. Usually this constitutes a resistance and not infrequently may result in a significant disruption of the therapeutic alliance. The involvement of all others, particularly other therapists, should be closely examined for elements of resistance to treatment.

Denial of Multiplicity and/or Flights into Health

Flights into health or disavowals of multiplicity are common and often occur as the therapy begins to get down to serious uncovering work. Following a difficult session, a multiple may present on the next occasion stating that he or she is fused and appearing calm and confident. David Caul (1985a) observes that a "therapist should be cautious in accepting such happy news" (p. 5). Spontaneous total fusion may *rarely* occur in MPD patients, but is highly unlikely to occur in the middle of a turbulent therapy that is beginning to work with unrevealed trauma. Caul (1985a) recommends that the therapist carefully seek out the reasons why this "fusion" has occurred. In particular, the therapist should ask about how the "fusion" has occurred: the circumstances, the reports of other personalities, and the mechanism of final decision making. The patient may be acting out the therapist's unconscious wish to be rid of the other personalities.

Disavowal of multiplicity also commonly occurs in the same context. The patient "admits" that he or she "made it all up." Frequently, however, this disavowal is immediately preceded or followed by some clear demonstration of the patient's multiplicity as one or more alters break through the internal suppression to demonstrate their continued existence. Neither "spontaneous fusion" nor disavowal of multiplicity constitutes grounds for discontinuation of treatment. Even if the patient has truly fused, there remains the important postresolution stage that is necessary to successfully conclude the patient's treatment.

Personalities Not in Treatment

"Don't give me any of that therapy bullshit! She's the patient, not me. I just bring her here," one alter told me. Some patients will have alters who steadfastly maintain that they are not in treatment. They will claim that they do not have any problems and that it is the other personalities (particularly the host) who are in need of treatment. Such an alter is not unlike the patient who says, "I don't have any problems. It's my wife [mother, boss, etc.] who should be seeing you." The therapist's position is that all of the alters have got to learn to live together in some form or other, and therefore they are all in treatment, without exception.

Requests for Medication or Other Interventions

Requests for medication, shock treatments, or other forms of somatic intervention usually represent a major resistance to the work of uncovering, re-experiencing, and metabolizing past trauma. It is an understandable wish, and many patients hope that such measures can blot out the remembered pain from the past. Usually it is the host who asks for these interventions. The host may also be seeking ways to suppress alters who are experienced as tormentors or otherwise troublesome. These requests should be carefully explored with the host and other personalities, since a refusal may be experienced as a rejection and deprivation. Guidelines for the use of medications are discussed in Chapter Ten.

Information without a Context

In therapy with a multiple personality patient, much of the initial information provided by the patient will exist without a clear context. Memories, feelings, and behaviors will appear to come from nowhere, and the patient will have great difficulty in connecting them to past events or present situations. This is largely the result of the fragmentation and discontinuity of memory produced by dissociation. This process becomes a resistance when the patient repetitively produces significant material but avoids any attempt to help the therapist place it into a larger context.

When this situation develops, the therapist should explore it with the personality system. It is difficult to engage in useful therapeutic work without a context, and, as Langs (1974a) points out, "all effective psychotherapeutic work ultimately begins with the reality precipitate and ends with its intrapsychic repercussions" (p. 285).

Working with Resistances

Focusing on resistances should *not* become the central work of psychotherapy with MPD patients. The core therapeutic work is, first, stabilizing the patient; next, developing increased internal communication and cooperation; and then uncovering and reintegrating dissociated memories and affects. Resistances should be explored and confronted only when they begin to obstruct the core work. The first step in working with a resistance is for the therapist to recognize that there is a resistance and that it is interfering with the core work of therapy. The therapist must then clarify as best he or she can the nature of the resistance and what may be driving it. The resistance should be discussed with the patient in plain and simple language, in an attempt to make the personality system aware that there is an impediment to the core therapeutic work. The therapist should identify the therapeutic context in which the resistance is expressed and the manner in which the resistance is blocking the therapeutic work. The therapist should then make a statement about the "cost" of the resistance to the patient.

SUMMARY

This chapter discusses a number of psychotherapeutic techniques and interventions with the personality system and specific alter personalities. Talking through, an extremely useful tool, allows the therapist to work with the personality system as a whole, at the same time challenging the patient to open up channels of internal communication. The process of assembling whole memories is one of the major reconstructive tasks in therapy. The therapist must help the patient fit the pieces together, integrating content with affects. Cross-inventorying is useful as a background technique, slowly building an awareness of the complementarity of the alters. Dreams may be important avenues into unremembered trauma and can be used to demonstrate the common ground shared by the alters. The use of journals, diaries, or autobiographies can help the patient organize his or her life history in a displaced manner so that it can be internalized more easily. The patient can also be asked to map the personality system, providing a schema that is useful as a model and metaphor for his or her internal world.

The ISH can be helpful in guiding the therapist, though these alters are not universally present in MPD patients, and imposter ISHs exist. The persecutory alters, while destructive and dangerous, hold important affects and energy that must be enlisted in the service of the patient as a whole. Many persecutors are simply resisting exploration of trauma and can be won over by allowing them to ventilate. Multiples exhibit all of the usual resistances to treatment, plus a number of unique variations that make therapy with these patients always interesting.

CHAPTER NINE

The Therapeutic Role of Hypnosis and Abreaction

Despine's successful treatment in 1837 of Estelle, an 11-year-old Swiss girl with dual personality and a paralytic conversion disorder, is the first recorded case in which hypnosis was used to treat MPD (Ellenberger, 1970). It remained for Janet (1889), however, to first make the connection between hypnotic trance states and multiple personality. Clinicians working with multiple personality patients continue to be impressed by the high hypnotizability of these subjects (Bliss, 1986; Brandsma & Ludwig, 1974; Braun, 1984c; Kluft, 1982). Brende and Rinsley (1981) are the only authors, to my knowledge, who have reported working with an MPD patient who was *not* a good hypnotic subject. Bliss (1984b) has systematically investigated the issue of hypnotizability in MPD subjects and presents data indicating that the anecdotal reports cited above appear to be accurate.

CONCERNS ABOUT IATROGENIC HYPNOTIC CREATION OF THE DISORDER

Historically, the concern that the use or misuse of hypnosis could create MPD can be traced at least as far back as Janet's (1889) and Morton Prince's (1890/1975) writings. This possibility remains a concern for many therapists beginning to work with MPD patients. Articles by Harriman (1942a, 1942b, 1943), Leavitt (1947), and Kampman (1974, 1975, 1976) are often cited as "proof" that hypnosis can be used to create MPD. Braun (1984b), Kluft (1982), and Greaves (1980) have critically reviewed these papers and concluded that the "personalities" induced by such hypnotic manipulations are not "multiple personalities by any reasonable criteria" (Braun, 1984b, p. 194). Kluft (1982) concludes that "the literature generally overstates the risks of hypnosis" (p. 232). I agree with the independent assessments by Greaves, Braun, and Kluft of these experimental creations. The descriptions of hypnotically induced experimental entities fall far short of what one encounters clinically in patients with MPD.

A number of authors warn of the possibility that the therapist, with or without hypnosis, may unintentionally shape or reinforce the behavior of the patient and thereby exacerbate the dissociative process (Bowers *et al.*, 1971; Gruenewald, 1977; Horton & Miller, 1972). A statistical comparison of the presenting symptoms and the phenomenology of the alter personalities (e.g., numbers and types of alter personalities) in MPD patients treated with hypnosis and in those not so treated indicates that there are no significant differences between these two groups (Putnam *et al.*, 1986). The appearance of personalities created during the course of therapy—as opposed to previously existing personalities who were discovered during the course of therapy—was reported in approximately 30% of the cases in the NIMH survey (Putnam *et al.*, 1986), as well as by experienced therapists in the clinical literature (Bliss, 1980; Brandsma & Ludwig, 1974; Herzog, 1984). There is no statistical difference in the reported incidence of newly created personalities between patients treated with hypnosis and those not so treated (Putnam *et al.*, 1986). The evidence to date indicates that whereas hypnosis is an effective tool for the treatment of MPD, its use does not appear to contribute to an exacerbation of dissociative psychopathology.

INDUCTION OF TRANCE IN MULTIPLES

Spontaneous Trances

The existence of spontaneous trance states has been described since the observations of De Boismont in 1835 (Bliss, 1983). Breuer and Freud (1895/1957) commented on the existence of spontaneous hypnoid states in the case of Anna O. Subsequently, a number of psychoanalysts have noted the existence of similar hypnoid states in patients suffering from early childhood trauma, particularly sexual abuse (Putnam, 1985a). Fagan and McMahon (1984), Kluft (1984b), and I (quoted in Elliott, 1982) have all independently reported the existence of spontaneous trance-like states in the childhood dissociative disorders. Spontaneous trance states have also been reported to occur in normal subjects (Wilson & Barber, 1982).

Spontaneous trance phenomena are responsible for many crises in the lives of MPD patients (Kluft, 1983) and may represent a major psychopathological mechanism in MPD, according to Bliss's (1986) theory. An MPD patient will frequently move in and out of spontaneous trances during a psychotherapy session. Bliss (1983) describes two major modes of spontaneous trance states in his patients. The first is one in which the patient seeks refuge in a quiet, relaxed repose of internal focus. The second type of induction comes from overwhelming traumatic experiences when the subject feels "trapped, terrified and unable to cope—the situation where personalities are usually invoked or created" (p. 115). Spiegel and Spiegel (1978) also identify the existence of a fear-induced trance mechanism.

During spontaneous trance states, it is possible to use the same types of hypnotherapeutic techniques used during therapist-induced trance states. It is generally better, however, to induce hypnosis formally with an MPD patient. The formal hypnotic induction, with overt permission given by the patient, allows better control over the process. Multiples, with their exquisite sensitivity to issues of control and manipulation, rarely do well with informal or Ericksonian types of hypnotic induction.

Patient Resistance to Hypnosis

Despite their generally high hypnotizability, many MPD patients are fearful of and resistant to a therapist's first attempts at hypnosis. They may react with feelings of panic to the mere suggestion that hypnosis be tried. Usually they are not able to verbalize clearly why they are afraid. Fear that they may lose control seems to be at the root of many host personalities' resistance to hypnosis. They fear that they will lose control to other personalities or that they will lose control to the therapist. With regard to the latter concern, Braun (1984c) notes that "no matter how much these patients are reassured that they cannot be 'controlled' via hypnosis, [their] fear of loss of control will persist until they have experienced formal trance" (p. 36). The best method for helping a patient overcome his or her fears of being controlled by the therapist is to provide some initial, benign, rapport-building trance experiences such as those described later in this chapter.

The fear of losing control to other personalities is more complex and difficult to work with. In many cases, the host personality is unwilling to relinquish control and enter into a trance because he or she is afraid, at some level, that another personality will take over and never allow the host back into control. Allowing another personality "out" also undercuts the host's denial of multiplicity. In addition, the process of switching to another personality may be experienced by the host personality as akin to death or oblivion. Many host personalities describe such switching as a sensation of being sucked down into a terrifying vortex or black hole. A host may experience a variety of disturbing somatic sensations during the induction of hypnosis, typically including feelings of intense, bursting pressure in the head or chest, often accompanied by fluttery sensations in the gut. Sometimes MPD patients report seeing terrifying images as they enter into a trance.

The therapist must prevail upon the host to ride out these disturbing, but transient, experiences. The therapist must also assure the host that he or she will return to full control at the end of the session. In the beginning, it is important to bring the host back at least 15 minutes before the end of the session, to allow for reorientation and processing of the experience. It may require several attempts before a successful induction occurs. Often the patient will bolt out of trance in a terrified state during the first several attempts at induction. Such behavior does not mean that the patient cannot be hypnotized. On the contrary, it indicates that the patient is highly hypnotizable and has begun to directly experience the existence of the other alters or dissociated traumatic material in the trance state.

Horevitz (1983) describes a number of other sources of resistance to hypnosis. He mentions a need to protect the system as a whole. Some multiples who are "not hypnotizable" are simply resisting hypnosis because the personality system has no wish to allow the therapist to see what lies beneath the surface. It is my impression that such stonewalling is a poor prognostic sign. Horevitz (1983) notes that the fear of violation of long-protected secrets and the fear of the immense loss that getting well represents may also be sources of resistance to hypnosis. These resistances need to be explored and dealt with so that the patient can permit himself or herself to go into trance.

Multiples may fake hypnosis without going into trance. As Orne (1977) has demonstrated, it is difficult even for an experienced hypnotist to distinguish a simulated trance from a real one. When a patient fakes hypnosis, it indicates a significant resistance coupled with a lack of trust. Such deception, although nominally in the service of protecting the patient from contact with traumatic material, is usually a poor prognostic sign. It is likely that this degree of deception extends to other areas of the therapy and the patient's life.

Induction Techniques

There are a wide variety of techniques to aid in the induction of hypnosis. Most standard hypnotic induction techniques have been successfully used with multiple personality patients, and there is no evidence that one technique is clearly superior to another. A therapist should use whichever techniques are familiar and comfortable.

Bliss (1986) expresses a preference for brief and simple techniques with his patients. He describes using a request for relaxation, coupled with visual fixation on a point and repetition of statements to the effect that the subject's eyelids are getting heavier and heavier. If he has difficulty with this form of induction, he will ask the patient to talk about where he or she enjoys being. He will then ask the patient to picture the experience and mentally go there to relax. I have found this latter technique to be particularly useful in patients wtih a strong resistance to the idea of hypnosis. A patient can choose a safe and relaxing place and mentally go there. Trance can be deepened by having the experience become more and more vivid for the patient.

Braun (1980) believes that the choice of hypnotic technique is relatively unimportant, but suggests staying away from "confusion techniques." He stresses that the main goal early in treatment is the creation of a "calm, relaxed and pleasant psychological and physiological state in association with the therapist and treatment" (p. 211). He makes a point that can be easily overlooked in the chaos of a hypnotic abreactive session, which is that whenever hypnosis is employed, the therapist must formally "remove" the trance before the session ends and reserve some time for reorientation and processing of the experience. In his experience, patients will complain of a "hangover effect" if a trance has not been properly removed (Braun, 1984c).

THE USE OF HYPNOSIS IN DIAGNOSIS

In Chapter Four I have discussed the principles of diagnosis of MPD; these are a knowledge of the dissociative process and its varied manifestations, informed history taking, and careful scrutiny of the patient's intra-interview behaviors. A suspected diagnosis of MPD can only be confirmed by meeting one or more alter personalities. In most cases, this can be accomplished by simply directly asking to meet with suspected alters. In some instances, particularly where time is limited such as in a clinical emergency or a consultation, hypnosis may be useful in facilitating the emergence of an alter personality.

The principal advantage of hypnosis in diagnosis is that it diminishes the host personality's suppression of other alters and thereby allows an alter personality to emerge who might otherwise be unable to break through the host's resistance. In general, one induces and deepens a hypnotic trance and simply asks the patient "if there is another thought process, part of the mind, person or force that exists in the body" (Braun, 1980, p. 213). In my experience, a host personality in a hypnotic trance state has a more direct experience of an alter personality than when the switch occurs without a trance state. In the latter instance, the host may be completely amnesic for the events surrounding an alter's emergence and interaction with the interviewer. When in trance, however, the host may see and hear these events, and consequently may be more disturbed by the process. Braun (1980) suggests that another useful hypnotic diagnostic technique is age regression. He cautions, however, that one must be careful to distinguish between age regression with revivification (i.e., the realistic and intense re-experience of past events) and the appearance of true alter personalities. Age regression and age progression techniques are discussed later in this chapter.

HYPNOTHERAPEUTIC TECHNIQUES

The following is a review and discussion of hypnotherapeutic techniques used in the treatment of MPD. For heuristic purposes, I have grouped these techniques into three categories: (1) trance-inducing/rapport-building techniques; (2) techniques for penetrating amnesic barriers; and (3) abreactive/healing techniques. In actuality, most of these techniques will be useful across a range of problems in treatment.

Trance-Inducing/Rapport-Building Techniques

Rapport-building techniques are methods used to develop trust, facilitate the induction of trance, and enhance the therapeutic alliance. In this section I discuss the use of benign trance experiences, ideomotor signaling, ego strengthening, and cue word induction techniques.

Benign Trance Experiences

Benign trance experiences are a useful way to begin increasing a patient's trust and comfort with hypnosis. The principle of a benign trance experience is to allow the patient to directly experience hypnosis and perhaps achieve a sense of mastery or control over the hypnotic process or a troublesome symptom. The classic benign trance experience is an extension of the hypnotic induction technique, in which the patient mentally pictures himself or herself going to a safe and pleasant place and allows this mental image to become increasingly vivid. The therapist works with the patient to heighten the immediacy of the experience and to increase the sense of safety and relaxation. It is important to allow the patient to structure the image and its accompanying perceptions and sensations. For example, a patient may suggest picturing himself or herself at the seashore. A therapist who jumps in with suggested images of hot sun, warm sand, and rolling waves may be surprised to find that the patient's image is of a lonely windswept beach in winter and that his or her sense of safety comes from huddling among the rippling dune grass, out of sight of the booming surf. The therapist should be careful in suggesting images, because an incongruity between the image conjured up by the patient and one suggested by the therapist can produce a sense of distress and resentment in the patient, which translates into a resistance to hypnosis.

Horevitz (1983) notes that hypnosis can improve the therapeutic alliance when it is "offered as a tool helpful to the patient rather than as helpful to the 'treatment'" (p. 141). He suggests presenting hypnosis as a cognitive skill that the patient can master for anxiety management, relaxation, symptom relief, self-control, and mastery. Similarly, Braun (1980) describes teaching an MPD patient to use self-hypnosis for relaxation and reduction of anxiety. Herzog (1984) suggests demonstrating some aspect of hypnosis (e.g., visual imagery or posthypnotic suggestion) to the patient as a rapport-building technique. He states that this works best when the hypnosis is included as an "incidental" exercise rather than being the focus of the session. There is a clear consensus that exploratory work, such as attempting to elicit alter personalities or to recover traumatic material, should not be attempted during this initial rapport-building stage of hypnosis (Braun, 1980; Herzog, 1984; Horevitz, 1983; Kluft, 1982).

Ideomotor Signaling

The use of ideomotor signaling is generally most helpful when it is introduced at an early stage in the course of hypnotic interventions. The technique itself is widely applicable to many hypnotic situations and is not simply a rapport-facilitating method. The principle of ideomotor signaling is to establish a set of prearranged signals that provide the patient with a way to answer questons nonverbally and to exercise some communication and control with the therapist during the course of hypnosis. Most commonly, a set of finger signals is used. Braun (1984c) suggests that the movement of the index finger stand for "yes," that movement of the thumb mean "no," and that movement of the little finger mean "stop." The stop signal gives the patient some measure of control over the process and prevents a forced-choice situation. It is recommended that all of the agreed upon signals be confined to one hand, rather than shared by both hands (Braun, 1980). This is due to the change in dominant handedness that can occur across alter personalities and can cause confusion about the meaning of signals divided between two hands.

Ideomotor signaling can be used to contact alter personalities without directly eliciting the overt emergence of the alter. Many patients who are reluctant to go completely into a trance will be willing to relax and relinquish control of one or more fingers. The introduction of ideomotor signaling techniques allows alter personalities some form of communication with the therapist and relieves some of the immediate pressure to emerge following hypnotic induction of the host. This decrease in internal tension often increases the patient's willingness and/or ability to relax, which in turn aids the induction process. Ideomotor signaling remains a useful technique throughout the course of treatment in MPD. Kluft (1983) has described allowing different alters to use different fingers as signals, which permits him to gather a "wealth of data" from a single question.

Ego Strengthening

In his lectures on MPD, David Caul has described the use of an "ego-strengthening" hypnotic technique with depleted or frightened host personalities. This involves having the host personality mentally rehearse difficult tasks or imaginarily confront phobic or frightening objects or situations while in trance. One example offered by Caul was that of a patient who was frightened of construction equipment. While in trance, he had her imagine approaching a crane, climbing into it, and eventually controlling it. I have used this technique, which is very similar to the relaxation/desensitization techniques used by some behavioral therapies, to help MPD patients prepare for situations that are anticipated to be difficult or frightening (e.g., visits to a dentist or the driver's license bureau).

Key or Cue Words

Morton and Thoma (1964) first described using key words to elicit specific alter personalities. The use of "cue words," as they have come to be known, is an important technique for facilitating the hypnotic process.

Caul (1978b) originally utilized cue words for rapidly inducing trance as a protective measure for patient and/or therapist. In his original paper, he described several episodes in which the instant induction of trance prevented harm to the patient or the therapist. Both Braun (1980) and Kluft (1983) describe using cue words to elicit the emergence of a previously agreed-upon alter personality who can come out and take over if the need should arise. Cue words can be used in routine hypnotherapy as a means of decreasing the time spent on induction. This is especially useful if the therapist is doing multilevel trance work (Braun, 1984c).

Cue words do not always work and should not be depended upon as the only safety precaution to protect the therapist or patient. One therapist in our local MPD study group described having her patient undo an induction cue word by self-hypnosis. The therapist found that a previously effective cue word suddenly lost its ability to induce trance. Later, the patient reported that she had gone into self-induced hypnosis and by auto-suggestion had blocked the cue word's effect. In spite of this caution, cue words remain useful for the rapid induction of trance.

I have had good results with cue words that the patient and I have selected and agreed upon for the rapid induction of trance. I have the patient or a specific alter personality suggest an appropriate cue word. We then pair the cue word with the experience of a deep state of trance produced by a standard induction. I suggest that the patient can reach this state instantly when he or she hears the cue word. We then spend some time using the cue word to deepen trance. This technique is presented to the patient as a means of rapidly inducing trance, to save us time during the therapy session. The cue word, however, can be used in an emergency situation if needed. The emergence of a predesignated alter personality can be arranged in a similar fashion.

Techniques for Penetrating Amnesic Barriers

Caul (1978b) has stated that the first and most obvious use of hypnosis in MPD is to penetrate amnesic barriers. There are many ways to do this, and I discuss a variety of techniques, ranging from simple "talking through" to multilevel hypnosis.

Talking Through

Talking through, a technique described in detail in Chapter Eight, is particularly effective when combined with hypnosis. One talks through the hypnotized host personality to the alters presumed to be listening in the background. Braun (1984c) notes that it is important to carefully observe facial expressions, posture changes, mannerisms, and other responses to the topics under discussion. These signs may signal covert switching induced by the content of the discussion. Kluft (1982) also uses talking through to challenge amnesic barriers by addressing personalities who are not "out," commenting that his most common hypnotic instruction is "Everybody listen." He believes that this technique promotes inward listening on the part of alters who are not "out," and thereby facilitates the development of internal dialogues.

In general, talking through works best when directed to the personality system as a whole, rather than to specific alters who may not be available to hear the comments. Caul (1978b) observes:

> It is possible under hypnosis to speak to them all simultaneously or to target two or more personalities for specific therapeutic contact in order to reinforce the bargaining process. The technique would appear to be relatively simple but requires a great deal of care and attention on the part of the therapist so that the message is presented as clearly as possible and that all those "receiving" the messages do so in language that is both understandable and clear regardless of the personality differences . . . (p. 3)

Beahrs (1983) also endorses the use of talking-through techniques with MPD patients and notes that it is "not necessary to separately call forth an alter personality for it to hear what we want to tell it" (p. 107).

Contacting Alters

Hypnosis is a useful tool for contacting alter personalities directly. Kluft (1982) reports that he has used hypnosis to contact alters in over 95% of his MPD patients. After the induction of trance, alters may be asked to emerge, to speak inwardly to the currently dominant personality (who perceives this as an auditory hallucination), or to use ideomotor signals to communicate with the therapist. Under hypnosis, personalities may be asked for directly if their names are known, or by description of an act that they may have been involved in (e.g., "I would like to speak to whoever was responsible for destroying all of Jane's paintings"). If no alters can be elicited by these requests, the hypnotized patient can be asked to look around within his or her mind for painful or frightening experiences. If any are found, the patient can be asked to remember one of his or her choosing. If a painful experience is recalled in the hypnotized state, the patient can be instructed to remember only as much as he or she can tolerate after emerging from trance.

Age Regression

Age regression, a well-studied hypnotic technique, is useful in the recovery of repressed or "forgotten" memories and for initiating controlled abreactions of traumatic experiences. Janet used age regression in his therapeutic work, as illustrated by his treatment of Marie for "great hysterical crises" associated with menstruation. The interrelation between age regression and hypermnesia (i.e., heightened memory) has been described by Hilgard (1965). This hypermnesia appears attributable to the vivid reliving of past events in the age-regressed state of consciousness. Memories recovered in this way are not always veridical and can be created by suggestions from the hypnotist under certain conditions (Hilgard, 1965; Spanos *et al.*, 1979; Rubenstein & Newman, 1954; Zolik, 1958). In spite of this caveat, age regression has proved to be a powerful technique for the penetration of amnesic barriers in MPD patients.

Age regression is most effective in highly hypnotizable individuals, such as the vast majority of MPD patients. Reseachers have found that some individuals retain a layering or stratification of memories, responses, and reflexes, and that these appear sequentially as the individual is age-regressed backwards in his or her life history. The appearance of developmentally primitive neurological reflexes, such as the Babinski, rooting, and grasp reflexes, has been documented by investigators (Spiegel & Spiegel, 1978). The reversion of subjects who are not native speakers of English to their native languages at an age-regressed point corresponding to the appropriate age in their life history has been reported (Hilgard, 1965; Spiegel & Spiegel, 1978). In the age-regressed state, non-MPD subjects often manifest a duality of awareness, so that the age-regressed part may respond in childlike fashion and an observing adult ego may respond in another. For example, the age-regressed part of a subject whose native language is not English may not understand English commands, but the adult observing part may understand and comply fully. Hilgard (1965) has likened this process to a type of dissociation similar to MPD.

Age regression for the recovery of memories can be done with the MPD patient as a whole (i.e., through the host personality) or with a specific alter personality. In the latter case, a multilevel hypnotic technique is frequently useful (Braun, 1984c). In consultation with the patient, it is important to identify a "target" beforehand and to direct the age regression back to that point in time. Examples of targets include important life events (e.g., birthdays, Christmases, school grades, births of siblings, deaths and losses) or the first appearance of specific symptoms or troublesome behaviors.

After an appropriate hypnotic induction, the patient is walked backwards through time by the therapist to the preidentified target. For example, the therapist may say, "It is no longer the present; you are going backwards in time; you are getting younger. You are now 22 years old . . . 18 years old . . . 12 years old . . . 7 years old. Now you are 5 years old. Today is your fifth birthday. When I touch your hand, you will open your eyes and talk with me. Later, when I touch your hand again, your eyes will close." The therapist may now proceed to explore with the patient or alter personality the events associated with the chosen target. The patient or personality is returned to the present time by a reversal of the sequence described above. An adequate response to age regression is manifested by the patient's making age-appropriate responses and speaking in the present tense (Spiegel & Spiegel, 1978).

Affect Bridge Techniques

The affect bridge, a special form of age regression first described by John Watkins (1971), can be an effective technique for recovering dissociated memories. In the affect bridge procedure, the patient moves along a chain of affect or sensory/somatic associations rather than "idea" associations. This procedure is most appropriate when the patient reports recurrently experiencing a major affect or sensation that is troublesome in the present. Under hypnosis, the affect or sensation is heightened by suggestion until it blots out other aspects of the situation. The patient is then taken backwards as in age regression, except that the therapist allows the patient to choose the termination point. For example, if the troublesome somatic symptom is a sensation of queasy nausea that overwhelms the patient without a clear precipitating stimulus, the therapist will heighten this experience by suggestion and then move the patient backwards in time over this bridge: "You are going back . . . back . . . back into the past over a bridge of nausea. Everything is changing except the nausea. The nausea remains the same as you become younger and younger. You are going back to the first time that you felt this sensation. Where are you? What is happening?" The therapist does not know the termination point; he or she only indicates a belief that the patient will move back to the original time and place.

The affect bridge, like age regression, can be used with the patient as a whole or with specific alter personalities. Braun (1984c) has described a variant of this procedure in which he allows the affect to change. The therapist may begin by tracing back anger and finding an event where it changes into fear; this new affect is then traced backwards in the same manner. Allowing the affect to change often leads to a better understanding of the interconnection of the complex, multilevel affects associated with specific traumatic events. Tracing affects or somatic sensations, which are often uncoupled from recall of events and segregated in specific alter personalities, aids in the unification of emotions and memories necessary for the integration of MPD patients.

Multilevel Hypnosis

It is widely acknowledged that MPD subjects are "naturals" at hypnosis and readily enter into deep trance. Multilevel hypnosis takes advantage of this capacity by inducing trance at several levels in the personality system (Braun, 1984c). In a typical application of multilevel hypnosis, the host personality undergoes an induction, and an alter personality is elicited. This alter then undergoes a second hypnotic induction. This method of induction for the alter personality can be the same as for the host or can take advantage of special prearranged cue words specific to that alter. Multilevel hypnosis is useful for working with individual alter personalities in combination with techniques such as the age regression and affect bridge procedures described above. It is important to terminate trance in the *reverse* order in which it was induced (i.e., the alter personality is brought out of trance first, and then the host).

Abreactive/Healing Techniques

For MPD patients, the recovery of hidden memories is usually traumatic. In many instances, the act of remembering will produce a florid abreaction that can cause considerable distress for both patient and therapist. Revivification, the experience of vividly reliving an event, is in some ways more traumatic than the original experience. As many patients have commented to me, remembering is worse than actually being there. I cover the principles of abreaction in more detail later in this chapter. This section deals with specific hypnotherapeutic techniques that can be applied during abreactions and that can promote psychological healing.

Screen Techniques

Screen techniques can help the patient obtain sufficient psychological distance from a traumatic event, while at the same time being able to see, relive, and describe the experience. The patient or specific alter personality is helped into trance and asked to visualize a huge screen. This can be a movie screen, a television screen, or even a section of clear blue sky that acts like a screen. The events or experiences that need to be explored are projected onto this screen so that the patient can watch them from a distance with a sense of detachment. Events seen on this screen can be slowed down, speeded up, reversed, or frozen by suggestion as needed. The screen can even be split or subdivided so that more than one event can be viewed simultaneously, if this is necessary. The patient can also be instructed to zoom in on details, or zoom back and pan for a larger perspective. This repertoire of camera techniques greatly facilitates the recovery of memories by allowing the patient to "see" more than would be possible from a single point of view.

Screen techniques work well in conjunction with age regression or the affect bridge for the exploration of potentially traumatic experiences. When an abreaction is triggered, the therapist reminds the patient to keep the experience up on the screen, where it can be viewed and described. Often the patient mentally splits at this point, with one part of him or her reliving the experience in a visceral way while another part views it on the screen and is able to give a detached commentary on the events. Sometimes the patient is not able to keep the memories up on the screen, and the experience degenerates into an unstructured abreaction. With practice and persistence, however, patient and therapist can use such screen techniques to great advantage in the recovery and integration of traumatic memories. In many instances, patients learn to use screen techniques to continue abreactive work outside of therapy sessions. This is an important ability, because most MPD patients have such an extensive history of terror and trauma that if they were not able to continue abreactive work outside of sessions, their treatment would be prolonged for many additional years.

Permissive Amnesia

Permissive amnesia is a useful technique for the titration of painful memories and affects recovered during hypnotic explorations and abreactions. In some cases, the patient or host personality cannot bear the full brunt of the recovered traumas without becoming acutely self-destructive or transiently psychotic. When traumatic material is recovered in a hypnotic state, the therapist can give the patient, the host personality, specific alter personalities, or the personality system as a whole permission to remember only as much of the material as can be tolerated. The therapist may also suggest that the recovered memories can "trickle" back slowly at a rate that the patient can absorb and process. In this manner, the full content of a recovered memory can be built up in the patient's awareness over a period of hours to months.

Patients seem to be intrinsically capable of regulating this seepage of traumatic material so that the pain, horror, revulsion, and sadness are bearable. During the period when traumatic material is entering into a patient's conscious awareness, there may be such transient reactions as catatonia, strong emotional responses, miniabreactions, and suicidal/homicidal ideation. The therapist and significant others need to be sensitive to this process and alert to potential problems caused by these transient reactions.

Symptom Substitution

Symptom substitution can sometimes be useful in defusing dangerous or self-destructive behavior. The therapist, using hypnotic suggestion, replaces the dangerous behavior with one that is symbolically equivalent but not harmful. For example, Kluft (1983) describes transforming a physical struggle between two alters, each controlling a flailing arm, into a fight between the patient's nondominant fourth and fifth fingers.

One can use hypnotic suggestion to put some alters to sleep in order to weather a specific crisis, or to leave them in a fantasized safe place. A number of multiples whom I know spontaneously use the latter metaphor whenever they come to participate in research projects, leaving their alters who would be frightened or do not wish to participate in the research at home or in an imaginary safe place. When using hypnotic suggestion to send an alter to a safe place, it is important to enlist the patient's personality system in defining that place. MPD therapists must come to know the topography of the patient's internal world and draw on this knowledge for therapeutic metaphors and interventions. As noted earlier, one should not forcibly suppress or "bury" troublesome alters. Kluft (1982) has reported that in his experience, attempts at hypnotic extrusion or suppression of troublesome alter personalities may produce temporary relief through the transient suppression of a difficult alter, but may extract a painful price when the alter retaliates at a later date.

Age Progression

Age progression techniques are useful in the "growing up" of infant and child alter personalities after therapeutic work has been accomplished with them. Via hypnotic suggestion, the infant or child alter can be helped to grow older. The amount of age progression depends on the goals of each specific intervention. Frequently age progression is used to help alters "grow up" prior to their fusion with other personalities. Various metaphors or images can be used to help the alter progress in time. Kluft (1982, 1984b) describes using "time machine" fantasies in the age progression of alter personalities. Other metaphors or images, such as riding along a river through time, flipping calendar pages, or speeding days and nights, are equally useful if the personality being age-progressed finds them compelling. In this technique, as is true in most instances, allowing the personality to make suggestions or collaborate in creating the image or metaphor used greatly enhances the power of the hypnotic intervention.

Autohypnosis

The relationship of the dissociative process in MPD to that seen in self-induced hypnosis or autohypnosis has been a matter of conjecture for over 100 years. Autohypnosis, irrespective of its relationship to the larger dissociative process in MPD, is a technique that can be used to help the patient increase control over his or her life. Autohypnosis is most commonly employed for symptom control. Caul (1978b) describes teaching autohypnosis to his patients so that they may enter into trance and trigger prearranged hypnotic suggestions to terminate or control anxiety attacks or psychosomatic symptoms. In addition, he describes using this technique to facilitate dental analgesia with a multiple who was unable to tolerate conventional anesthesia. Braun (1980) and Kluft (1982) also describe teaching patients self-hypnosis for symptom control or to facilitate inner dialogue.

Some difficulties with self-hypnosis have been reported. Kluft (1982) describes the use of autohypnosis as a resistance to treatment in three patients. One patient used autohypnosis to block therapy; another used it to avoid conflict; and a third caused problems by creating a new personality based on the therapist. Miller (1984) has also described the use of autohypnosis to block fusion and avoid anxiety. As mentioned previously, one therapist in the Washington MPD study group has reported that her patient used autohypnosis to undo hypnotic suggestions made by the therapist. Because of this potential for misuse, Kluft (1982) recommends that autohypnosis not be taught to a patient until the therapeutic alliance "is solid and has already weathered strenuous testing" (p. 237).

Facilitation of Coconsciousness

Hypnosis can be used to facilitate coconsciousness, which most authorities believe to be a necessary precondition for successful fusion/integration, as well as being extremely important in promoting day-to-day cooperation within an unintegrated multiple personality system. "Coconsciousness," a term coined by Morton Prince (1906), is a state of awareness in which one personality is able to directly experience the thoughts, feelings, and actions of another alter (Kluft, 1984c). Caul (1978b) reports that coconsciousness can be facilitated by placing the patient in a trance, directly addressing the targeted alters, and instructing them to blot out all issues and distractions except this process. The therapist then suggests that the alters will become aware of each other and that they will be able to see and hear all of the things that any one of them sees or hears. The therapist can suggest that during times of minimal stress, they will continue to maintain this coconscious state. Caul (1978b) cautions that this procedure is not always predictable and may result in increased anxiety due to the loss of amnesic barriers among alters. He concludes, however, that when used as the therapy approaches a resolution of multiplicity, this technique can result in significant benefit for the patient.

Deep Trance

Deep trance appears to have a nonspecific healing effect in MPD patients, as well as increasing the porosity of the amnesic barriers (Kluft, 1982). Both Kluft (1982) and Braun (1984c) refer to early unpublished work in this area by Margaretta Bowers. Bliss (1980) also reports MPD patients describing the good feelings induced by deep trance experiences. Braun (1984c) describes placing the patient into deep trance and increasing the depth of trance over time. The patient is told that the mind will remain blank until a prearranged signal is heard. Kluft (1982) specifies that this deep trance experience must be shared by all of the personalities. I have found deep trance experiences to be soothing and healing in patients with and without MPD.

ABREACTION

An abreaction is defined as follows:

> Emotional release or discharge after recalling a painful experience that
> has been repressed because it was consciously intolerable. A therapeu-
> tic effect sometimes occurs through partial discharge of desensitization
> of the painful emotions and increased insight. (American Psychiatric
> Association, 1980b, p. 1)

The term "abreaction" dates from the earliest work of Breuer and Freud
on hysteria, when they observed that patients were helped by "just talking
it out" (Shorvon & Sargant, 1947, p. 47). Later they used this process in
combination with hypnosis to facilitate an emotional catharsis (Breuer &
Freud, 1895/1957). shortly after the publication of *Studies on Hysteria*,
Freud rejected the use of hypnosis in favor of free association and the
psychoanalytic technique.

During World War I, however, it rapidly became apparent that
abreaction was an important therapeutic tool for the treatment of "shell
shock" or acute traumatic neuroses (Shorvon & Sargant, 1947). Culpin
(1931) observed:

> Once a man's conscious resistance to discussing his war experience
> was overcome, great mental relief followed the pouring out of emo-
> tionally charged incidents. It was as if the emotion pent up by this
> conscious resistance had by its tension given rise to symptoms. The
> memory, usually of a nature unsuspected by me, then came to the
> surface, its return being preceded perhaps by congestion of the face,
> pressing of the hands to the face, tremblings, and other bodily signs of
> emotion. (p. 27)

Culpin noted that although the details of an event may be remembered,
the emotional content is often split off and repressed. It is the latter that
must be recovered and re-experienced to produce therapeutic benefit.

Following the end of World War I, abreaction as a therapeutic tool
declined in popularity. During the 1930s, Blackwenn and others in the
United States pioneered the use of sodium amytal and related drugs in
conjunction with psychotherapy (Shorvon & Sargant, 1947). Their work
received little attention until the outbreak of World War II, when Sargant and Slater (1941) first reported on the value of drug-facilitated
abreaction in the treatment of psychiatric casualties following the evacu-
ation of British troops from Dunkirk. Many of these soldiers suffered
from amnesias and gross conversion symptoms. Grinker and Spiegel

(1943) also made significant contributions to the use of drug-facilitated abreaction, which they called "narcosynthesis," during the North African campaign. These dramatic successes quickly led to the widespread adoption of drug-facilitated therapeutic abreaction for the treatment of psychiatric casualties in all combat theaters.

Following World War II, attempts were made to apply wartime experiences with drug-facilitated abreactions to a wide variety of psychiatric conditions, without notable success (Kolb, 1985). The abreactive treatment of chronic posttraumatic stress reactions, such as those found in victims of the Holocaust, was also largely unsuccessful (Kolb, 1985). These failures, together with work by Redlich *et al.* (1951), which cast doubt on the veracity of material recovered during drug-facilitated recall, led to a virtual abandonment of abreactive therapeutic work for several decades. Kolb (1985) has recently reintroduced drug-facilitated abreactions in the treatment of chronic posttraumatic stress disorder in Vietnam veterans, and the Israeli success with abreactions in short-term psychotherapy of acute stress reactions (Maoz & Pincus, 1979) has led to renewed interest in this therapeutic tool. The value (and inevitability) of abreaction in the treatment of MPD has also led to a resurgence of interest in the therapeutic uses of abreaction.

This section focuses on the principles, techniques, indications, and contraindications of therapeutic abreaction, with special attention to unique aspects and issues raised in the treatment of MPD and related major dissociative disorders.

Principles of Therapeutic Abreactions

Spontaneous abreactions or abreaction-like phenomena are common in victims of trauma. The most familiar examples are the "flashbacks" seen in combat veterans, but similar phenomena have been reported in association with victims of many other forms of trauma, including natural disasters, brutal crimes such as assault and rape, fires, airplane crashes, and automobile accidents. Blank (1985) identifies four types of intrusive recall in posttraumatic stress disorder: (1) vivid dreams and nightmares of the traumatic events; (2) vivid dreams from which the dreamer awakens still under the influence of the dream content and has difficulty making contact with reality; (3) conscious flashbacks, in which the subject experiences intrusive recall of traumatic events, accompanied by vivid multimodal hallucinations, and may or may not lose contact with reality; and (4) unconscious flashbacks, in which the individual has a sudden, discrete experience that leads to an action that recreates or repeats a traumatic event, but the subject does not have any awareness at the time or later of the connection between this action and the past trauma.

All of these four forms of intrusive recall are typically present and active in MPD patients. Flashback and intrusive-recall phenomena are often responsible for the regressed and psychotic-like behavior witnessed at times in MPD patients. The spontaneous, uncontrolled, and largely unconscious nature of these abreaction-like phenomena prevent or impede any emotional relief that might occur from the discharge of memory and affect accompanying the flashback. The therapist and patient must learn to induce, control, and process these experiences if the patient is to derive therapeutic benefits from abreactive episodes.

Induction of Abreactions

The induction or initiation of an abreaction is triggered by the recall of suppressed, repressed, or dissociated memories and affects. As discussed above, this process frequently occurs spontaneously in victims of trauma. Spontaneous abreactions can be utilized for therapeutic purposes by an alert therapist. In addition, many MPD patients can learn to use spontaneous abreactions occurring outside therapy to do self-healing work. In general, however, in the early stages of treatment, more work can be done and fewer complications ensue when the patient and therapist work together to elicit and process a controlled abreaction.

Externally Cued Abreactions

Recall of traumatic material that is wholly or partially out of conscious awareness can be facilitated and controlled by a variety of techniques. The power of external cues to trigger vivid recall has long been recognized by clinicians and has been utilized in both therapy and experimental studies of the neurophysiology of abreaction (Putnam, 1988c). The external cues may be sights, sounds, smells, behaviors, or any combination thereof. In many instances, the cues are normal, everyday objects or experiences that appear to be innocuous to an observer. The power of external cues to cause discomfort and trigger intrusive recall may produce avoidance and phobic behavior in trauma victims. Sounds and smells are particularly potent triggers and are more difficult to avoid. For Vietnam veterans, helicopter noise, increasingly common in major urban areas, is frequently mentioned as an unpredictable trigger of flashback experiences (Sonnenberg et al., 1985).

Therapists have long learned to exploit the effects of cued recall for therapeutic purposes. Janet used to provide external cues or play roles to facilitate induction of abreaction in his patients (Ellenberger, 1970). Maoz and Pincus (1979) describe the utilization of sound effects (e.g., bombing) in facilitating recall. They also describe allowing the therapist to become a participant in the "drama of battle" by playing the role of a comrade or officer. They found that the "mere mention" of relevant cues was often sufficient to reactivate repressed traumas. In MPD patients, the effect of an external cue is frequently to trigger the emergence of a specific alter personality who embodies the traumatic material. This alter will usually vividly relive the traumatic experience. In some instances, a group of alters will relive the experience simultaneously.

External cues are most useful for the induction of abreaction in cases where they are highly situation-specific, relatively commonly experienced, or associated with traumatic experiences. In multiples, external cues tend to be highly idiosyncratic and can be unreliable and unpredictable. They are most useful in situations where there is a specific phobia or avoidance behavior that needs to be worked with. Externally cued abreactions will, however, occur spontaneously in therapy with multiples from time to time. The patient may see an object in the room, or the therapist may unknowingly use a cue word, assume an expression or posture, or otherwise provide an unintentional cue to the patient. Abreactions triggered in this fashion can be disconcerting for therapists, who at some level recognize their role in precipitating such patients' distress.

Abreactions Induced via Suggestion

Once an appropriate therapeutic context has been established (e.g., the creation of a hypnotic viewing screen and the identification of alters to observe and report what they see), suggestion, combined with hypnosis or drug facilitation, is a more controllable stimulus for triggering and structuring abreactive recall in MPD patients. Specific experiences or periods of the patient's life can be targeted for therapeutic work and approached in a directed fashion. Age regression techniques are useful in this context, because they allow the therapist to take the patient back to a moment in time preceding an event, to establish some form of psychological distance for the patient (e.g., using the screen techniques described earlier), and then to proceed with a sequential revivification of the trauma. This structuring of the abreactive experience allows both patient and therapist to exert more control over a powerful psychophysiological process. Structure and control enhance the feeling of safety for both patient and therapist and will increase the willingness of all parties to do further abreactive work. This structuring also facilitates a more coherent recovery of traumas, which aids in the psychotherapeutic processing and integration of this material.

HYPNOSIS-FACILITATED ABREACTIONS

Hypnosis and the use of drug-induced relaxed states of consciousness are the therapeutic modalities most frequently used to structure abreactions. Therapists working with MPD patients strongly favor the use of hypnosis over drug induction (Putnam *et al.*, 1986). Hypnosis can be rapidly induced in cooperative MPD subjects, does not have any medical contraindications, and is readily structured. Drug-facilitated abreactions, on the other hand, usually require medical/anesthesia backup; they may be contraindicated in certain medical conditions; and the patient's level of alertness can be difficult to control, with excessive sedation often interfering with the conscious processing phase of the abreaction. Rosen and Myers (1947) have compared the results of hypnotically induced and drug-facilitated abreactions in a military setting and concluded that hypnosis is the method of choice, except in rare instances where the individual is unusually resistant or medical–legal reasons preclude the use of hypnosis.

Under hypnosis, abreactions can be elicited in MPD patients by a number of hypnotherapeutic techniques. Not infrequently, simply using hypnosis to contact and bring out specific alter personalities is all that is required to initiate an abreaction. Age regression and affect bridge techniques, discussed earlier in this chapter, are also highly successful avenues for exploring traumatic material and triggering therapeutic abreactions. Other hypnotherapeutic techniques can then be used to help structure the recovery of traumatic material and to reintegrate this material into the patient's larger awareness.

DRUG-FACILITATED ABREACTIONS

Drug-facilitated abreactions have been used since the work of Hurst and his colleagues with "etherization" of hysterical conversion symptoms during World War I (Shorvon & Sargant, 1947). They can be rapidly induced (under battlefield conditions if needed) and do not require the level of trust or rapport necessary for hypnotic work. Sodium amytal and sodium pentothal are the most commonly used medications, though a wide range of drugs have been reported to be capable of inducing abreactions. Horsley (1943) coined the term "narcoanalysis" for treatment using drugs. Other terms to describe this process that are used more or less synonymously in the literature include "narcosynthesis," "narcosuggestion," and "narcocatharsis."

Sodium amytal is reported to have a wider range between the therapeutic effects and sedative effects than sodium pentothal, and therefore allows better control of the depth of sedation. It is also longer-acting and may interfere with the processing phase of the abreaction (Walker, 1982). Sodium pentothal, on the other hand, has a faster onset of action, a shorter duration of effect, and less postabreaction sedation (Walker, 1982). Porphyria is an absolute contraindication to the use of these drugs, and severe cardiac, respiratory, liver, or kidney disease or barbiturate addiction are relative contraindications (Marcos & Trujillo, 1978). Horsley (1943) reports a mortality rate of zero in over 2000 interviews, and Hart *et al.* (1945) report only 1 instance of respiratory arrest, due to too rapid administration, in 500 interviews.

Induction is by intravenous drip or infusion into a superficial arm or hand vein of a reclining patient. Marcos and Trujillo (1978) recommend a 21-gauge butterfly needle with a 10% solution containing 500 mg of sodium amytal in distilled water. Perry and Jacobs (1982) recommend a 5% solution of sodium amytal. The rate of injection is 1 cc per minute for the first 2 minutes, and then the rate is varied according to the patient's response. Typically, 400 mg is sufficient, and 1 gram is the usual maximum upper limit for a successful interview (Marcos & Trujillo, 1978; Perry & Jacobs, 1982). The drug is usually administered until sustained, rapid lateral nystagmus is noted or drowsiness occurs. A mild slurring of speech may be noticeable at this point. The usual dose required to achieve this level is 150–350 mg of sodium amytal (Perry & Jacobs, 1982). The patient should not be allowed to become so drowsy that it is difficult to make contact. After a suitable lowering of consciousness is achieved, this level is maintained by infusing 25–50 mg of sodium amytal approximately every 5 minutes.

The interview is usually divided into an introductory phase, during which the clinician begins with reassuring remarks, suggestions that the patient will soon feel like talking, and neutral questions as the needle is inserted and the infusion is begun. The exploratory phase follows after the patient has reached a suitable twilight state of consciousness. The patient can be taken back to the past by age regression, and exploration is begun. The therapist should approach affect-laden or traumatic material gradually, working through a traumatic episode several times to recover additional details. During the recovery of traumatic material, the therapist can work with the patient on two levels, the past and the present. The therapist helps the patient re-experience and work through the feelings of pain, anger, guilt, horror, shame, fear, isolation, hopelessness, and helplessness evoked by the past experience, and provides support and reassurance in the here-and-now (Maoz & Pincus, 1979).

Typical drug-facilitated interviews/abreactions last 30–60 minutes and are terminated when sufficient material has been uncovered to occupy one or more waking psychotherapy sessions. In the termination phase of the interview, the patient is "accompanied" back to a state of full alertness and awareness of the present place and time (Maoz & Pincus, 1979). The therapist may also include remarks and suggestions that the uncovered material will be processed more completely in the following psychotherapy sessions, as well as supportive and encouraging remarks. The patient should remain reclining for 15 minutes or more until he or she can walk with close supervision (Perry & Jacobs, 1982). The processing of the recovered material in psychotherapy is mandatory for therapeutic benefit and is discussed below.

Regression/Revivification

Irrespective of the method of induction, regression and revivification are almost inevitable concomitants of abreactions. The regression is secondary to a number of factors. Trauma that overwhelms normal psychological defenses tends to produce behavioral regression in most individuals. In MPD patients, the trauma usually occurred during early to middle childhood, so that alter personalities created to absorb this trauma are frequently frozen at the age a patient was at the time the trauma occurred. It is often these child and infant alters who are activated by the abreaction and who behave in a fashion that appears to be markedly regressed for an adult. Age regression and other techniques used in the induction of abreactions also promote behavioral regression in the most hypnotically susceptible subjects, even in the absence of trauma.

The differentiation between the beneficial regression associated with therapeutic abreaction and pathological regression can be difficult to make at times. In doing narcoanalytic work with soldiers suffering combat reactions during the 1973 Arab–Israeli war, Maoz and Pincus (1979) found several cases who displayed repetitive "regressive behavior," such as infantile crying or self-pity, which tended to become fixed without any further progress in treatment. In these instances, the authors discontinued the narcoanalytic sessions. I have also found that fixity of repetitive regressed behavior, together with an absence of therapeutic progress, is a reasonable indicator of pathological regression. One must be careful, however, not to judge regressed behavior as pathological too soon. Many traumatic experiences require repeated abreactions to uncover the full extent of the patient's ordeal and to discharge multilayered affects. If, however, a therapist repeatedly finds that a given alter becomes stuck in a stereotypic regressed state without recovery of additional material, it is best to plumb the system for other alters who may provide the insight necessary to work through the traumatic experience.

Revivification, the vivid reliving of past experiences, is a hallmark of abreaction. The clinical literature on abreaction, flashbacks, and post-traumatic stress disorder is filled with vignettes illustrating the graphic reliving of past traumatic episodes experienced by victims. Confusion between the past and present is common during these episodes, although some patients report reliving the event on a split screen, with one half in the past and the other in the present. The vividness of these experiences is due to the multisensory hallucinatory and illusory phenomena that accompany them. The individual may see, hear, feel, smell, and taste the past experience. An abreacting individual can also incorporate surrounding objects and people into the abreaction. Having once narrowly escaped the murderous assault of a former long-range reconnaissance patrol leader, who mistook me for one of his North Vietnamese captors and the tile-floored, cabinet-lined Veterans Administration examination room for his bamboo-barred jungle prison camp, I can testify to the ability of an abreacting individual to incorporate present surroundings into the site of past terror.

The affects that accompany an abreaction can be equally vivid and intense. They have all of the freshness of the traumatic moment and are concentrated by years of repression and dissociation. In my judgment, it is the re-experiencing of these affects rather than the contents of the memory that most patients, whether or not they have MPD, find so painful. In some instances, recall of the details of a traumatic event has been consciously available to the individual for some time, and the affects associated with the event are what must be uncovered and abreacted before therapeutic progress can be made. The expression of these affects can be explosive and frightening for patient and therapist. When traumatic material is close to conscious awareness, the patient may immediately enter into an abreaction with hypnotic or drug-facilitated induction. In my experience, this happens more often with the latter. The instantaneous appearance of an intense affect, particularly when it is not clearly related to current circumstances, should alert the therapist to the possibility that the patient has entered into an abreaction.

Recovery of Traumatic Material

The recovery of dissociated and repressed memories and affects is necessary so that this material may be worked through by the patient on several levels. Patient and therapist must work together to structure the abreactive process so that the appropriate material is recovered in a form that can be processed in psychotherapy. There are a number of principles or suggestions that can aid in the structuring of these experiences.

In most instances, it is useful for the abreactive process to have a beginning, middle, and end, and for these points to lie along the temporal sequence of the traumatic experience. Of course, nothing as complex as an abreaction is necessarily going to run a simple linear time course! In addition to the confusion between past and present, the patient will jump around in time within the past. MPD patients may rapidly switch among several alters who are all connected to the traumatic experience in some fashion. Each alter may believe that he or she is in a different time and place. A patient may also jump around and abreact other traumatic experiences that are thematically connected with the targeted traumatic experience. This has been noted in combat veterans, who may abreact prewar trauma while undergoing treatment for combat-related stress reactions.

Yet the therapist must do what he or she can to move the patient through the reliving experience in as sequential a manner as possible. Part of the reason why the spontaneous flashbacks experienced by a trauma victim are ineffective in discharging the traumatic episode is that the victim tends to pop in and out of the flashback but is not able to work through the experience from beginning to end in a more linear fashion. It is my experience that more linearly experienced abreactions are more easily worked with in psychotherapy and more easily integrated into conscious awareness by the patient.

A therapist can help structure the linearity of an abreaction by age-regressing the patient to a point before the trauma and moving forward in time from there. Unfortunately, the therapist often does not know where one trauma begins or another ends. Still, the patient generally can manage to find this point if directed to go back to "just before the event happened." The therapist can then have the patient "look around" and describe the place, the circumstances, and himself or herself (i.e., how old the patient is, what he or she is doing, etc.). This helps orient both the patient and therapist and establishes a jumping-off point. The therapist then can ask the patient to move forward in time, while watching and describing the events on a mental screen. If the patient jumps around in time or the therapist becomes confused about what is happening, the therapist can tell the patient to "freeze" the action and to describe the circumstances. It may be helpful to have the patient "zoom back" or "zoom in" and scan the frozen moment, in time to better orient himself or herself and the therapist.

The therapist should try to stay oriented to the time, place, and circumstances of the abreaction. Sometimes this is just not possible. Within a single session, it is often useful to go through the abreactive sequence several times. The patient may be instructed to view each pass through the trauma from another perspective or camera angle. In multiples, different personalities can make separate passes through the sequence of events. With each pass, the therapist and patient will gather new details, and contradictory perceptions and emotions will begin to emerge. The therapist should pay close attention to any points where the linearity of the time line is disturbed. If the patient suddenly jumps to a later point, says that things are "difficult to see" or the "screen goes blank," or gives other evidence of a break in the continuity of sequence, the therapist should note this point and return to it again in the next pass through the sequence of events. Breaks in the continuity of an abreactive experience generally indicate a deeper level of trauma that may be further suppressed, repressed, or dissociated.

The observation that repeated abreaction is often necessary for the full uncovering of traumatic material has been repeatedly reported in the literature on treatment of combat-related casualties (Rosen & Myers, 1947; Shorvon & Sargant, 1947; Walker, 1982). Kluft (1982) has extended this observation to MPD patients and states, "A single intervention (abreaction), no matter how intense or prolonged, rarely allowed sufficient ventilation and relief. Sometimes several personalities had separate abreactive experiences of the same event or affect" (p. 235). The therapist and patient may have to repeatedly abreact a given experience in a number of separate sessions, interspersed with psychotherapy focused on the material that was recovered. Often it is only during the integrative psychotherapy phase following an abreaction that the therapist or the patient first becomes aware of a gap or discontinuity that indicates missed material.

Abreactions must be allowed to run their full course whenever possible. An abreaction that is interrupted in midstream by the therapist or by an external distraction will often resume with full intensity later at an inopportune moment. This may cause serious problems for the patient, and even when it does not, it will heighten the patient's natural resistance toward uncovering traumatic material. Unfortunately, abreactions do not fit neatly into a 50-minute psychotherapy hour. Even when the abreaction has run its full course one or more times within a session, the patient is likely to experience aftershocks of miniabreactions, flashbacks, intrusive imagery, and traumatic nightmares. Such is the nature of the process.

Intuitively, patients know that once they let the traumatic material out, it is difficult or impossible to completely re-repress it. There is now a hole in the dike, and incompletely abreacted or additional dissociated traumatic material will continue to leak into conscious awareness. The therapist should anticipate this process and prepare the patient. Patients should be told to use the screen techniques that they have already learned to observe and take note of any flashbacks or intrusive recall, so that this material can be brought back to the next therapy session.

Repeated abreaction of a given traumatic event will produce contradiction. The patient may relate very different versions of the same event and express widely divergent emotions. In MPD patients, different alters will often embody these contradictory perceptions. In some cases, specific events or specific versions of an event will have clear fantasy components; in many other cases, the therapist and patient will never be sure what actually occurred and what was fantasy. I do not know of any way to sort out truth from fantasy in these cases. One may argue that "it is all real to the patient" and therefore the actual veracity does not matter, but as Maoz and Pincus (1979) observed in their abreactive work with Israeli soldiers, "there are times when it seemed to be of prime importance to ascertain the truth" (p. 95). When contradiction does occur, it is important to focus on it during the integrative psychotherapeutic processing of the abreactive material. The understanding and resolution of contradictions are often instrumental in the patient's acceptance and integration of the uncovered material.

Termination of Abreactions

The process of terminating an abreaction depends in part upon the technique used to initiate it. In drug-facilitated abreactions, the termination is initiated by stopping the infusion and allowing metabolism to lower the drug level to the point where the patient becomes fully conscious and is able to walk without help. Some advocates of amytal-facilitated interviews suggest that the patient be given an extra bolus of medication at the termination to induce sleep (Marcos & Trujillo, 1978). In most instances, I think that this is not useful; rather, it is preferable to bring the patient back to a fully waking state, to aid in the conscious retention of material recovered during the interview.

In hypnotically induced abreactions, the therapist must remove the hypnotic state in the reverse of the order in which it was induced. If the patient was first hypnotized, and then a specific alter was elicited, hypnotized, and then age-regressed, the termination should be effected by age-progressing the alter to the present, ending the alter's trance, and then ending the patient's trance. Permissive amnesia or other posthypnotic suggestions may be made before the termination of trance with the alter, host, other personalities, or some combination of alters. After an abreaction, I usually terminate hypnosis by bringing the patient out of trance slowly, using a reversal of whatever metaphor or image was used to deepen the trance. Although some therapists unfamiliar with hypnosis worry that the patient will become "stuck" in trance or locked into an interminable abreaction, this does not happen.

As the patient returns to waking consciousness, the therapist should deliberately and repeatedly orient him or her to place and time and to situation (i.e., the fact that the patient has just had an abreactive experience). The therapist should also ask the patient about what he or she is feeling at that moment. Abreactions often leave strong residual affects, and taking some time to identify and process these will aid the patient in achieving the necessary closure. Ideally, there should be sufficient time left in a session after an abreaction to orient and ground the patient in the present, identify residual affects, and do some preliminary processing of the recovered material. The last may be postponed until the next session, but the reorientation, grounding, and identification of residual affects are absolutely necessary to achieve sufficient closure to allow the patient to re-enter day-to-day existence without significant disruption. Adequate closure is often overlooked by neophyte therapists who may feel overwhelmed by the intensity of an abreactive experience. It is, however, essential to the therapeutic effects of an abreaction, and failure to provide adequate closure will heighten resistance to further abreactive work.

Reintegration of Abreacted Material

The need for ongoing, concomitant psychotherapy to process material recovered through abreaction has long been recognized by virtually all clinicians working in the area (Rosen & Myers, 1947). Grinker and Spiegel (1943) stated, "The idea that narcosis therapy or any form of abreaction is all that is necessary for the treatment of acute war neuroses is erroneous, as proven by the fact that if nothing else is done for the patient he relapses. . . . Psychotherapy must be instituted as soon as possible" (p. 23). The role of integrative psychotherapy, while first recognized in the context of drug-facilitated abreactive work, has been incorporated and extended by clinicians doing hypnotherapy with Vietnam veterans (Brende & Benedict, 1980; Spiegel, 1981). If traumatic material, relived through abreaction, is not brought into waking conscious awareness within a short time after the abreactive experience, much of it will be redissociated, re-repressed, or otherwise blocked from conscious recall.

The therapist can aid the patient in recalling this highly charged material in a number of ways. The first and perhaps most important intervention is to help the patient organize the material into some sort of coherent form. The attempt to provide a time line, discussed above, is one example of a therapeutic structural intervention that can help the patient organize the material for future waking recall. This will work with some patients but not all. Different organizing structures—perhaps based on affect bridges, for example—may be more useful in some cases. In MPD, patient and therapist will get a lot of practice in doing abreactive work together, and over time they can hit upon some individualized solutions to minimize their mutual discomfort and maximize the results.

Many therapists have independently initiated the use of audio- or videotaping to provide direct feedback to the patient of material recovered during an abreaction. Hall *et al.* (1978) first described this approach in their single case study; subsequently, David Caul (1984) has creatively expanded the use of videotaping in the treatment of MPD. As with many other techniques for the treatment of MPD, the empirical proof of videotaping's clinical efficacy rests on its independent discovery and widespread adoption by therapists with vastly differing professional orientations (Putnam, 1986b).

"Permission to feel" is also a therapeutic intervention that aids in the integration of affects and somatic sensations. In many instances, painful injuries were inflicted on the person during abuse or other traumatic events, but the physical pain from these experiences was dissociated and not fully felt at the time. Later this dissociated pain may resurface in the form of psychosomatic complaints or be triggered in therapy (Brende & Benedict, 1980). Similarly, powerful affects such as fear, rage, helplessness, and hopelessness were also generated by the events but dissociated, so that they were not directly experienced at the time, but later periodically surface in response to life stresses. During the abreactive episode, the therapist should help the patient "feel" these dissociated affects and physical sensations. This can be done by simply inquiring periodically during the abreaction about what the patient is feeling, in addition to asking for the details of the experience. The therapist should make every effort to help the patient recover, re-experience, and reintegrate split-off affects and somatic sensations, as these are probably the most potent sources of everyday discomfort and dissociative behavior.

The therapist can help the patient reintegrate repressed or dissociated material by working through in psychotherapy the contradictory versions that arise when a traumatic experience is abreacted several times. In some instances, the patient may have told the therapist one version of the events in therapy and revealed a very different version during an abreaction. The "same" event, when abreacted by several alter personalities of an MPD patient, will typically be experienced very differently. For example, an episode of incest was experienced by several alters as a brutal rape, by one alter as if it were happening to an unknown person, and by one alter as an expression of paternal affection. As long as such an experience has several unintegrated representations for the patient, it cannot be accepted and worked through.

The therapist must help the patient recognize the simultaneity and validity of mutually exclusive representations, and must work with the patient toward a resolution of the contradictions. The alters must hear one another's versions of the events and come to accept in a nonjudgmental way that each version has its own validity, and that these separate versions can be collated into a larger understanding of the event without denying the specific experiences of any alter. The lines of internal communication must be well developed within the personality system before the give-and-take among alters that is necessary to effect an integration of traumatic material can occur. This is one reason why a premature attempt to work with abreactive material is usually ineffective.

Resistance to Abreactive Work

Uncovering work, such as therapeutic abreaction, naturally elicits a high level of resistance to treatment in MPD patients. A patient's personality system of dissociated traumatic memories and painful affects exists as a global defense against conscious awareness of these experiences. All of the usual defense mechanisms that serve to keep unacceptable material out of consciousness are present, and additional phenomena unique to MPD are also active (e.g., persecutor personalities who punish the host for revealing "secrets").

The patient's concerns and fears of abandonment by the therapist, which are already at a high level, become greatly magnified when the therapy moves into more active uncovering work. This is understandable in the context of the typical patient's childhood history, during which the patient was abandoned to neglect and abuse by his or her caretakers. Consequently, the patient's sensitivity toward rejection and abandonment will markedly increase during this phase of therapy. Once the abreactive work has begun in earnest, most patients are terrified that the therapist is going to leave them to re-experience these traumas in the same awful isolation that accompanied them originally. For this reason and others, most multiples will not allow serious uncovering work to begin until they have tested the therapist's commitment many times. The usual scenarios that stir up feelings of rejection and abandonment (e.g., vacations) can be expected to have an increased effect during this phase of treatment. They must be anticipated and worked with by the therapist.

The incomplete abreaction of traumatic material has been cited by many authorities as a major cause of failure of therapeutic abreaction (Kline, 1976; Kluft, 1982; Maoz & Pincus, 1979; Rosen & Myers, 1947; Shorvon & Sargant, 1947). Signs and symptoms indicating a failure to completely abreact a traumatic incident include the following: (1) gaps in continuity of the conscious recall of the episode; (2) intense abreactions, flashbacks, and intrusive recall of the incident occurring outside of therapy; (3) failure in psychotherapy to work through contradictory versions of the event; (4) failure of partial integrations involving personalities containing the incompletely abreacted material; and (5) increased resistance to doing further abreactive work. When a therapist suspects that there may be an incomplete abreaction, he or she should carefully work through the event step by step with the patient, looking for incongruities, discontinuities, intense affects without a clear relationship to content, and other signs of hidden material. This can first be done in the integrative psychotherapy of the incident and then followed up with additional abreactive sessions if necessary.

The sheer volume of trauma sustained by the typical MPD patient also affects the patient's level of resistance. Once uncovering work has begun to open the closed doors, the patient will have increased difficulty in keeping painful material out of conscious awareness. This process seems to gather a momentum of its own; it often begins to breach repressive and dissociative barriers at inopportune times and to create significant problems in the patient's daily life. The patient and therapist must strive to find a rate at which the patient can recall and integrate trauma in therapy so that the patient is not left with large amounts of unprocessed material for long periods. Ideally, a balance is achieved between the amount of trauma that the patient can recover and the working through and reintegration of this material.

the Therapist in Abreactive Work

therapist does many things to help a patient, and most of these are ineffable. In working with abreactions, the therapist should be aware of trying to create a situation of safety, support, and structure for the patient. A sense of safety is absolutely necessary before MPD patients will begin serious work. The personality system will test the therapist's commitment, ability to tolerate graphic details of traumatic episodes, and willingness to work with noxious alters in an even-handed fashion before allowing the therapist to dig deeply into the past. The patient must believe that the therapist can keep the situation under control and protect all parties from real harm. The patient must experience the therapist as caring and sensitive to the recovered material and its effects on the patient. Fear of a judgmental response by the therapist fuels resistance to uncovering work, as does confirmation or denial of specific self-representations (particularly confirmation of those with components of shame and humiliation).

The physical setting of the therapy has a great deal of impact on the patient's sense of safety. Privacy must be guaranteed, external intrusions must be minimized, and the environment should not offer any objects that make convenient weapons (e.g., scissors, letter openers) or present dangerous possibilities (e.g., open windows in high-rise buildings). The patient is about to surrender control to powerful forces, and although dangerous acting out is infrequent, many patients are acutely fearful of this possibility. Protector and helper alters should be consulted about safety concerns and solutions early in the course of treatment. Some therapists conduct abreactive work in special settings, such as furniture-free rooms filled with pillows and stuffed animals. Young (1986) describes placing the patient in voluntary restraints to ensure safety. Although I have not worked in such settings, I think that they may be useful with some patients.

In addition to safety and support, the therapist must provide a structure that contains and channels the abreaction for therapeutic purposes. A sequential time line or other framework provides a continuity for the experience and helps ensure that it is more completely discharged. The therapist helps the patient hunt for missing details by orchestrating several passes through the material and stopping and backtracking when evidence of hidden material surfaces. The therapist also aids the patient in moving backward and forward between the past and the present. Abreacting patients, particularly MPD patients, become lost and disoriented and depend on the therapist to ground them at crucial points in the process. Maoz and Pincus (1979) give a description of the process of moving back and forth between the traumatic memories of battle and a therapeutic dialogue in the present during the course of an abreaction. At the end of an abreaction, the therapist reorients the patient and helps him or her achieve a degree of closure necessary to re-enter the here-and-now of daily life.

Should Every Trauma Be Abreacted?

Authorities disagree on whether or not it is necessary to abreact every major trauma. With most MPD patients, it is probably not possible to formally abreact every major trauma in the course of treatment. Many MPD patients will, however, develop the ability to do abreactive work on their own as treatment proceeds. The sheer volume of accumulated trauma in many MPD patients probably precludes the abreaction of every episode. In some instances, abreaction of a single episode or a "generic" episode of a specific form of repetitive abuse may serve to discharge the dissociated material from a series of episodes. Unprocessed or incompletely processed trauma is, however, the main reason for the failure of fusions of alter personalities. My best guess is that a therapist should anticipate having to abreact or otherwise specifically process most of the major trauma experienced by the patient if the patient is to achieve an adequate therapeutic resolution.

SUMMARY

This chapter has focused on using the altered states of consciousness induced by hypnosis or drugs to work with the traumatic affects and memories driving dissociative behavior. It begins by examining commonly expressed fears that hypnosis may "create" MPD, and concludes that there is no evidence to support these concerns. Multiples are, however, widely recognized to be hypnotic virtuosos and often spontaneously move in and out of trance states during therapy, though they may be resistant to suggested formal hypnotic inductions. Formal trance induction is, however, the best way to proceed. The fearful patient can be helped to accept hypnosis if it is offered as a tool and if some benign trance experiences can be provided. Fears about being controlled by hypnosis should be acknowledged, but will not disappear until the patient has experienced formal trance.

Although the manner of induction does not appear to be important, a range of specific trance techniques are recommended for providing benign trance experiences and building rapport. Much of the work in treating MPD revolves around the recovery of dissociated traumas. Hypnosis has proven exceptionally useful in contacting alters and uncovering hidden memories. Age regression, affect bridge techniques, multilevel hypnosis, screen techniques, permissive amnesia, symptom substitution, and other techniques can help patient and therapist manage this task.

The second half of this chapter has explored the principles of abreaction. Although spontaneous abreactions often occur, they are a source of discomfort and provide little therapeutic relief. It is only when abreaction is coupled with specific techniques for induction and control that progress can be made. Therapeutic abreactions may be induced through age regression, affect bridges, or other hypnotic or drug-facilitated techniques. In general, hypnotic management of abreactions is preferable to the use of drugs, which requires medical support and may be contraindicated by medical problems.

Abreactions are accompanied by vivid recall and reliving of events. The therapist must help to structure the course of this chaotic process in order to facilitate the psychotherapeutic working through of recovered material. This is done by establishing a linear chronology of events and providing a supportive, reality-based anchor in the present while the patient relives the past. Often a specific trauma must be abreacted several times, and contradictory versions of the event must be reconciled before therapeutic effects occur. Abreactions should be allowed, whenever possible, to run their full course. The patient should be intensively reoriented as the abreaction terminates.

Following an abreaction, the therapist helps to provide closure by identifying residual affects and doing some preliminary processing of the material. Often several psychotherapy sessions are required to work through the recovered material adequately. Incomplete abreactions are a major cause of therapeutic failure. Signs of incompletely abreacted traumas include (1) gaps in the continuity of recall of the episode; (2) intense flashbacks and intrusive thoughts, affects, or images outside of therapy; (3) failure to reconcile contradictory versions of the event; (4) failure of fusions of alter personalities; and (5) increased resistance to further abreactive work. Although abreactive work can be intense, few psychiatric interventions offer such dramatic relief to a suffering patient.

CHAPTER TEN

Adjunctive Therapies

PSYCHOPHARMACOLOGY

Introduction

There are no controlled studies of the use of medication to treat multiple personality patients. A body of empirical knowledge, however, has accrued and been shared by practitioners in the field over the years. It is unlikely that any large-scale, controlled studies of psychopharmacology in the treatement of MPD will be attempted in the near future. There are a number of thorny methodological and ethical issues associated with the design and implementation of such studies (Putnam, 1986b). Unless, and until, appropriate methodology can be devised, the psychopharmacology of MPD will remain a pragmatic art. We may draw some guidance, however, from the results of controlled studies in patients with posttraumatic stress disorders.

When using medication with dissociative disorder patients, one should be cognizant of which symptoms you expect the medication to treat. There is no good evidence that medication of any type has a direct therapeutic effect on the dissociative process as manifested in MPD (Barkin et al., 1986; Kline & Angst, 1979; Kluft, 1984d; Ross, 1984). In fact, Ross (1984) and others (Barkin et al., 1986) have suggested that the use of medications may actually reinforce the dissociation by isolating the dissociated personalities and blocking their reintegration. There is, however, evidence that medications may at times serve as a useful adjunctive treatment in the therapy of MPD. In this role, medication is primarily used for controlling or ameliorating specific nondissociative symptoms (e.g., depression and anxiety) that may interfere with psychotherapy. The clinician must be careful, however, not to depend too heavily on the use of medication to treat symptoms that are largely psychosomatic and usually provide important psychodynamic clues to the patient's past trauma.

General Principles for Medication Use in Multiples

Anecdotal reports, together with two unpublished case studies involving double-blind medication administration, suggest that nonspecific placebo-like responses often occur from the use of medications in MPD patients (Putnam, 1986b). In following well over 100 MPD cases in treatment, I have often heard clinicians wax ecstatic about the beneficial effects of some medication or other for their MPD patients. These positive responses rarely last more than 1 or 2 months. Kluft (1984d) reports observing a similar pattern in his large series of cases.

Anecdotal reports of different responses and sensitivities to medications or allergens among alters are common among clinicians who work with these patients (Barkin *et al.*, 1986; Braun, 1983a; Kluft, 1984d; Putnam *et al.*, 1986). One alter may demonstrate a beneficial response to a given medication, while another has an apparently life-threatening side effect, and still other alters exhibit little or no response at all. To date, no one has actually documented such differential sensitivities beyond reporting clinical observations, but the widespread nature of these reports—for example, 46% of therapists surveyed by the NIMH study reported observing differential medication sensitivities across alter personalities (Putnam *et al.*, 1986)—indicates that alter-personality-specific medication responses are a clinical factor in the psychopharmacology of MPD.

In general, my experience suggests to me that MPD patients as a group are more likely to develop disabling side effects from a given medication than are other psychiatric patients. In many instances, the side effects involve somatic complaints that are subjective and cannot be verified, but blood dyscrasias and other observable signs seem relatively common, compared to their expected incidence. The onset of side effects does not appear to be as clearly dose-related as is often observed in other psychiatric patients.

There are no data on medication compliance in MPD patients, but experience and common sense suggest that MPD patients have a difficult time with any activity that requires keeping track of time and behavior. Anyone who has been on oral medication for any length of time understands that it is difficult to remember to take the medication on time, and on occasion one has trouble remembering whether or not the medication was even taken. MPD patients, with their disordered sense of time, frequent amnesic behavior, and fragmented sense of responsibility, appear to have a particularly difficult time in maintaining any semblance of a medication schedule. In addition, one or more alters are usually actively opposed to the medication and either sabotage compliance or hoard pills in anticipation of overdosing themselves or other alters. In my experience, most MPD patients only take their medication on a sporadic p.r.n. (as-needed) basis. Barkin *et al.* (1986) note that extreme over-compliance problems may occur when more than one alter personality assumes responsibility for taking the medication. An additional compliance-related issue is the possibility of unwitting iatrogenic drug interactions caused by alters separately seeking therapy with different physicians (Putnam, 1985b).

The high rate of substance abuse noted in MPD patients suggests that physicians must take this possibility into consideration when pre-scribing medications with abuse potential, such as benzodiazepines, bar-biturates, and analgesics. In addition to all of the usual reasons for drug abuse, multiples may abuse prescription medications because a given drug suppresses certain alters or activates others.

Demands for medication are common from MPD patients, and a therapist should neither accept nor reject them without careful considera-tion. Richard Kluft (1984d) first enumerated a number of questions that one should ask when contemplating the use of medication in an MPD patient. The first point is to determine whether any of the patient's symptoms are likely to be medication-responsive. If potentially respon-sive symptoms such as anxiety or depression are present, are they causing sufficient distress across the personality system to counterbalance the possible adverse consequences of medication? If the patient's distress is caused by dissociative or nonspecific symptoms that are not medication-responsive, is the therapist simply attempting to "do something" or to treat the anxiety of others involved with the patient? Are there other, nonpharmacological interventions that may be equally effective without the risk? For example, many chronic pain syndromes in MPD can be successfully managed by hypnotherapeutic interventions. What is the patient's past track record with regard to medications? Has he or she overdosed in the past? In the end, Kluft (1984d) asks, "After weighing all considerations, do the potential benefits outweigh the potential risks?" (p. 53).

Medication Classes

Neuroleptic Medications

MPD patients are frequently misdiagnosed as suffering from schizo-phrenia or some form of psychosis, and consequently often receive neu-roleptic medication. There is no evidence that neuroleptic medication has any beneficial effect on the dissociative process, though at times it may produce a transient suppression of disturbed behavior. Kluft (1984d) and Barkin *et al.* (1986) have reported a high incidence of adverse physiological and psychological effects with neuroleptic medications in MPD. The physiological effects commonly include an extreme sensitivity to tardive dyskinesia and extrapyramidal syndromes, as well as autonomic and antimuscarinic effects.

The psychological effects involve a selective suppression or weakening of rational and/or protector alters, a disturbance of the patient's reality testing, and increased alter personality switching in an effort to regain control. There are anecdotal reports of the creation of new alter personalities as a response to neuroleptic medications (Barkin *et al.*, 1986). The use of a neuroleptic can be interpreted as an assault or an abuse by the therapist. I recommend that, in general, neuroleptic medications should not be used with MPD patients. The major exception is the use of low doses of neuroleptics for sedation, which at times may be preferable to hospitalization (Barkin *et al.*, 1986; Kluft, 1984d). The extended use of neuroleptics is uniformly discouraged by experienced therapists.

Often the diagnosis of MPD is made after the patient has been treated with neuroleptic medication for a period of time, sometimes for years. In such cases, I recommend that the therapist first begin to establish a therapeutic alliance with the personality system before starting to wean the patient off the medication. The medication may well have been suppressing certain alter personalities who will erupt as the suppression is lifted. The clinician should discontinue the medication gradually while frequently checking with a number of alter personalities as to the effects of this process. Many of the alter personalities will dislike the experience of being on an antipsychotic medication, but the host personality may experience the medication as stabilizing and may be fearful of losing control if it is discontinued. A marked increase in the host personality's anxiety level, as well as increased acting out by previously suppressed alters, often accompanies the initial discontinuation of a long-term neuroleptic medication.

Antidepressant Medications

Antidepressant medications do have a role in the treatment of multiple personality. These drugs probably do not directly affect the dissociative process per se, but can make a useful contribution to reducing the patient's distress from the depression often associated with major dissociative disorders. Other concurrent conditions that may be responsive to antidepressant medications include agoraphobia, panic attacks, anorexia, bulimia, and chronic pain syndromes. When the host, presenting personality, or other prominent personality is the only alter who is depressed, antidepressant medication is not indicated. Only when the signs and symptoms of depression are manifest in the host and a large percentage of other alters is antidepresant medication a useful adjunctive treatment. In these situations, polycyclic antidepressants may produce a marked elevation in mood and facilitate psychotherapy (Barkin et al., 1986; Kluft, 1984d). Premature withdrawal of the medication can lead to a relapse, with an exacerbation of both depressive and dissociative symptoms.

Barkin et al. (1986) report that polycyclic antidepressants produce inconsistent results across the alter personalities of MPD patients and that an antidepressant effect may not be obtained for all of the depressed personalities in the patient's system. The use of monoamine oxidase (MAO) inhibitors for the treatment of depression or other symptoms in MPD patients is strongly discouraged (Barkin et al., 1986; Putnam, 1985b). The MAO inhibitors can interact with other drugs and with foods containing a high content of tyramine to produce a potentially lethal hypertensive crisis. Anecdotal accounts of alter personality conflicts involving dietary sabotage in MPD patients taking MAO inhibitors have made the rounds on the therapists' grapevine for years. Even where overt sabotage is not thought to be a problem, inadvertent dietary indiscretions by child or other alters remain a serious risk.

Although a substantial percentage of MPD patients are diagnosed as having a bipolar disorder, in most cases the superordinate diagnosis is actually MPD (Putnam et al., 1984). Some cases of MPD with genuine concurrent affective disorder have been reported, however (Kluft, 1984d). Experience with lithium in MPD patients is limited, and the scanty data available suggest that most MPD patients do not respond to lithium (Barkin et al., 1986). There is some suggestion that lithium may suppress personality switching in a few MPD patients (Barkin et al., 1986).

Anxiolytic Medications

Like the antidepressant medications, anxiolytic medications (e.g., benzodiazepines, hydroxyzine, meprobamate) have a role in alleviating some of the symptoms of generalized anxiety, panic, and phobic states seen in MPD patients. These medications can be used at times to help the patient weather anxiety associated with major crises. Barkin et al. (1986) recommend the circumspect use of a benzodiazepine in cases where a high anxiety level is manifested across all of the alters or where anxiety is seriously interfering with the functioning of a major personality (e.g., an executive or work personality). They also state that these medications can be used to calm the overall patient during early treatment interventions; to decrease anxiety during periods of intense treatment or during fusion; and to help the patient in developing nondissociative methods of coping during the postintegration period. This is the class of medications that I prescribe most often for MPD patients, and I have found them useful in reducing nightmares and night terrors in some patients.

Anticonvulsants

The higher-than-expected apparent incidence of abnormal EEG findings in MPD patients (Benson *et al.*, 1986; Putnam, 1986a), and disproportionately high number of case reports of MPD and concurrent epilepsy in the clinical literature, have led a number of clinicians to try anticonvulsant medications. Mesulam (1981) and Schenk and Bear (1981) separately reported a decrease in dissociative episodes in the same handful of patients with MPD-like dissociative symptoms or clear-cut MPD and concurrent temporal lobe abnormalities when these patients were treated with anticonvulsants. These findings do not represent controlled studies and have limited follow-up. I have followed a number of MPD patients in whom anticonvulsants, particularly carbamazepine, have been tried (Devinsky *et al.*, 1988). In my experience, sustained beneficial responses to anticonvulsants in MPD without clear EEG evidence of concurrent epilepsy are nil. In addition, I have seen a number of life-threatening side effects occur with the use of carbamazepine in MPD patients. Kluft (1984d) reports similar observations.

Sedatives and Hypnotics

Sleep disturbances are common in MPD patients (Barkin *et al.*, 1986; Putnam *et al.*, 1986). Typically the disruption is similar to that seen in posttraumatic stress disorders, with nightmares, night terrors, and hypnagogic and hypnopompic phenomena, and benzodiazepines may be helpful. Requests for "sleeping pills" are commonly made by tormented host personalities, and many clinicians find it difficult not to accede to these demands. The success of these medications in controlling patients' sleep disturbance is transient at best, however. Sedative and hypnotic medications are notorious vehicles for suicide attempts and generally should not be prescribed to MPD patients unless and until appropriate contracts have been negotiated and tested. A patient must be educated to accept the long-standing sleep disruption, and work can be done with specific alters to allow the host personality some peace at night.

Other Medications

Analgesic medications, frequently prescribed for the pain syndromes found in MPD patients, may lead to abuse and addiction in some patients (Coons, 1984; Barkin *et al.*, 1986). In many instances, these pain syndromes are functional and represent the somatization of abusive experiences. Careful evaluation of the etiology of the pain should be undertaken before a clinician resorts to analgesic medication for pain control and management. Tracing the pain backwards to its origin, using hypnotic techniques such as the affect bridge, may be useful.

Adequate surgical and dental anesthesia appears to be difficult to achieve in some MPD patients (Barkin *et al.*, 1986; Putnam, 1985b). Again, anecdotal reports making the rounds suggest that some alters may go under, but others may wake up on the table, causing problems and consternation among the surgical team. Excess doses of an anesthetic may be necessary to achieve sufficient depth of anesthesia across all alters. If an MPD patient is scheduled for elective surgery or a dental procedure requiring anesthesia, the clinician should inform the surgical team or dentist of this possibility. It is advisable to acquaint the postoperative recovery room team with the patient's multiplicity, because child alters often are the first to wake up after general anesthesia.

GROUP THERAPY

Heterogeneous Group Therapy

Heterogeneous group therapy with MPD patients is, in the words of David Caul (1984), "a difficult and little studied area" (p. 50). Caul (1985b) reports that in his experience, the placement of a multiple into a heterogeneous group proves to be disastrous for the multiple and highly disruptive for the group process. Although he believes that better preparation of the group and the multiple may mitigate this outcome, there are strong dynamics that may make it inevitable. I worked for 3 years with a ward group that contained one or more MPD patients and found that my experiences were similar to those described by Caul. Other group members tend to see the multiples as "self-centered, attention-seeking, faking, lying, pretending and in general, guilty of 'one upsmanship' by displaying the special nature of their illness to group members who could scarcely understand or tolerate what they saw and what they were told" (Caul, 1984, p. 50). These other group members are often frightened by the dramatic changes exhibited by MPD patients. For a number of reasons, non-MPD group members tend to band together in attacking MPD patients. Caul (1984) observes that the hostility between multiples and nonmultiples occurs even though the same patients have good one-to-one relationships outside of the group setting. For these and other reasons, I would strongly recommend against knowingly including an MPD patient in a general therapy group.

Homogeneous Group Therapy

A number of therapists have worked with homogeneous groups of multiples. Although no published reports have examined the effectiveness of group work as an augmentation to individual psychotherapy, most therapists that I have spoken with about their experiences claim modest to moderate benefits. The responses of some of the group members with whom I have spoken is, however, more positive. Coons and Bradley (1985) found that their group members described the group treatment as extremely helpful and attributed the curative benefits to the commonality of diagnosis and dynamics. A number of all-multiple peer support groups, initiated and run by multiples, are also springing up around the United States. Similar groups have been found to be of value by other trauma victims, including combat veterans, rape victims, incest survivors, abuse victims, concentration camp survivors, cancer patients, and families of suicide victims (Smith, 1985).

Therapists working with homogeneous groups of multiples describe a number of similar experiences. One of the most common is the attempt of group members to "out-multiple" each other (Caul, 1984). Focusing on dissociative symptoms is part of the early group process (Coons & Bradley, 1985). Frequent, rapid switching among all group members can produce chaos at times, though Coons and Bradley (1985) found that their patients on the average switched only once per group session. Multiple abreactions triggered off in patients by one another have been commonly reported. Herman (1986) has described a similar process in her group work with incest survivors. Attempting to contain and work

simultaneously with several abreacting patients is one of the most difficult aspects of working with a homogeneous MPD group.

Rivalry among the patients for the therapist's attention can become
intense, according to therapists' accounts (Coons & Bradley, 1985). The
emergence of certain alter personality types in one patient may elicit
similar alters in other group members; for example, child alters can elicit
other child alters, and hostile alters will trigger the emergence of other
members' angry alters. Conflicts between dissimilar alters may also occur
(Coons & Bradley, 1985). Attempts to split cotherapists are common and
often are initiated outside of the group setting. Not surprisingly, therapists tend to report feeling outnumbered and overwhelmed at times.
Sachs and Braun (1985) have made use of videotaping to help them keep
track of group process and to record events that they missed at the time.

Therapists inexperienced in the individual psychotherapy of MPD
should not try to run an all-multiple therapy group. It is difficult enough to
track one MPD patient in a one-to-one psychotherapy. Therapists experienced in individual psychotherapy with MPD patients may want to try
small homogeneous therapy groups when demand for treatment outstrips
available resources. Such therapists must strive to create a group atmos-
phere in which trauma and its attendant affects can be uncovered, explored, consciously examined, and transformed. Despite the turbulent
dynamics associated with such groups, Caul (1984) believes that homogeneous therapy groups for multiples can make significant progress, provided
the patients and therapist make a sustained commitment.

Internal Group Therapy

Internal group therapy (IGT) is an innovative and promising treatment
technique originated by David Caul (1984). Although Caul is the first to
admit that the technique per se is less important than the underlying
process, he has found a means of sensitively rechanneling pathological
behavior into a constructive and therapeutic outlet in selected cases. In
IGT, selected alter personalities of a single MPD patient constitute and
function as a formal therapy group focusing on the patient's problems.
Caul states that IGT is most appropriate for MPD patients who have
come to a reasonable acceptance of their diagnosis, but are not making
significant therapeutic progress. In my experience, this is a particularly
useful intervention well worth trying in the later phases of treatment.

The therapist begins by explaining the purpose and process of IGT
to the patient, speaking to the personality system as a whole. The person-

ality system is asked to select an alter to function as the group leader, to select alters to form the group, and to decide the length of the session and the manner in which the session will be ended. The patient is told that the therapist will be present as an observer and is available for consultation or intervention if the group should request it. The therapist should not intervene without the internal group's request except in an emergency. Whenever possible, a videotape should be made of internal group sessions for later review by patient and therapist. When the patient has understood and agreed to these stipulations, a session may be undertaken. Generally, each IGT session should have a specific problem-solving focus determined ahead of time.

Patients who are appropriate for IGT will often have acquired the ability to bring out the selected alters spontaneously when an internal group session starts. When a patient is unable to manage this task, the therapist can place the patient in trance, deepen the trance, and then ask for the group leader and other group members. The therapist reiterates the instructions that he or she will be available upon request for consultation and emergencies, but will not be an active participant in the therapy. The therapist then withdraws to the side and allows the group to proceed.

The personality designated as a group leader, often an ISH, usually determines which other personalities will be active in the group and where they will "sit." The videotapes that I have seen of Caul's internal group work show that he uses a circle of chairs to constitute the group setting, and the group leader will often tell the selected alters to "sit" in specific chairs. Such a formal group setting is not always necessary, and the alters can participate in a group process from a single chair. In my experience with this technique, the patient usually switches back and forth among the group members as they speak in turn. One of my patients alternated between two chairs, moving back and forth between them as different alters appeared and addressed each other.

VIDEOTAPE TECHNIQUES

The use of motion pictures or videotape to capture the phenomena of multiple personality dates back to the silent film era. C. C. Wholey (1926) made a classic silent film of a female MPD patient who switched into a small child and adult male alters, which he presented to the meeting of the American Psychiatric Association in 1926. The patient's dissociative behavior and the actions of patient and physician on camera more than half a century ago are strikingly similar to the videotapes shown today. Many

clinicians have independently discovered the usefulness of video- or audio-
tapes in the treatment of MPD. Again, David Caul (1984) has elucidated
the principles of using videotapes with MPD patients and has pioneered
their more systematic use in therapy. In certain situations, the use of video-
or audiotaping and replay can have a significant impact on a MPD patient.
It is important for therapists using videotaping to do everything possible to
ensure that this impact is therapeutic.

General Principles of Videotape Use

I think that all too often videotapes are made just to have some sort of a
record or proof of the patient's multiplicity. Very little consideration is
given to how the tape is actually going to be used afterwards and to
whom it will be shown. With today's equipment, videotapes are simple to
make, and consequently little thought may be given to the reasons for
making them. A therapist considering the use of videotaping should have
a clear idea of how the tape will be used, whether or not it will be shown
to the patient, and who else may be allowed to see the tape. The answers
to these questions should be shared with the patient as part of the consent
procedure.

The patient should be informed as to why the tape is being made,
how it will be used, who will be allowed to see it, whether or not the
patient will be allowed to see part or all of it, whether or not the patient
may have a personal copy, and the guarantees the therapist can provide
about maintaining the confidentiality of the recording. It is not realistic
to expect to obtain individualized signed consent from each alter, so as
long as the personality system as a whole agrees to the taping, the patient
may sign a single consent form (Putnam, 1984b). A copy of the consent
form should be provided to the patient.

Although some therapists have access to elaborate television studios
for making videotapes, most are limited to the use of simple home
equipment in an office setting. This is sufficient for making tapes useful
in therapy, but is inadequate for teaching or research purposes. Most
MPD patients rapidly habituate to the presence of a video camera or tape
recorder (Caul, 1984). I have used a camera operator at times, but find
this unnecessary and intrusive. When making a therapy tape, I usually
just set up the camera with a wide-angle lens in the corner of the room,
center the patient in the frame, turn the recorder on, and commence the
session without prolonged manipulation of the camera. I then try to
forget the camera and do not spend session time fooling with it. If the

patient, for whatever reason, moves off camera, the audio portion of the tape will still record what is happening and provide sufficient feedback for therapy purposes.

Effects of Viewing Videotapes on Patients

The therapeutic results of using videotapes are predicated on patients' viewing the tapes and incorporating new information about themselves into their ongoing sense of self. In actuality, the impact of viewing a videotape can run the gamut of possibilities. Caul (1984) stresses that videotape work should not be done early in therapy because of the frightening effects the tapes may have on the patient. Fisher (1973) points out that most people who walk into a room and are unexpectedly confronted with their own image in a mirror will momentarily feel as if they are face to face with an unknown and somehow alien person. Given this normal reaction, the effects of seeing living proof of oneself as a number of very different and contradictory selves understandably has a profound impact on an MPD patient. Increased dissociative behavior may result as part of the patient's defense against accepting this new image. Episodes of depersonalization, fugue behavior, and panicked flight can occur and must be anticipated as possible reactions to seeing a videotape. Most patients do not have such strong reactions, however, and typically switch personalities when the material becomes too anxiety-provoking.

I usually do not show a patient a videotape immediately after it has been made. Instead, I view it first myself and often select some part of it to show to the patient initially. Before we view a tape, I go over the contents of the section to be replayed, and describe and discuss the material with the patient. Often we view only a few minutes of the tape at first. As the patient becomes used to seeing alters, it is possible to view longer sections, and on occasion I have made copies of tapes for a patient to view at home. I do not edit therapy tapes, because the distortions and discontinuities produced by editing detract from demonstrating to the patient the continuities of self that persist in spite of the switching of alters. I do not believe that videotherapy techniques such as self-modeling, which are appropriate with physical disabilities, are useful in MPD because of the distortions in continuity produced by extensive editing. When properly used, videotaping can help the patient see and accept what others already know about him or her, and can provide a powerful channel for internal communication across dissociative barriers.

FAMILY THERAPY

The clinical literature on the use of family therapy models and treatment interventions in multiple personality is limited. There are no articles to date that describe work with the family of origin in adult MPD patients. There are a few reports on family-of-origin treatment interventions with child MPD patients (Fagan & McMahon, 1984; Kluft, 1984b, 1985b; Sachs & Braun, 1986). Several papers address the use of family treatment models to guide interventions in marital and family therapy (Beal, 1978; Davis & Osherson, 1977; Kluft *et al.*, 1984; Levenson & Berry, 1983; Sachs & Braun, 1986). These papers generally describe limited family treatment, rarely lasting more than a half-dozen sessions, with minimal follow-up. Roberta Sachs (Sachs & Braun, 1986) and others with extensive clinical experience in MPD have observed that family or social-environmental treatment interventions are inadequate as primary treatments but are important adjuncts to a patient-oriented therapy. The following discussion of family therapy in multiple personality is based on the premise that the primary treatment is a patient-centered psychotherapy for which family therapy serves as an important supportive work.

Family-of-Origin Therapy

Although therapists have not yet reported on working with the family of origin in MPD, the characteristics of these families have been of considerable interest to clinicians, reviewers, and theoreticians concerned with MPD. Extreme inconsistency in parental behavior and contradictory expectations of the child by the parents have been repeatedly identified in the literature as characteristic of the childhood home situations of MPD patients (Allison, 1974b; Greaves, 1980; Saltman & Solomon, 1982; Braun & Sachs, 1985). Parents frequently alternate between loving, nurturing behavior and extremely sadistic abuse. The child may be praised and punished for the same behavior on different occasions. Often one pole of parental behavior is marked by extreme fundamental religiosity and perfectionism, while the other may involve substance abuse and promiscuity. The relationship between the parents is usually polarized and often places the child in double-bind situations (Allison, 1974b; Greaves, 1980). The child's elaboration of different alter personalities is thought, in part, to be an adaptive response to the inconsistent and radically different demands made upon him or her.

Secrecy, denial of abuse, and presentations of a "united front" characterize the family of origin's style of dealing with the outside world

(Kluft *et al.*, 1984; Sachs & Braun, 1986). The child is exposed to one standard of behavior within the family and expected to exemplify another very different image with respect to the rest of the world. In MPD patients, the incongruity between these opposite images is resolved by the creation of specific alter personalities appropriate to the different contexts. The united-front dynamic, in which the family of origin maintains that all is well except for the problems of the identified patient, is powerful and may be quickly re-erected when a therapist seeks to probe family behavior even decades later.

In cases where the patient is an adult and is separated from the family of origin, patient and therapist may wonder about the value of involving the family of origin in the therapeutic process. Although the urge to include the family of origin in the primary treatment is especially pronounced in therapists with an extensive theoretical or clinical background in family work, this issue will come up at some point in treatment with most MPD patients.

Two dynamics contribute to the raising of this concern in therapy. The first is the wish on the part of the patient and/or therapist to confront parents and abusers with the results of their behavior and to "punish" them in some fashion. In the patient, there will also be some personalities who are seeking reconciliation, love, or other positive responses. Therapists often want to see "justice" done. A second dynamic is a wish on the part of the patient and/or therapist to have an external source of validation for the remembered accounts of abuse. The need to know "what really happened" is always a forceful undercurrent in the process of uncovering therapeutic work. Both patient and therapist will find themselves wondering, doubting, disbelieving, and intensely believing the accounts of the trauma. At some point in their treatment, many multiples will seek directly or indirectly to obtain information about "what really happened." In addition to contacting siblings or relatives not involved in their abuse, they may visit their hometowns or contact childhood friends, teachers, doctors, ministers, and other people outside the family who might remember certain events. Direct confrontation with abusers usually occurs much later, if at all.

I have included extended-family-of-origin members in special therapy sessions on occasion with mixed results. Validation and reconciliation were the two primary agendas for most of these sessions. In my experience, extended-family members are not good sources of validation for abusive episodes. Either they are outside of, and therefore believe, the united front, or they are part of the united front. They may be able to recall specific events that lend circumstantial support to the patient's memories, but often give very different interpretations of the events in question. Attempts at reconciliation are generally more successful. In truth, much of my work around family-of-origin issues is spent helping the patient separate and protect himself or herself from further intrusion or abuse.

Siblings often remain part of the united front throughout adult life and seek to emphasize the patient's illness and lack of stability while denying memories of abuse. Sometimes a sibling will acknowledge the abuse privately, but will remain part of the united front publicly. More than one multiple has been told by a sibling, "Yes, you were abused, but the family reputation is worth more than you!" I have never attempted to include a patient's abusers in joint therapy with a patient, and accounts of other therapists' attempts lead me to believe that this is not likely to be useful, particularly early in the course of treatment.

It is not uncommon for MPD patients to be in contact with their abusers, but confrontation over abuse and its results is avoided by all parties. In the worst situations, the adult patient still periodically returns to the abuser and reverts to a child alter, who is abused. It is impossible to treat such cases successfully while this is going on. The abuse must be stopped before any further interventions are undertaken. In several cases on which I consulted, adult patients were continuing incestuous relationships begun in childhood. These patients would become manifestly more symptomatic, depressed, and suicidal following an incestuous encounter. This possibility should be kept in mind when an MPD patient has a sudden dramatic deterioration in function after contact with a past abuser.

Early in the course of therapy, confrontation with abusers is, in my opinion, not fruitful and may be seriously detrimental to treatment. The family may bring all of its influence to bear on the patient in an effort to suppress long-hidden secrets. No therapist can adequately protect his or her patient from the effects of such a traumatizing family. The patient often responds with an exacerbation of dissociative behavior, depression, and self-destructive or murderous impulses. The patient may drop out of therapy at the request of the family or in flight from the internal and external uproar caused by such a confrontation. Open rejection of the patient by the family can occur (Kluft, 1984d). Late in the course of therapy, when some form of unification has been achieved, the patient may wish to do some work with his or her abusers as part of the process of the renegotiation of relationships that accompanies the patient's evolving self-representation. At this point, the patient may feel secure and safe enough to confront his or her abusers, though not without strong trepidation. Even confrontation at this late date will usually prove traumatic and often unproductive in effecting any useful response from the abusers, but some patients need to do this as part of postresolution work.

Marital/Family Therapy

Several therapists have reported on their experiences in doing marital and family work with spouses, lovers, and children of MPD patients (Beal, 1978; Davis & Osherson, 1977; Levenson & Berry, 1983; Kluft *et al.*, 1984; Sachs & Braun, 1986). There is no question that the symptoms and behaviors of most MPD patients have a strong impact on other family members. Coons's (1985) finding of a significantly higher incidence of psychopathology in children of MPD patients compared to the children of non-MPD psychiatric patients can be interpreted as one effect of having a parent with MPD. Since their immediate families often provide the main system of social support for MPD patients, including family members in the therapeutic work is often necessary and desirable. The family work should encompass interventions for the welfare of the patient and of other family members.

Working with Spouses and Lovers of Patients

Sachs and Braun (1986) state that for married patients, marital therapy is an essential adjunct to the primary treatment approach. The therapist can work with the couple to promote a stronger marital relationship while addressing specific marital/family issues that evoke dissociative behavior in the MPD patient. The therapist may also identify and intervene with respect to pathological behavior in a spouse who seeks to use the patient's illness for self-gratification.

Not surprisingly, MPD patients often marry spouses with a significant amount of psychopathology. Anecdotal accounts suggest that depression, alcoholism, character pathology, and gender identification problems are not uncommon in the spouses and lovers of MPD patients. A disturbed marital partner may get a great deal of gratification from encouraging dissociative behavior in the patient. Women who have been abused as children often marry abusive husbands, and Sachs and Braun (1986) point out that the therapist must be alert to the possibility that the patient has merely moved from one abusive context to another.

Another dynamic that I have seen operative in men knowingly married to MPD patients is the promotion of dissociation for sexual gratification. As one such husband explained to me, "It's better than having a harem. You only have to feed one!" Many of these husbands have learned to elicit specific alters for their sexual pleasure by using cues or situations reminiscent of earlier sexual abuse. In such a case, the spouse will deliberately sabotage the therapy. Sachs and Braun (1986) suggest that the sabotaging spouse be confronted with the negative consequences of his behavior. Despite confrontation, my experience is that the behavior often continues unabated because the spouse has no investment in the patient's progress. Only when the patient has achieved sufficient internal cohesion to be able to actively differentiate her pathology from that of the spouse is the patient able to collaborate with the therapist in addressing the spouse's pathology. Less pathological spouses may still resist therapy because they fear the loss of favorite personalities or the unmitigated influence of hostile personalities. A healthy spouse usually can work out a relationship with those alters who do not believe that they are married to the spouse or who are otherwise hostile. The spouse should be counseled that with resolution, many of the characteristics of the favorite personalities will emerge (Sachs & Braun, 1986).

Couples therapy should focus on the here-and-now issues in the relationship. Sachs and Braun (1986) recommend that the spouse be well educated about the nature of MPD and prepared to expect significant changes in the patient during the course of therapy. The couple should be encouraged to communicate about all issues related to MPD. Many spouses report that with the diagnosis of MPD, the patient's behavior suddenly becomes understandable. I find that shortly after the diagnosis and dynamics of MPD are explained to a spouse, I receive a letter or call in which the spouse re-examines a number of "unexplained" experiences that now "make sense." Working through some of these examples with a spouse can go a long way toward enlisting the spouse in support of the therapy.

Working with Children of Patients

Interviews and interventions with an MPD patient's family have an important role in the treatment of MPD. By seeing the family, a therapist can evaluate the impact of the patient's disorder on the family and the family's contribution to the patient's dissociative behavior. Although most MPD patients who are parents will have nurturing parental alters, in some cases there may well be other personalities who are hostile or actually abusive toward their children. Experienced MPD therapists make it a rule of thumb to evaluate the children of *any* MPD patients that they treat (Braun, 1985; Kluft, 1985b; Sachs & Braun, 1986). If evidence of abuse is found, the therapist must take whatever steps are necessary and required by law to stop the abuse of the patient's children. MPD patients will ultimately respect strong interventions on behalf of their children. The incidence of abuse by MPD parents toward their children is not known; it may not be any higher than that of any other group of formerly abused children who have become parents (Brown, 1983; Coons, 1985; Kluft, 1984b).

Children of MPD patients are usually exquisitely attuned to the changes in their parents. They are aware of having several "mommies" or "daddies" and often alter their behavior to adjust to the parents' personality switches. In some instances, the children may promote dissociative behavior because it gratifies their own needs. The account of family therapy with an MPD patient, her children, and her lover by Levenson and Berry (1983) documents the extent to which family members can encourage switching and dissociation for their own ends. The children, for example, learned to make use of more permissive personalities to get approval for activities or to use their mother's amnesia to cover misbehavior. Levenson and Berry (1983) found that the "quality of individual family members' superego functioning appeared . . . contingent upon which personality was present" (p. 79).

It is important for a therapist working with the children of an MPD patient to confirm and explain the children's perceptions of changes and inconsistency in the parent. The children must be helped to understand that the parent's behavior is part of an illness and not something to be imitated or manipulated. In times of crisis, the therapist should have discussions with the children concerning their fears and fantasies, ambivalence, confusion when confronted with bizarre behavior, and guilt over wished-for removal of the parent. The therapist should provide the children with reality-oriented discussions, emphasizing realistic attitudes and behavior. The therapist can also help to demystify the parent's behavior and decrease magical or superstitious interpretations by the children.

INPATIENT TREATMENT

Reasons for Inpatient Treatment

Most diagnosed multiples are admitted to inpatient psychiatric units because of ideation or behavior that threatens to harm or overwhelm the patients. Suicidal impulses are the single leading cause of inpatient admission, followed by depression and threats of violence (Caul, 1985c; Kluft, 1984d; Putnam et al., 1986). A variety of other reasons may lead to hospitalization, including fugue behaviors, self-inflicted injury (nonsuicidal), and lack of logistical resources to support outpatient treatment (Caul, 1985c; Kluft, 1984d). MPD patients may also be admitted to inpatient units as part of the treatment plan for the facilitation of specific procedures (e.g., protracted abreactions) or provision of structure and safety during certain phases of treatment (Kluft, 1984d). In the future, this option will probably become an increasingly important part of the treatment of MPD. Multiples may end up in the hospital through another major route, however: They are often admitted under another diagnosis, and the correct diagnosis is made while they are in the hospital. In some cases, multiples have been chronically hospitalized for years.

Patient–Staff–Milieu Issues Raised by Inpatient Multiples

The presence of a multiple on an inpatient unit, whether or not the patient has been diagnosed as suffering from MPD, usually results in significant splits and conflicts among the ward staff. At St. Elizabeths Hospital, we discovered a number of MPD patients who were chronically hospitalized with other diagnoses; in every case, there was a long history of difficulty and staff conflict surrounding the patient. This was often reflected in the transfer of the patient to another unit. In one instance, the patient had been on three different long-term units in less than 2 years. Each time, he was transferred after causing severe staff conflicts that prevented further effective work on the unit.

If a ward staff is not split over the diagnosis, then there will be other issues. The patient's lack of participation in the milieu, special status conferred for any number of reasons, effect on other patients, apparent manipulative behavior, or many other issues will serve as a focus for staff tensions. It may sound as if I am overstating the case, but I have been impressed by the havoc a single MPD patient can wreak on staff relations. As a consultant, I have seen this phenomenon repeated in a wide range of settings, from back wards in rural state institutions to elite, psychoanalytically oriented private hospitals.

Multiples' Responses to the Inpatient Environment

It is not uncommon for an MPD patient to ask or even plead for hospitalization at some point in the course of treatment. From afar, the hospital may be perceived as a safe place. The patient may believe that the wearying internal vigilance required to keep dangerous alters from causing harm can be relaxed and replaced by the hospital staff's external watchfulness. Patients may believe that the hospital is a place where they can get "rest" or be "put to sleep" for a while. They may see it as a place of refuge from intrusive family members or other external threats. They may be seeking a safe place to let out the most dangerous of the alters, who dare not emerge in the therapist's office. These and other reasons often prompt a patient to request hospitalization.

Once a patient is admitted, perceptions of the hospital can change dramatically and rapidly. Within a short time, most multiples will have alters emerge who experience the hospital as a frightening and traumatizing place. Normal hospital procedures and routines, such as medications, milieu activities, privilege status, pass restrictions, and other unit rules, are perceived as coercive and traumatizing. Confinement on locked units is particularly difficult for multiples, many of whom have experienced childhood confinement abuses. Multiples require a great deal of personal privacy and do not easily tolerate the round-the-clock scrutiny given them by staff members and other patients. Many covert alters, who emerge only when the patient is alone, cannot or will not come "out" on the unit. As time passes, the patient will experience an increasing sense of internal pressure on the part of these alters to emerge. Whatever some alters want, such as hospitalization, other alters will angrily reject. Personalities hostile to the hospitalization and its purposes will often displace those who begged to be hospitalized. Not uncommonly, the patient who as an outpatient was pleading to be admitted now feels trapped and is fighting the institution and the therapist.

The major patient–staff dynamic involved in inpatient crises with multiples is "splitting." A number of factors contribute to the apparent divisiveness of these patients. Their chameleon-like abilities to bring out the personality who is most congruent to a given situation usually results in different alters' having relationships with different staff members. Each staff member may sincerely believe that he or she "understands" the patient, and yet each may be seeing a very different side of the patient. This process is further complicated by the ability of multiples to make the people involved in their care feel "very special." Multiples have an uncanny ability to activate grandiose and self-righteous feelings of rescue. Not surprisingly, the staff members may find themselves in conflict over who knows what is "best" for the patient or what the patient "really wants" in a given situation. Comparison by the staff of different versions of the patient may lead them to feel deceived and manipulated.

Multiples can, in fact, be manipulative, particularly when they feel threatened. Their basic coping strategy has been "divide and conquer," and in certain situations they attempt to externalize the process. They have an exquisite sensitivity to staff schisms and often catalyze latent staff conflicts. A multiple may feel safer when the staff members are fighting one another over what is going on with the patient or what the patient really "needs" than when he or she has a unified staff to deal with.

The hospital environment, with its many social interactions, also allows hostile alters a large and immediate arena within which to sabotage or complicate the patient's life and treatment.

Staff Responses to Multiples

Most staff members will have a strong reaction to a multiple. The form that the reaction takes depends on many factors, but multiples almost always have a significant impact on people and their surroundings. Commonly, staff members express this impact by either strongly accepting or rejecting the diagnosis of MPD. Those who accept the diagnosis often exhibit an extreme fascination with the multiplicity. They may seek special relationships with the patient or specific alters. They may also seek to use the patient in some inappropriate fashion (e.g., writing term papers on MPD using the patient as an example).

Those staff members who reject the diagnosis of MPD are likely to do so vehemently. They usually make this fact very clear to both therapist and patient. Often this is manifested in struggles around calling the patient's alters by different names. These staffers will steadfastly refuse to make any distinctions among alters and will deny all differences, treating all of the alters as though they were the same. The multiple, of course, feels as if his or her very essence is being rejected and denied. Crises will abound. Another scenario is for disbelieving staff members to deny the patient's history of abuse. They will cite this history as an example of outrageous lying by the patient. In small-town hospitals, staff members may even know the patient's abusers and use their personal relationships to call into doubt the patient's veracity (Quimby et al., 1986). Again, the multiple is likely to feel challenged at the very core and can be expected to react strongly in turn.

Skeptical staff members point to the multiple's behavioral inconsistencies as proof that the patient has control over specific symptoms or behaviors. They accuse the multiple of "making it all up" and being "able to turn it on or off" as needed. In one instance, the alters who primarily emerged on the ward either were regressed children, who soiled themselves, or were catatonic. At times, however, an alter who was interested in expensive clothes would emerge. The patient would go from a catatonic state to sophisticatedly ordering clothes by telephone and then back into catatonic trance. This apparent ability to go in and out of catatonia "at will" enraged many of the staffers who were responsible for the patient's hygiene and bodily functions. Staff members who disbelieve a diagnosis of MPD have a marked inability to see such behavior as being due to different alters, and perceive it instead as due to deliberate manipulation and deception. Consequently, they resent the multiple and other staff members who "cater" to the patient.

Multiples can activate primitive fears among staff members. One slender female multiple had a deep-voiced, blasphemous, hostile male alter who emerged late at night and paced the corridor. Whenever this happened, members of the night shift, believing that she was demonically possessed, would lock themselves in the nursing station and pray. They experienced genuine terror during these incidents and could not respond to her as a psychiatric patient, but only as a Satanic monster. Although this may appear to be an extreme example, these often unspoken fears are not uncommon.

Effects of Multiples on the Ward Milieu

Multiples make extensive demands on an inpatient unit's resources. They take far more staff time than most other patients and are often accused of monopolizing attention. As one state hospital administrator told me, "We have over 300 patients here and I'll bet she [the multiple] takes 10% of our total staff time." Resentment is often expressed about the time, attention, and effort that many multiples require and demand when hospitalized.

Other patients may be fascinated and/or frightened by a multiple. On occasion, a patient may legitimately believe he or she has, or may deliberately feign, MPD (Coons, 1980; Kluft, 1983). Resentment of the multiple's special status and monopoly of the staff's attention is common among other ward patients. They resent what appears to be a ploy on the part of the multiple to escape responsibility for his or her behavior by blaming different personalities, while the staff continues to hold the other patients responsible. They may also feel hurt and confused by the multiple's shifting responses toward them. Attempts at friendship with the multiple may be initially reciprocated, but later angrily rejected without apparent cause. Kluft (1983) notes that MPD patients also disturb other patients by openly manifesting conflicts or acting out behaviors that the other patients are seeking to suppress.

Effects of Hospitalization on the Therapeutic Alliance

A host of alter personalities that the therapist does not know well or does not know at all are likely to emerge in the hospital. Hostile and angry alters are triggered by the perceived abuses of hospital life. Frightened and traumatized alters are elicited by the recapitulation of trauma experienced in the hospital. Alters who are perceived as too powerful or dangerous to be let out in the therapist's office may now be unleashed. Protector alters, social alters, and others who are usually unnecessary in the outpatient treatment setting now come forth to deal with the many intense and complex social interactions that occur on any ward. In addition, many of the personalities with whom the therapist has a good relationship appear to weaken or disappear. *In toto*, the therapist may find himself or herself dealing with a different constellation of personalities in the hospital than were active outside the hospital. The combination of a radically changed patient and the complexities of trying to treat a multiple "publicly" while often critical staff and colleagues peer over one's shoulder can unnerve or deskill even the best of therapists.

Not surprisingly, the impact a multiple makes on a unit gets fed back to the therapist in many ways. The staff members frequently direct their anger and frustration with the patient toward the therapist, complicating an already difficult management situation. If the therapist is doing intense abreactive work in the hospital, the staff will accuse the therapist, directly or indirectly, of making the patient worse. This issue may be obliquely expressed as concern about the use of hypnosis with the patient. Some staff members will attempt to undo any special management arrangements the therapist makes. These issues are sometimes couched in terms of "fairness" or the patient's special status. The therapist will be seen as undermining the ward milieu and norms. The staff may question the therapist about whether or not the patient "belongs" on the unit or should be hospitalized elsewhere.

In some cases, the patient will have sought hospitalization as a way of terminating treatment with the therapist. In situations where the therapist does not have hospital privileges, hospitalization automatically disrupts or terminates the therapeutic relationship and interposes other parties, with all of the attendant complications. If a patient is seeking to use hospitalization to terminate treatment with a therapist who does have admitting privileges, then the patient may do so by drawing large numbers of other staff members into the therapy and creating a crisis over who is responsible for the patient's treatment. The converse is also true: Some therapists may seek to "dump" difficult or dangerous patients by hospitalizing them and legally turning over all responsibility to another party. Multiples will be acutely sensitive to this process, and grave difficulties are likely to arise as a result of this rejection.

In spite of the caveats discussed above, hospitalization can also strengthen the therapeutic alliance. The patient may experience a hospitalization that was imposed because of self-destructive behavior as a caring and life-saving act. When a therapist hospitalizes a patient because a satisfactory contract to control dangerous behavior cannot be negotiated, the limit setting implicit in this act will contribute to a healthier therapeutic alliance in the long run. An improvement in the therapeutic alliance is, in fact, one of the best indicators of when the patient is ready for discharge.

Recommendations for Inpatient Management of Multiples

1. If at all possible, prior to the hospitalization, a contract should be negotiated to cover the following: the reasons for admission, an agreement to cooperate with the rules and regulations of the unit, and the criteria for discharge (e.g., a contract with the personality system covering self-destructive behavior).

2. An MPD patient should have a private room whenever possible (Caul, 1978a; Kluft, 1984d). The patient's room serves as a refuge from ward turmoil and allows certain alters to emerge inconspicuously. Several alters will need to be informed about where the room is and even about the location of specific objects or possessions in the room (Caul, 1978a). Child alters, in particular, can use the room as a place to safely emerge and play or do abreactive work. A private room also eliminates many potential problems that can arise with roommates who do not have MPD.

3. The staff should be informed of the diagnosis as soon as possible. This is the time to do some anticipatory work with the staff about MPD and the multiple's potential effect on the unit. Staff concerns should be aired and addressed as much as possible. The staff members should be told that strong disagreement about the diagnosis of MPD is not unusual (Kluft, 1984d). They should also be told to anticipate that each of them will have a different perception of the patient and what is happening with the patient. It is worthwhile to predict the likelihood of staff splitting, so that if and when this occurs, the therapist can remind the staff that the multiple is behaving in an expectable fashion. The therapist should outline potential crises that may occur, and encourage staff members to call him or her with any concerns or during any crisis. Caul (1978a) also suggests that the staff be informed of any posthypnotic suggestions that the therapist has arranged for controlling crises.

4. The staff members should also be told that it is not necessary for them to acknowledge or interact with the alters as separate entities. The patient should be told not to expect that the staff will relate to the alters as separate and different. Although some narcissistic alters may be provoked by this lack of recognition, it is important to treat this "social"

situation like any other in which the alters are going to have to deal with people who do not know about MPD. This also serves to dampen staff fascination with the separateness of alters and discourage alters' investment in separateness for its own sake.

5. Caul (1978a) suggests that the ward use a "case manager" to coordinate the patient's care. There should be an identified person on each shift who will serve as the patient's main contact. The personalities should be introduced to these people and encouraged to use them, especially in times of crisis. The case manager, or primary nurse, can be included in therapy sessions that occur on the ward.

6. The therapist should take responsibility for explaining the ward rules and procedures to the personality system, requesting that all of the alters listen. Expectations and limits should be reviewed. When an alter breaks the rules, the consequences must be enforced in a nonpunitive manner. Caul (1978a) notes that it is usually a good idea to restrict home visits and off-ward privileges until the patient has been stabilized on the unit and is not a suicide or elopement risk.

7. It is strongly recommended that the patient not be included in any general group therapy sessions (Caul, 1978a; Kluft, 1984d). As noted earlier in the chapter, a multiple is likely to be disruptive to the ward group, and the benefits for an MPD patient are limited at best. The multiple should participate in nontherapy ward group meetings. A multiple may benefit from nonverbal group therapies, such as art, music, occupational, or movement therapy (Kluft, 1984d).

8. Caul (1978a) stresses the role of the ward in documenting the multiple's behavior. Alter personalities unknown to the primary therapist may be discovered by members of the ward staff who have the opportunity to observe the patient continuously over days. In one of my cases, for example, hospital staff were able to document the nonneurological nature of the patient's motor weakness through careful observation. This patient had undergone repeated workups for these symptoms. The ward staff should be informed of any specific symptoms or behaviors that are of interest, and arrangements for their documentation should be agreed upon.

Discharge Strategies

Acute Hospitalizations

In the case of acute, short-term hospitalizations, the multiple is usually admitted for control of self-destructive behavior or some other crisis situation. The resolution of the crisis or the reinstitution of internal control over dangerous behaviors is usually a sufficient criterion for discharge. The precipitants of the crisis may have been identified and worked through. Previously unsuspected alters who were responsible for self-destructive behaviors or fugue episodes may have been met and brought into the therapeutic process. Contracts may have been negotiated that allow the therapist to feel comfortable in returning the patient to outpatient status. Social supports may have been put in place that remedy problems or protect the patient from intrusion by pathological significant others. These or other solutions to the patient's crisis allow the multiple to return to his or her previous situation and resume therapy as an outpatient. In cases where a patient was admitted for specific therapeutic interventions, such as prolonged abreactive sessions, the therapist should allow sufficient time to evaluate the impact of the intervention before proceeding with discharge.

Probably the single most important criterion for discharge is the state of the therapeutic alliance. The therapist should feel comfortable in his or her relationship with the personalities before allowing the patient to leave the relative safety of a hospital ward. Adequate contracts should be in place, and protector or helper personalities should believe that it is safe for the patient to leave.

Chronic Inpatients

The growing awareness of MPD is leading to the recognition of these patients in a variety of settings, including chronic care psychiatric facilities. Bliss and Jeppsen (1985) found, for example, that 13% of the inpatients in their survey met DSM-III criteria for MPD. The recognition of an MPD patient in a long-term psychiatric setting may come after years of institutionalization and usually presents significant difficulties in addition to the usual problems. At the present time, most chronic care facilities are overburdened and understaffed and have only marginal resources available to devote to the intensive psychotherapy required by MPD patients. The effects of chronic institutionalization may also have taken their toll, making such patients doubly difficult to treat. Yet experience has shown that some of these patients can respond with a dramatic increase in functional level when treated as multiples for MPD (Quimby et al., 1986).

In a team treatment setting such as a chronic inpatient unit, the issue of the acceptance of the diagnosis of MPD takes on even greater complexity. Not only does the patient have to struggle with this question, but many other parties are involved, including the immediate treatment team, the ward/milieu staff, social services, and ultimately the hospital administration. To treat a patient effectively as a multiple, a therapist usually must win acceptance of the diagnosis from the majority of those involved directly and indirectly with the patient's care. It is particularly important to communicate an understanding of the diagnosis, dynamics, and treatment goals to the administration. Firm administrative support is crucial during the turbulent process of preparing the patient for outpatient treatment. Often it is useful to bring in an outside expert to confirm the diagnosis and educate the staff. There is something magical about having someone from outside the institution pronounce the patient a multiple. The expert should meet with key staff members after seeing the patient and, if circumstances permit, should give a lecture or grand rounds on MPD.

As soon as some institutional support for the diagnosis has emerged, a treatment plan for the patient as a multiple should be drawn up and initiated. The long-term goal should be the stabilization of the patient to a degree sufficient for discharge, with continuation of treatment as an outpatient. At first this may appear to be a wildly impractical objective, but it should be pursued nonetheless. I have seen a number of chronically institutionalized MPD patients make extraordinary progress when treated as multiples (Quimby et al., 1986). Shorter-term treatment goals may include moving the patient off a locked unit, placement in a sheltered workshop situation, or the like. The expectation should be that the patient can function at a significantly higher level than he or she has previously manifested.

The major goal of the treatment at this point should be the fostering of communication and cooperation within the personality system. Although some abreactive/trauma work is inevitable, deep probing for traumatic experiences should be postponed until contracts and channels of communication are firmly in place, and ideally the bulk of this work should occur in outpatient therapy. Social services need to be involved early, and sources of income and outpatient living situations should be identified.

Chronically hospitalized MPD patients are difficult to place in a supportive living situation. Typically, they do not do well in group living situations and can cause as much trouble in a halfway house as they do on a ward. Most halfway houses, with their emphasis on group process and limited staff coverage, find it difficult to tolerate multiples for prolonged placements. Apartments or other living situations that provide a greater degree of privacy are often more successful. Alas, finding funds to provide for this can be difficult. The patient will probably require weaning from the hospital. Sometimes arrangements can be made for the patient to spend days on the ward engaged in hospital-based therapies and nights outside of the hospital. Administrative understanding and support is necessary for such nonstandard arrangements. The patient may require several discharges and readmissions before a "stable" outpatient status can be achieved.

SUMMARY

This chapter has surveyed adjunctive therapies helpful in the treatment of MPD. Many therapists and patients first look to medication for symptom relief. Unfortunately, there is no magic pill for dissociation. Rather, medication is most useful for the reduction of depression or anxiety when these symptoms are widely distributed across alter personalities. Medication management is difficult in MPD patients, however. Alters may experience different effects from the same drug, compliance is poor, and misuse or abuse is common. Medication should be directed at specific symptoms. Hallucinations and psychotic-like symptoms are notoriously unresponsive to neuroleptics, which are largely contraindicated in MPD patients. Depression and anxiety can be reduced by judicious use of the appropriate medications, and traumatic sleep disturbances may respond to benzodiazepines in some cases.

Various forms of group therapy have evolved by trial and error. Experienced therapists concur that placement of MPD patients in mixed groups with non-MPD patients is not helpful. Groups composed exclusively of MPD patients may be useful as supplemental and supportive therapy. Such groups should only be attempted by experienced therapists. David Caul's IGT techniques have proven useful for selected MPD patients in the latter stages of treatment. Videotaping is useful with IGT and may provide important face-to-face feedback among alters in individual psychotherapy. The therapist needs to think carefully through the purposes and provisions of making videotapes, however, as the impact can be devastating if used too early or inappropriately.

Family therapy has a limited role in the treatment of MPD. In general, work with the family of origin is too traumatic to be undertaken until very late in treatment, if at all. Confrontation of abusers, validation of memories of abuse, and attempts at reconciliation with abusers have limited success at best and may seriously disrupt other aspects of treatment. Most patients need help in separation from the family of origin rather than re-entry. Marital therapy can be important in increasing support for patients from spouses or significant others. Spouses and children can be helped to understand the dynamics of dissociation, and any manipulation of patients for secondary gain can be addressed.

Hospitalization is an important therapeutic option to control self-destructive behavior or facilitate intensive abreactive work. Multiples will, however, create significant staff tensions on most units. Therapists would be wise to do some anticipatory work with both patients and staff prior to hospitalization. Chronically hospitalized MPD patients constitute a special case, but dramatic improvement can occur when the institution is successfully enlisted in the service of returning them to an outpatient status.

CHAPTER ELEVEN

Crisis Management and Therapeutic Resolution

CRISIS MANAGEMENT

Crises are frequent and almost inevitable occurrences in the treatment of MPD. Even the best of therapists cannot avoid them on occasion (Kluft, 1984d). In fact, crises can be expected to occur with dismaying regularity! To a certain extent, however, specific crises can be anticipated and planned for. A crisis develops when some event or pressure, internal or external, occurs that unbalances the personality system, and the patient's usual coping mechanisms are unable to restore homeostasis. Crisis intervention attempts to restore equilibrium. The minimal goal is the resolution of the crisis and the restoration of the patient's previous level of function and homeostasis. A more desirable goal is the improvement of the patient's level of functioning beyond what was present at the onset of the crisis (Kluft, 1983).

Numerous factors contribute to crises in MPD patients. Their amnesias, precipitous psychophysiological shifts, split self and object perceptions, absence of an observing ego function, and vulnerability to environmentally cued abreactions and flashbacks are direct results of the dissociative process. Struggles for control and dominance among the alter personalities are frequent sources of internally generated crises. Persecutor personalities may provoke crises by abusing the host or punishing alters who reveal secrets about past trauma. Despite their often impressive individual accomplishments MPD patients as a group suffer many of the stigmatizing features of chronic illness, including few social supports and depleted financial resources. Alcoholism and substance abuse are not uncommon and generate their own crises. And treatment, even by the best of MPD therapists, is traumatizing in its own way.

General Principles

Prevention

In the treatment of MPD, as in many things, a few minutes of prevention is worth hours of a therapist's time during a crisis. One should try to anticipate and head off crises whenever possible, and when that is not possible, it still may be possible to mitigate the intensity of a crisis by being prepared ahead of time. Certain situations are very likely to precipitate a crisis, and therapist and patient can work together to anticipate the effects of such perilous experiences as a trip home to the family of origin, viewing a tape of a hostile alter, and the recovery of long-hidden memories of trauma.

Prevention involves advance exploration and planning. The patient's resources and vulnerabilities need to be assessed. The potential contributions of specific alters, either to the chaos or to the resolution, needs to be evaluated. Helper alters can be identified ahead of time; often they can provide some advance warning of impending conflicts or aid in the assessment of the impact of specific situations. It is well worth the therapist's time to query these alters on a regular basis about any possible problems the patient may be facing. I am always amazed by the ability of MPD patients *not* to mention during therapy sessions major upheavals happening in their day-to-day lives. Access to identified helper alters through the use of pre-established hypnotic cues can be arranged, so that they may be elicited quickly or over the telephone if necessary. The therapist should also be versed in the personality system's metaphors and structure. Often there will be a "cave" or a "safe place" where personalities can be sent when they are frightened or are causing trouble.

The frequency of crises can be reduced by proceeding slowly and cautiously with the course of therapy. The therapist should not attempt to begin serious abreactive work until after the initial interventions discussed in Chapter Six have been implemented. The early therapy should be focused on increasing internal communication and taking advantage of the patient's strengths and abilities to improve self-esteem and the patient's life situation. Some practical experience with contracting needs to be in place early in the treatment. A viable therapeutic relationship will develop slowly, replacing the often intense and unrealistic initial fusion, which is driven by the patient's desperate needs and hopes. The therapist must also help provide structure for the patient and work with the personality system around limits and boundaries.

Therapy should move forward gently. The personality system's ability to tolerate stressful work should be explored. Whenever work in new areas is contemplated, the therapist should explain what steps need to be taken and should assess the responses of the alters to the plan (Kluft, 1983). The advice of helper personalities is particularly useful at these times. The patient needs to be taught that the difficult and painful responses to therapy are expectable and represent a form of progress; patients often interpret the disorganizing effects of painful emotions and memories as proof that they are deteriorating. Early hypnotic work should include a number of positive experiences designed to increase the willingness of the alters to accept hypnosis. Cue words, discussed in Chapter Nine, should be established early.

Crisis Intervention

Crises, in my experience, typically begin with a frantic phone call from either the patient or a significant other that serves to alert and involve me in the process. Often there is the unrealistic explicit or implicit demand that I do something instantly to resolve the situation or save the patient from imminent destruction. One of the difficult aspects of working with multiples is the frequency with which these patients abdicate responsibility and leave the therapist to carry the treatment (Kluft, 1984d). This tendency is particularly evident in times of crisis. The therapist is often saddled with the burden of being identified by the patient or significant others as the only one who can save the patient. And, of course, crises will occur at the most inopportune times.

The ability of MPD patients to modulate the frequency and/or intensity of their crises is a point of debate among therapists. Certainly some patients demonstrate an ability to "tone it down" at times and seem to exercise some modicum of control even when they appear to be raging out of control. Kluft (1984d) has observed that therapists who either fear or relish crises are likely to have more of them. Not all multiples have a capacity for modulating their crises. Very disorganized and/or fragmented patients, often with psychotic alters, may not have the resources to exert control during a crisis. Many MPD patients, however, can regain self-control if and when necessary.

Crises demand greater availability and involvement from the therapist. Unusual hours, long sessions, daily sessions, and even several daily sessions may be required at times. The therapist must be willing to give this time and energy, but it should not be expended unreasonably. Sheer volume of involvement will not resolve a crisis by itself; in fact, it may perpetuate it by gratifying the alters' wish to have the therapist all to themselves. Boundaries and limit setting must be scrupulously maintained, especially in times of crisis. Many crises are, in fact, a form of limit testing. The therapist must make it clear how far he or she is willing to go and when it will become necessary to transfer or hospitalize the patient. The patient should be kept informed of these limits and the alternatives the therapist is considering.

When a crisis develops, the therapist should attempt to gather as much information as possible about the precipitating circumstances and the responses of the alters. Alter personalities may be contacted directly or through hypnosis. The therapist should inquire of each alter what is known about the crisis, what that alter thinks is happening, and what might happen. The alters should be asked whether they are losing time during the crisis and whether they are aware of any personalities who are active or in control during these times. The therapist should poll as many alters as can be reached. In some instances, all of the alters will indicate that they have lost time and are not aware of what has happened. In this event, one or more personalities who have not yet been overtly met are likely to be involved in the crisis. An attempt should be made to contact the unknown alter(s) and start a dialogue. One can ask for the alter by description (e.g., "I would like to speak directly to whoever was responsible for bringing a man into the apartment last night"). In addition to direct or hypnotic inquiry, the therapist can instruct the patient to listen inwardly for internal dialogues, or can use automatic writing, fantasy techniques, or age regression within a single alter to obtain information about the crisis and its causes.

Every effort should be made to locate alters responsible for symptoms and behaviors contributing to the crisis. When these are found, the therapist should attempt to involve them in dialogue, negotiate with them to defuse the crisis, and engage them in the ongoing therapeutic work. If this is not successful, with the personality system's help and with hypnosis, the therapist can put them to sleep or send them to special safe places in the personality system's topography. Attempts at forced fusions, exorcisms, extrusions, or other suppressive techniques may buy a little time, but are more likely to backfire and lead to increased system conflict and crisis, as well as to seriously disrupt the therapeutic alliance.

Symptom and target substitution may be useful. Self-destructive behaviors can be rechanneled into nonharmful activities. This is particularly useful with self-mutilating alters. Attacks on the body can be transferred to nonliving substitutes, such as pillows, clay models, or whatever seems appropriate. A red Magic Marker can be substituted for a razor blade to permit discharge of self-mutilatory impulses. The therapist can suggest under hypnosis that certain troublesome symptoms contributing to the crisis be replaced by other lesser symptoms. In some cases, the therapist may suggest symptoms such as paralysis or amnesia to protect the patient from self-destructive behavior or painful memories. These last interventions have limited utility but may prove useful in crisis. Kluft (1983) describes hypnotically moving the patient or specific alter personalities backward or forward in time so as to "leapfrog" a crisis that the patient is not ready to handle. Carefully selected alters may also be taught the use of autohypnosis for themselves or the use of hypnosis to control other alters.

The Management of Specific Types of Crises

Self-Destructive Behavior

Suicidal or self-destructive impulses or actions lead the list of crisis events in MPD. Patients' feelings of being overwhelmed by the pain and chaos in their lives, fears of being rejected and abandoned by the therapist or significant others, and anger and dysphoria that they cannot express outwardly are all common precipitants of suicidal urges. In most MPD patients, the background level of suicidal ideation is high even during the calmer moments of their lives. It takes little to tip the balance into a more active expression of these thoughts. The host personality may become suicidal or depressed; suicidal alters may be attempting to take control; or alters seeking to harm other alters may be threatening to emerge. Often the personalities who serve as counterweights to more pathological alters report losing control or becoming "too tired" to prevent the dangerous alters from gaining control. The therapist is thrust into this breakdown of internal control and disequilibrium, with the mandate of preventing disaster and restoring order. Frequently the therapist's hands are tied by other constraints (e.g., lack of hospitalization insurance), which severely limit the range of responses.

Suicide attempts and gestures are frequent. Over 61% of the NIMH sample of clinicians reported serious attempts in their patients, and 71% reported nonlethal gestures (Putnam *et al.*, 1986). The usual methods such as wrist cutting and overdoses are frequent, but bizarre methods are not uncommon. Suicidal alters may grab the wheel when another alter is driving and attempt to crash the car, or seek to turn some other innocuous everyday activity into a self-destructive act. The mortality rate of multiples as a group is unknown. The lethality of these attempts/gestures in the NIMH survey was very low, but successful suicides of MPD patients are known to have occurred. Anecdotally, there are frequent reports of suicide attempts' being aborted by other alters, who seize control at the last moment and avert disaster; Kluft (1983) describes this dynamic as a dissociative version of compromise formation, in which the self-destructive act by one alter is then followed by another alter's attempts to get help.

The "internal homicide" is another form of suicide attempt, in which one alter attempts to kill another alter. The alter attempting to murder another alter always fails to grasp the obvious fact that if the attempt is successful, the first alter too will die. Attempts to point this out are almost always futile. Kluft (1984d) has called this phenomena a "pseudo-delusion" of separateness. The intensity and fixity of this conviction of separateness can, however, easily qualify as frankly delusional in many patients. This conviction of separateness will slowly yield over time to frequent statements and interpretations by the therapist to the effect that whatever happens to one alter ultimately happens to all. Attempted internal homicides were reported in over half of all patients in the NIMH survey and were driven by the usual dynamics of internal conflict (Putnam *et al.*, 1986).

In some cases, the internal homicide attempt is a direct act in which one alter tries to kill another or to set up the death of another. In other instances, the attempt may be indirect: The homicidal alter urges or commands a suicidal alter or the host personality to kill himself or herself. An internal homicide attempt may be accompanied by copresence phenomena, so that the alter who is the intended victim watches helplessly as the homicidal alter attempts to carry out the act. One patient told me, for example, of watching herself phone her boss to tell him that she would not be in because there was a "death in the family," then watching in helpless horror as she attempted to suffocate herself with a plastic bag. She, like many other MPD patients, was saved at the last minute by a protector alter.

The therapeutic interventions one chooses when faced with a crisis involving self-destructive behavior depend on a number of factors that are difficult to specify and must be determined individually for each patient. The patient's track record with respect to a number of issues should be reviewed by the therapist. What has worked in similar situations in the past, and what has not worked? What is the patient's degree of lethality? All of the usual suicidal predictors are relevant, as well as some factors specific to MPD.

The personality system's track record with respect to honoring contracts is critical. Can the system or specific alters be trusted to make and keep contracts? What is the level of internal communication among the alters? Breakdowns in internal communication during a crisis are common and need to be addressed early in the process. The strength of the protector personalities is important. Are they able to contain or abort the self-destructive behavior, or to alert the therapist in sufficient time that action may be taken to ensure the patient's safety? What do the protector and helper personalities think? Are they frightened by the power of the self-destructive alter? Do they foresee periods of danger? Are the self-destructive personalities inexorably committed to the destruction of the patient, or do they show willingness to compromise? Do the self-destructive personalities manifest delusional ideas of separateness? If the answers to these questions suggest that the patient is a poor risk, then hospitalization or other protective measures should be initiated.

The particulars of the crisis itself will suggest some interventions and eliminate others. Is this an acute crisis or one more round in a more chronic crisis? In the latter cases, the therapist should choose interventions that he or she can sustain over a long period without exhausting therapeutic resources and energies. In the former case, intense and highly focused short-term interventions can be used. What is the role of outside factors in precipitating and perpetuating the crisis? Are abusers or pathological significant others playing a major role that must be directly addressed by the therapist?

The therapist's experience and comfort with possible interventions are also crucial factors. For example, if a therapist is inexperienced in the use of hypnosis, a crisis is not the time to begin hypnotic work with the patient. The state of the therapeutic alliance is likewise critical. Early in the course of treatment, when patient and therapist do not know each other well, the preferable response is one of extreme caution and over-reaction. Later, therapist and patient can more realistically evaluate the seriousness of the crisis and the degree of response required. The therapist's ability to tolerate anxiety and uncertainty is another crucial element. Feeling responsible for a self-destructive outpatient multiple can be a harrowing experience that depletes the therapist and seriously weakens the therapeutic alliance. Each clinician has a threshold that he or she must take into account when contemplating the pros and cons of various interventions.

A number of therapeutic interventions are available to a therapist working with a self-destructive MPD patient. Among the first that should come to mind is hospitalization. As noted in Chapter Ten, inpatient treatment of MPD is a complex and difficult task that often creates its own subset of crises, but it is clearly necessary at times with some patients. Contracting is an important intervention that can be used to control dangerous behavior. The basis statement, "I will not hurt myself or kill myself, nor anyone else, external or internal, accidentally or on purpose, at any time," is the starting point for negotiations. Contracts can be made that cover specific ranges of behavior or specific time periods. To reiterate the points made in Chapter Six, when contracting is used to control dangerous behavior, the therapist must be extremely cautious in choosing the wording and attentive to the expiration date of the contract.

Very often self-destructive behavior on the part of a specific alter can be addressed by allowing that alter to emerge, ventilate, and work through feelings (Kluft, 1983). This is particularly effective with persecutor alters who influence other personalities toward self-destructive acts. Validation of the feelings expressed by the alter, together with an emphasis on the alter's importance in the personality system and facilitation of negotiations between the self-destructive alter and others in the system, will often defuse a crisis. When delusions of separateness are not fixedly established, self-destructive alters may, on occasion, be persuaded of their own inevitable mortality. In some instances, the self-destructive alter can be convinced to relinquish control or responsibility to a nondestructive alter.

The utilization and strengthening of protector and helper alters are important interventions for chronic self-destructive crises. These alters can be recruited to guard the patient's safety and to intervene to stop self-destructive alters. Some multiple personality systems, typically the larger and more complex systems, have body protector alters whose function is to guard the safety of the body, irrespective of which other personalities are "out." These body protectors are usually more or less constantly monitoring the patient's status and situation, and are ready to emerge and take over if danger should arise. Prior to crisis situations, body protector alters need to be sought out and their abilities assessed. Some are very strong; others are considerably weaker and may need help in establishing a route of access to control over the body in times of crisis. Hypnotic imagery work, and, on occasion, teaching a protector to hypnotically control other alters, can aid in strengthening protectors. Helper personalities tend to be weaker and to have less of a mandate from the personality system to protect the patient. They are more useful as consultants and predictors of possible danger.

Kluft (1983) lists several other interventions for dealing with self-destructive alters. He suggests that "fantasy excursions with suggestions of mastery" may be helpful in some cases. I have found this type of intervention to be most useful with child alters who have phobic/avoidance behavior that triggers off panic attacks. Under hypnosis, alters can be helped to visualize and master the objects or situations that they fear. The ego-strengthening techniques developed by David Caul and discussed in Chapter Nine are applicable here. Self-destructive alters may be hypnotically "put to sleep" as a method of removing them from circulation for short periods of time. If this approach is used, it must be noncoercive and benign. Consequently, this technique appears to be most useful in alters whose suicidal ideation is driven by unbearable pain and who experience sleep as a respite.

Fugues, Amnesias, and Rapid Switching

Fugues, amnesias, and trances or depersonalized states are common expressions of crisis in MPD patients and are frequent responses to the recovery of painful, frightening, or disturbing memories that are too overwhelming for the patients to accept. Not infrequently, a patient may go into a dazed trance-like state in the therapist's office following a particularly intense abreactive session. The therapist is then left with the responsibility of getting the patient "back" so that he or she can safely leave the office. After a few of these episodes, the therapist may be reluctant to do any significant abreactive work. Similarly, fugue episodes frequently follow recovery of traumatic material or confrontation with a disavowed part. Not uncommonly, a panicked patient will call the therapist after finding himself or herself in some distant place.

These dissociative experiences are disturbing for patients. Fugue episodes, in particular, will cause panic and confusion and will increase resistance to uncovering work. These episodes frighten patients because they find that they have done something—often something dramatic, such as traveling a great distance—with little or no memory for what happened. Many patients are fearful that they may have done something terrible during these prolonged blank periods. One patient, for example, was afraid that she was responsible for a series of murders occurring in her city. Patients may, in fact, find evidence that during these episodes they are behaving in ways that are morally repugnant to them. They will also fear fugue episodes because they often "wake up" in some frightening or messy situation and are left to deal with the consequences.

Direct or hypnotic inquiry can often elicit the alter(s) responsible for seizing control and taking off. Sometimes these are frightened alters seeking to flee from trauma relived in therapy or other intrusive phenomena. Sometimes the alters responsible are persecutors who are punishing the patient, often by setting up situations that recapitulate earlier trauma. Kluft (1983) notes that the cause of such fugue episodes is usually readily apparent; if it is not found after a few hours of inquiry, the patient may require a protective setting.

Often the therapist is plunged into the middle of this type of crisis by a phone call from a frightened and confused host or other alter who has just found himself or herself in the middle of nowhere. Telephone interventions are tricky, but usually the therapist has no choice but to try them. Kluft (1983) has offered a number of valuable recommendations for working over the telephone with a multiple in crisis. He advises that the therapist keep the patient talking; just hearing the therapist's voice provides a calming effect. Given time and the therapist's telephone presence, protector or helper alters may be able to regain control. The therapist should talk through the specific alter on the phone to the larger personality system. Confrontation or provocation of hostile personalities should be avoided.

The therapist should not invoke formal hypnotic induction ceremonies over the telephone, as these may evoke fears of dyscontrol in some alters. Hypnotic induction through prearranged cue words or through a nonspecific soothing dialogue is possible. Sometimes, frightened alters can be calmed by reminding them of the next session and providing reassurance that the therapist is available if necessary. Kluft (1983) notes that in his experience, multiples with borderline, masochistic, or narcissistic tendencies may not respond to these interventions. When this is the case, the therapist should try to elicit sufficient information to allow the authorities to locate the patient.

Rapid switching or the revolving-door syndrome usually occurs when the patient is in the midst of a highly anxiety-provoking situation or when he or she is caught between two intensely conflicting demands. Levenson and Berry (1983) describe a classic example of rapid switching that occurred when their patient presented in the emergency room with her two lesbian lovers, both of whom were insisting that they were married to her. The patient "began to switch quickly between personalities, and the rapidity of these changes became frightening to her, her children, and her lovers" (p. 76). When a patient is in a rapid-switching crisis, either no personality wants to be "out" and therefore various alters are pushed "out" by other alters and immediately seek to retreat, or two or more personalities are struggling for control of the body and each is displacing the other in a circular fashion.

Patients caught in a revolving-door crisis look exceedingly disturbed and not infrequently appear psychotic. The rapid alternation of personalities produces extreme lability of affect as frightened, laughing, angry, and depressed alters whiz by. The patient will not be able to carry on a coherent conversation, and his or her speech will be akin to the "word salad" one would get from rapidly changing the channels on a television set. The therapist needs to look behind this disturbed behavior to determine whether a series of alters is involved or whether the rapid switching is limited to two or three alters. In the latter case, it is likely that this represents a struggle for control over the body and behavior. In the former case, it is more likely that no personality wants to be "out" and in control.

If the rapid switching is due to a struggle for control over the body, the therapist should try to get the alters to relinquish control to a neutral party and resolve their conflict through communication and cooperation. This crisis should be viewed as an opportunity to further the personality system's experience in negotiation and compromise. In some cases, the struggle between two alters involves a self-destructive alter and a protector seeking to prevent injury. In this case, provisions for the protection of the body should precede the relinquishing of control by the protector alter.

In cases where the rapid switching results from the unwillingness of any alter to be "out," the therapist should look for an immediate environmental cause. This pattern of rapid switching is usually a response to an acute situational precipitant, and the elimination of this stimulus and the creation of a safe environment will stop the rapid switching. In some instances, the rapid switching is an attempt to stave off an impending abreaction. One patient, for example, began rapid switching shortly after an unexpected visit from his father, who had just been released from jail, where he had been serving time for molesting the patient's sisters. His group home leader brought him to the hospital, where we were able to stop the rapid switching by abreacting a specific abuse episode triggered by his father's visit.

Acute Somatic Symptoms

Acute somatic symptoms are another manifestation of crisis in multiples. Many times these symptoms are blatantly hysterical, but sometimes they may closely resemble true medical emergencies, and in some instances they may actually be life-threatening. Headaches are the most common somatic complaint in multiples (Bliss, 1984b; Greaves, 1980; Putnam et al., 1986). Often they are migraine-like with unilaterality and scotoma, and are described as "blinding." Unexplained pain syndromes, particularly abdominal and pelvic pain, colitis, and other "functional" gastrointestinal disturbances, are common (Bliss, 1984b; Putnam et al., 1986). Classic hysterical paralysis, aphonia, psychogenic deafness, blindness, and pseudoseizures are not rare (Bliss, 1984b; Putnam et al., 1986). Patients may have cardiac, respiratory, and neurological crises that at times demand acute medical responses, even though the etiology is often later found to be psychogenic. Significant fluctuations in body weight often occur, particularly in females. Anorexic behavior is seen in a surprisingly high percentage of cases, with a lesser percentage exhibiting bulimia (Putnam *et al.*, 1986). In some patients, these symptoms can become life-threatening crises.

The causes of these crises are usually conflicts among alters, the recall and re-experience of prior trauma (this is a frequent cause of the unexplained pain syndromes), and self-destructive urges. The therapist should first determine, as much as possible, whether the symptoms are being experienced by only a few of the personalities or are shared by all or a large number of alters. In the former case, it is usually safe to assume that the symptoms are psychosomatic. In the latter case, a medical workup for the symptom(s) may be indicated to rule out any organic pathology and to allow the therapist to address the symptoms with a greater assurance that they are in fact psychogenic.

In seeking effective interventions for somatic crises, the therapist should try to differentiate between crises that appear to have acute causes and those that reflect chronic problems. Acute crises usually respond well to interventions directed at personality system issues. Seeking out alters involved in the crisis and allowing them to ventilate and work through feelings can be effective. Many times, acute somatic symptoms are a visceral expression of repressed trauma that is now close to conscious awareness and needs to be fully recovered and abreacted. Age regression of the patient as a whole or specific personalities back to the first time that the symptom appeared, or the use of the affect bridge (both techniques are discussed in Chapter Nine), is often effective in uncovering the source of somatic symptoms. Kluft (1983) notes that direct or indirect suggestions may be helpful in mitigating these symptoms.

Long-standing somatic symptoms often reflect deeply dissociated visceral memories of traumas, long-standing interpersonality conflicts, and chronic self-destructive behavior. These symptoms respond slowly to the improved level of internal communication that, one hopes, occurs as therapy progresses. Ventilation, inner dialogues, compromises, and the recovery of repressed traumas will wear away at these symptoms. Chronic headaches are a particularly troublesome symptom and often represent covert struggles over control of the body and behavior. They can be acutely dealt with by asking the personalities involved to "stand aside" and allow one another to possess the body in sequence. In the long run, as interpersonality communication and trust improve, alters will be more willing to "hand over" control of behavior, because they know that the other alters will give it back in an appropriate manner and place.

In some rare but not unheard-of cases, chronic medical symptoms are secondary to factitious induction by one alter inflicted on an amnesic host. Shelley (1981) describes a case of a woman who had severe and inexplicable dermatitis limited to her left arm. During hospitalization for a medical workup for a suspected vascular etiology, it was discovered that the patient was suffering from MPD and that an alter was applying fresh poison ivy leaves with a gloved right hand to the patient's left arm. This alter was also responsible for producing large, mysterious hematomas on two occasions. The possibility of a factitious etiology for mysterious symptoms needs to be kept in mind when one is medically working up somatic symptoms in multiples.

In some instances (e.g., severe anorexic crises), the psychosomatic symptoms become life-threatening and require medical interventions. However, medical interventions in such cases usually lead quickly to complicated chronic crises. These interventions run several risks. The first is that the interpersonality conflict fueling this type of crisis now can be played out between the medical staff and the patient. I have seen numerous protracted battles between self-destructive alters and medical staff members who are determined to "save" the patient even if they kill the patient in the process. These battles follow a pattern of cyclic escalation, with both sides pulling out all stops. The culmination of one such battle found the patient in four-way restraints, a nasogastric feeding tube taped in place, and a staff member detailed round the clock to sit by her bed to prevent her from removing the feeding tube. The anorexic/self-destructive alters, on their part, had made two very serious suicide attempts while on stringent suicide precautions, and had managed to lose weight to the point where the patient had severe anemia and general malnutrition. Both sides were exhausted, depleted, and grimly determined to "win."

The second difficulty involved with medical interventions is that some types of interventions (e.g., gynecological procedures) often symbolically represent a recapitulation of the original trauma. This can be gratifying to some alters at times and can drive the crisis to new heights. One should be alert to this possibility when a patient repeatedly has somatic symptoms that receive medical treatment. The third problem with medical interventions is that they are of limited value in the long run. They may be necessary to rule out possible serious organic illness or even to keep the patient alive in the short term, but they quickly become complicated by other dynamics and serve to derail the psychotherapy. Every clinician must do what is necessary to ensure that a patient is not suffering from a medical problem, but once some reasonable degree of assurance is possible, the interventions for somatic symptoms and crises should be psycho- or hypnotherapeutic.

Discovery of New Alters or Failure of Previous Fusions

The discovery of new alters can precipitate a crisis. Often this occurs when a whole new "family" of alters is uncovered in a patient who formerly believed that he or she already knew most of the personalities. This new group of alters—often perceived as alien and malevolent in comparison to the "known" personalities—overwhelms the patient with evidence of how much more work remains to be done, as well as with fears about these unknown entities. The balances and compromises that had been worked out among the previously known alters may now also be jeopardized, and the personality system can quickly slide into disequilibrium. Similarly, the discovery that personalities believed to have been previously integrated have in fact remained covertly separated may produce crises with themes of failure, betrayal, despair, and hopelessness.

Therapists too become despondent at the discovery of new groups of alters or the failure of previous integrations. "When is it ever going to end?" is a familiar question asked repeatedly in our local peer supervision group. The discovery of new alters, particularly new families of alters, should not be viewed as a setback, but rather as a statement that sufficient progress has been made in the therapy that these alters now are ready to emerge. Although the new alters will disturb the previous balance of the system, they are usually relatively easy to include in the ongoing work and hold many of the missing pieces that will make more stable fusions and integrations possible. They should be welcomed to the therapy.

This is one of the crises that is best handled by anticipation and preemptive work. The patient should be counseled to expect that new alters will be found as the therapy progresses. Some alters will remain hidden, but actively watch the therapist and the therapy until they feel ready to reveal themselves; other alters may exist in a dormant state and not be activated until the therapy moves into issues that energize them. The therapist should always assume that there are alters that he or she has not yet met. When addressing the personality system as a whole or using talking-through techniques, the therapist can specifically include such alters by making statements such as this: "I am talking to everyone I know, and also to those whom I have not yet met." When new alters are discovered or the failure of previous fusions is uncovered, and the patient responds with feelings of despair, agitation, and hopelessness, the therapist should remind the patient that these experiences are expectable and predictable events that have been anticipated and discussed in the past. Most patients will respond to explanation and reassurance, particularly if the therapist has also been prepared and is not mirroring feelings of despair and hopelessness.

Intrusion or Rejection by Family of Origin

Crises secondary to encounters with the family of origin are extremely common (Kluft, 1983). The dynamics and interactions among family members often closely resemble the patient's own personality system dynamics, so that family crises often create mirror-image crises within the patient (Kluft *et al.*, 1984). Contact with the abuser(s) or other family members, or even anticipated contact, can trigger massive regressions in the patient (Kluft, 1983). The families of MPD patients usually fit the descriptions coined for other abusing families, such as "united front" or "pseudonormal veneer" (Kluft *et al.*, 1984). This dynamic of maintaining a facade of extreme righteousness at all costs leads such families to intervene in the patients' lives and to sabotage or undermine any treatment that may reveal the family pathology. Often, alter personalities will slip into their old roles and collude with family members in denying past abuse and undermining any uncovering work in therapy (Kluft *et al.*, 1984). Crises are also created by the family's outright rejection of the patient, sometimes after appearing to be supportive of treatment efforts (Kluft, 1983). Actual abuse of adult MPD patients by family members does occur and can touch off devastating crises. This possibility should never be discounted. Even strong, young, athletic male patients can be retraumatized by their sickly old parents if they regress to helpless child alters in the face of the family dynamics.

Crises involving family intrusion, rejection, or other forms of family uproar are best dealt with by prevention. In a situation where the patient's trauma was inflicted or facilitated by family-of-origin members (in fact, this is true of most MPD patients), I advocate keeping the patient away from the family of origin (if this is the source of the past trauma) until at least well into the treatment course. Unfortunately, this is often difficult, and certain alters will sabotage any attempts to keep the patient and family apart. When contact with the family of origin is anticipated, the therapist and patient should do anticipatory work in therapy. Contingency plans with preidentified alters should be worked out to allow the patient to escape if abuse or other retraumatization appears imminent. The focus and limitations of the contact should be established, and the patient and therapist should try to choose and control the setting of the contact to prevent the patient from regressing into old patterns of interaction. The therapist should also preschedule a follow-up session soon after contact with the family, to aid in processing the events and reestablishing system equilibrium.

Copresence Crises

Copresence phenomena in multiple personality patients typically resemble the old descriptions of "lucid possession" states (Kluft, 1983, 1987). Lucid possession is a form of possession in which the individual remains constantly aware of himself or herself, but feels "a spirit within his own spirit" that cannot be prevented from speaking or acting (Ellenberger, 1970). Crises of copresence in multiples usually include some or all of the following phenomena: (1) states of extreme depersonalization; (2) disruption or impairment of normally autonomous ego functions; (3) perceptual alterations (e.g., auditory and visual distortions, illusions, or hallucinations involving alter personalities); and (4) cognitive disturbances (e.g., thought insertion, thought withdrawal, and intrusive commentaries) (Kluft, 1983). Early in the therapy, crises of copresence may be terrifying to a host personality who does not know about or accept the existence of alter personalities.

Crises of copresence are usually a manifestation of a struggle for control among two or more personalities. In most cases, they respond to some form of compromise that allows the intruding alter to express its opinions and communicate with the host, therapist, or important others. Kluft (1983) states that most crises of copresence respond to (1) persuading the host or other alter that is "out" to listen, and (2) making contact with the intrusive copresent alter. Often, negotiating a contract that gives the intrusive alter a chance to state his or her case and then withdraw usually resolves the crisis. The communication can occur through speaking, writing, or ideomotor signaling. In severe cases, hypnotic inquiry with the intruding alter(s) may be required. At times, deep trance may be useful to control dangerous behavior or reduce the fear of the host personality.

THERAPEUTIC RESOLUTION

Lack of Data on Treatment Outcome

A thorough reading of the many single case reports, reviews, and articles on treatment interventions for MPD will reveal that, with a few notable exceptions (e.g., Coons, 1986; Kluft, 1984a, 1985e, 1986b), there are no clear indications of treatment outcome for MPD patients. This lack of outcome data is both surprising and dismaying. Among clinicians who are experienced in working with multiples, it is generally accepted that

MPD has a good prognosis for those patients who remain in treatment (Kluft, 1985d; Putnam, 1986b). Yet there are only a few professional articles, together with a number of novelized or autobiographical accounts of treatment, that hint at favorable outcome. As Kluft (1984a) observes, these sources "offer tantalizing clues but hardly constitute a data base" (p. 9).

In part, the reason for the apparent discrepancy between the generally held belief of a favorable prognosis and the lack of published outcome data to support this position is that many successful clinicians have presented their results in meetings, courses, and workshops, or in other forums besides professional publications. The description of Cornelia Wilbur's treatment of Sybil, for example, had to be published in the lay press after her paper on the case was deliberately omitted from the proceedings of the professional symposium in which she first presented her work. In the context of this oral tradition on MPD, the outcome of the disorder is generally considered to be good. Kluft (1985d) states, "There is increasing agreement that the prognosis for most patients with MPD is quite optimistic if intense and prolonged treatment from experienced clinicians can be made available" (p. 3). He further observes that where there is a poor outcome, the logistics of providing treatment, rather than intrinsic intractability, are what prevent success.

I think, however, that the success of a few highly experienced clinicians should not yet be taken as representative of the overall treatment outcome of MPD. The follow-up study published by Coons (1986), examining outcome in patients treated by a variety of professionals at different levels of training, is probably a more realistic reflection of the overall prognosis of MPD. Although Coons's data generally indicate a significant improvement with treatment in MPD patients, they typically fall well short of the total integration of the patient so often held out as the usual outcome. It is my belief that the current lack of systematic outcome data has created a vacuum currently filled by unrealistic expectations and assumptions about integration such as those seen in *The Three Faces of Eve.*

Possible Treatment Outcomes

Remaining a Multiple Personality

A "between-the-lines" review of case reports in the literature suggests that many MPD patients probably leave therapy before achieving complete fusion/integration. The decision of whether or not to remain multiple or to attempt to achieve complete integration is faced by virtually every MPD patient at some point during his or her course of treatment. Usually this question surfaces covertly early on and more openly later, when the patient has achieved a modicum of internal communication and cooperation and is functioning at a higher level. At this point, a multiple may decide to terminate therapy and to remain multiple or to seek another therapist with whom to continue treatment. In some instances, a multiple will terminate therapy before any fusions/integrations have occurred; in other cases, a patient may undergo a number of partial integrations that reduce the overall size and complexity of the personality system, but leave the patient still psychologically organized as a multiple personality.

The reasons that multiples give for terminating therapy prior to the completion of fusion/integration and postresolution treatment are diverse. Some of the more commonly reported reasons are discussed below. The perceptions of multiples and their therapists will differ greatly, and what a therapist sees as a resistance to further work may be seen by a patient as the most "logical" thing to do. Too often, however, it is obvious that the termination of therapy is premature and that apparent increases in the patient's level of function have not been adequately consolidated, leading to another cycle of chaos and self-destructive behavior.

Many multiples appear to leave therapy because they do not wish to continue with the process of uncovering and working through past traumas. This work is painful and causes significant disruption in a patient's life outside of the treatment setting. The personality system is usually aware at some level of what lies ahead, and may at times elect to "protect" the patient from recovering further traumas. Not uncommonly, the patient exhibits a flight into health, rather than face particularly painful memories and affects.

The personality system as a whole or specific alters may be afraid of the loss of separateness or believe that fusion is equivalent to death. Many alters believe that to give up separateness is to die or, at the very least, to lose the capacity to uniquely express and enjoy themselves. The alters or the personality system may also fear that fusion/integration will lead to a loss of specific talents or abilities possessed by certain alters. Among patients who work in the arts, there is usually a great deal of concern about the possible loss of creativity with fusion/integration. Kluft (1984d) and other therapists with extensive experience with the results of fusion/integration report that although there may be a transient disruption in alter-specific skills or talents with fusion, this is not an enduring loss, and these abilities return with time. In some cases, the individual alters become so loved and cherished by the multiple that the patient does not wish to "lose" them through fusion/integration. The therapist must walk a fine line between urging the patient to respect the importance of each alter, which is necessary for the patient to come to terms with what each alter represents, and creating a situation in which the alters become so special that the patient is reluctant to give them up.

Patients may be concerned that fusion/integration will produce drastic changes in their relationships with the important people in their lives, including their therapists. Specific alters may be involved in relationships that the patients believe can only be maintained by those alters. The patients may be concerned that therapists or other important figures will lose interest in them if they "get better." A number of multiples have directly expressed these concerns to me as the primary reason why they will not permit final fusions to succeed. They believe that their therapists will lose interest in them if they stop being multiples.

In some cases, multiples discontinue therapy prematurely because of outside interference. Members of the family of origin, often but not always including the original abuser(s), will seek to sabotage the treatment. A multiple who succumbs to this outside interference has usually been enmeshed in the family of origin throughout the course of treatment. A multiple may also withdraw from treatment because of sabotage by a spouse or lover who does not wish to see the patient improve. In some instances, treatment has been terminated at the insistence of "friends" or fellow church members who seek to control multiples or see them as demonically possessed.

Some multiples terminate treatment short of final resolution because for them it is ego-syntonic to be multiples. These patients usually have developed a high degree of cooperation and communication across many (but not all) of their personalities and derive substantial secondary gain from publicly demonstrating their multiplicity. They will present themselves as superhuman, with repertoires of abilities that far outstrip those of mere "singles." Their extreme narcissistic investment in their multiplicity precludes any attempt at complete fusion/integration. Multiples may pass through a stage during the course of treatment in which they appear to become comfortable with their multiplicity, but usually this is a transient and self-limited phase. Of those patients who choose to remain multiples, some may do so overtly but others may do it covertly, deliberately concealing their multiplicity even from the therapist. A patient may also truly believe that he or she is fully integrated and may be unaware of alters who have remained hidden throughout the course of therapy. In either case, even experienced therapists may not detect any evidence of multiplicity unless they subject the patients to a systematic inquiry such as the protocol described by Kluft (1985e) for evaluation of the stability of fusion/integration.

Although there is a general consensus among experienced therapists that complete integration of the alter personalities is a desirable goal, this simply may be unrealistic with many patients. Kluft (1985d) is the first to acknowledge, "In a given case, it is hard to argue with Caul's pragmatism: 'It seems to me that after treatment you want a functional unit, be it a corporation, a partnership, or a one-owner business'" (p. 3). It is a mistake to make integration the focus of therapy. Treatment should be aimed at replacing maladaptive behaviors and responses with more appropriate forms of coping. Ideally, integration of the alters will emerge from this process, but even if it does not, the therapy may well be termed a success if the patient has achieved a significant improvement in his or her level of functioning.

Fusion/Integration

The terms "fusion" and "integration" are often used synonymously to describe the unification of alter personalities into a single entity (Kluft, 1984c). Experienced therapists, however, often distinguish between these two events. Integration is understood to be a "more pervasive and thorough psychic restructuring," while fusion is seen as an initial "compacting" process that lays the groundwork for integration (Kluft, 1984c). From this perspective, fusion can be understood as the process of removing the dissociative barriers that segregate specific alters. Integration occurs over a period of weeks to months and produces a synthesis of the previously separate elements of each alter into a more unified global personality structure.

Kluft (1984a) has enumerated a number of criteria that he believes constitute an operational definition of "fusion." He defines it as requiring at least 3 months of the following:

> 1) continuity of contemporary memory, 2) absence of overt behavioral signs of multiplicity, 3) subjective sense of unity, 4) absence of alter personalities on hypnotic re-exploration, 5) modification of transference phenomena consistent with the bringing together of personalities, and 6) clinical evidence that the unified patient's self-representation included acknowledgement of attitudes and awareness which were previously segregated in separate personalities. (p. 12)

Kluft makes the distinction between "apparent" fusion, which is the appearance of these criteria for a period of less than 3 months, and "stable" fusion, which is maintenance of these criteria for a period of at least 27 months.

These criteria really only apply to "final" fusions, in which all of the alters are included. Often MPD patients will undergo a series of "partial" fusions, which precede the final fusion and consolidate many of the personalities and personality fragments into a few discrete alters, who then participate in the final fusion process. Partial fusions may occur spontaneously, in or out of the therapy setting, as the dissociative barriers between alters erode following increased internal communication and cooperation. Partial fusions may also be deliberately performed as part of the therapeutic plan to reduce the number of alters and unify the patient. No operational criteria have been advanced for evaluating the success of partial fusions. Virtually nothing is known about either the process of fusion or integration, beyond phenomenological observation and the subjective reports of patients.

Spontaneous Final Fusion/Integration

The limited evidence available suggests that although spontaneous partial fusions of alters may occur in the absence of treatment, spontaneous final fusions do not occur, or occur only rarely in adult MPD patients (Caul, 1985a; Kluft, 1985a, 1986b). Kluft (1985a) has reported on 12 multiples who declined treatment and were subsequently re-evaluated 3 to 10 years later. All of these patients remained multiples, although the form of presentation was different on the second occasion compared to the first. Coons's (1986) data also support the interpretation that spontaneous fusions are extremely rare. Caul (1985a) notes that multiples' claims of spontaneous fusion occur in the midst of a difficult and anxiety-provoking therapy. Flights into health and claims of spontaneous fusion are to be expected from patients facing a long, difficult, and painful treatment course. The therapist should be sympathetic to the wish expressed and aware of the resistance manifested in these claims, but should take the position that even if the spontaneous fusion is real, it does not mark the end of treatment, only a milestone. Treatment does not end with fusion/integration; it only enters a new phase.

The Disappearance of Alters

Over the course of treatment, alters will "disappear" from time to time. With a few exceptions, the vast majority of alters who disappear will eventually reappear at a later point. The patient may be very distressed by these disappearances, and the therapist may share that distress when the alter who vanishes is perceived as a helper or protector. The alter involved, however, is not dead or gone, but merely dormant and inactivated by the larger dynamics of the personality system. The personality system of an MPD patient is a dynamic structure that is always undergoing developmental/evolutionary change. Like the rest of nature, it abhors a vacuum. When alters disappear, others will eventually fill the functions and roles of the missing ones.

Occasionally, a multiple may have a crisis in which all of the alters report that they are fading out and disappearing. Intense anxiety may result as the patient experiences a total dissolution of sense of self, accompanied by extreme feelings of depersonalization and derealization. Again, the patient's palpable anxiety is highly contagious, but the therapist should view and treat this event as part of the patient's larger dissociative disturbance of identity. Reasurance and support, communicated with the firm conviction that the patient will continue to exist irrespective of the existence or disappearance of any or all alters, will usually help the patient weather this crisis.

There are a few instances in which alters do seem to disappear for good. This process seems to involve alters, usually only very fragmentary entities, who cease to have a separate existence following the abreaction of the trauma associated with their creation. Kluft (1985e) reports a subgroup of MPD patients who appear to have a personality system composed of these "rather friable alters related to specific traumatic experiences" (p. 16). He reports that these patients are unified very quickly by hypnotically facilitated abreactions. In addition, patients who fall into the hypothesized "second-split" category of MPD patients—that is, patients who have a history of being multiple in childhood, who then appear to have achieved a spontaneous integration at an early age, and who much later in life appear to have a second split or breakdown of fusion/integration around a specific stress—may reintegrate spontaneously or with limited treatment after the stress is removed.

Forced Fusions

Although coercive or forced fusion techniques have been reported in the treatment of MPD (Brandsma & Ludwig, 1974), a number of authors clearly state that this practice is contraindicated except as a last-resort measure in extreme, life-threatening situations (Herzog, 1984; Kluft, 1983). Forced fusions either never "take" or come apart very rapidly, and often intensify the strife that they were supposed to stifle. I have never seen a forced fusion hold for more than a few weeks, and most come apart within days. There may be a significant disruption in the therapeutic alliance following a forced fusion.

Factors Influencing Prognosis

When there are such meager data on treatment outcome in MPD, it is difficult to determine the important factors that influence prognosis of the disorder. One must rely on clinical experience from experienced therapists to identify factors associated with poor prognosis. Caul (1985d) asks a series of common-sense questions. His first one is "Does the patient accept the diagnosis?" (p. 1). Failure to accept diagnosis generally leads to a stalemate early in therapy, with little productive work toward resolution. My own experience and Coons's (1986) data support the idea that acceptance of the diagnosis is one of the first issues that must be confronted and worked through for a successful treatment. If the patient has been previously diagnosed as having MPD, how long has the condition been known, and how many previous therapists has the patient had? Clinical experience suggests that the longer a person's career as a multiple, the poorer the prognosis. What is the maximum number of alters? Are there extreme or highly specialized functions among them, and is the patient preoccupied in focusing on the separateness of the alters throughout the therapy? Large numbers of alters, highly specialized functions, and long-term preoccupation with separateness all augur poorly for unification (Coons, 1986; Kluft, 1986b; Putnam et al., 1986). A related question posed by Caul (1985d) is this: "Throughout the therapy is the patient preoccupied with using the alter personalities as the exclusive means of problem solving?" (p. 1). Multiples who do not try nondissociative methods of coping with life stresses are not likely to give up their multiplicity readily.

Caul's next three questions are as follows: "Does the patient commonly attempt to dominate the nature, extent and course of the therapy?" (1985d, p. 1); "Does the patient attempt to control the therapist?" (1985d, p. 2); and "Does the therapy tend to focus on 'discovery' much more than therapeutic attitudes aimed at resolution?" (1985d, p. 2). The issue of control is an important therapeutic theme, discussed earlier in Chapter Seven. If the patient succeeds in controlling the therapy, either overtly or covertly, little progress can be expected in the area of uncovering and working through of painful memories and affects. Multiples will not trust therapists whom they can control, and this lack of trust will be reflected in a lack of substantive progress in treatment. Caul sees the patient's commitment to treatment as crucial in determining outcome. If the patient is not emotionally committed to change and is not working toward resolution, then the chances of achieving either are nil.

Kluft covers much of the same ground in a series of observations from his work with over 100 MPD patients. He notes that "patients whose personalities worked towards cooperation and integration fared better than those whose personalities tried to cooperate, but zealously guarded their separateness" (Kluft, 1986b, p. 36). Over time he has observed that in cases where apparent unity is achieved by suppression, extrusion, banishment or alleged departure of alters, there is almost universal relapse (Kluft, 1982, 1986b). Within limits, he notes a relationship between complexity and relapse, with three-quarters of his relapses occurring in patients with 18 or more alters. Beyond that, he feels that there is not a significant relationship between greater degrees of complexity and poor prognosis. He notes that male patients average fewer alters and have correspondingly shorter treatment times and fewer relapses.

With the exception of child and adolescent cases, Kluft (1986d) does not believe that age is a factor in prognosis. In children, age appears to be a potent prognostic factor, with younger children undergoing speedy unification. Kluft has not found that the existence of a concurrent medication-responsive affective disorder has a negative effect on prognosis. He cites unpublished data indicating that "problematic ego strength"—a high level of masochism and an extensive investment in separateness among alters—is associated with poorer prognosis (Kluft, 1986b). The reinforcement of multiplicity by the patient's significant others also bodes poorly for unification. Severe DSM-III Axis II psychopathology or the existence of an "extensive inner world of personalities in which alters interact with one another in relationships of great complexity and/or intensity," or both, complicate treatment (Kluft, 1986b, p. 55).

In summary, a good prognosis appears to be related to the patient's emotional commitment to treatment and resolution of separateness; a lack of investment in the separateness of the alters; the patient's willingness to try nondissociative coping skills; and the establishment of a therapeutic alliance in which the patient trusts the therapist sufficiently to relinquish control to him or her. Fewer alters, lesser degrees of internal complexity, and the absence of severe concurrent personality or developmental disorders (Axis II) psychopathology are also positive prognostic indicators. Coons's (1986) study would add one more issue: the role of retraumatization during the course of therapy. Coons found that patients who failed to integrate had twice as many traumatic events (e.g., deaths in the family, divorces, bankruptcy, revictimization, etc.) as those who achieved integration by Kluft's criteria.

Techniques for Fusion/Integration

Preliminary Work

It has been evident since the first comprehensive treatment plan put forth by Allison (1978a) that the therapy of MPD proceeds stepwise through a series of issues and stages (Braun, 1986; Coons, 1986; Caul, 1978a; Kluft, 1985d; Wilbur, 1984b). Although there may be minor disagreements on the order and emphasis of specific points, the majority of authorities on the treatment of MPD agree that the core therapeutic work includes (1) diagnosing the condition and helping the patient accept the diagnosis; (2) establishing communication and a working alliance with accessible alters; (3) gathering history about the origin, functions, attributes, relationships, and agendas of the alters; (4) contracting around problematic behaviors; (5) facilitating internal communications; (6) working through the alters' traumata, problems, and issues; (7) working toward increased unification, including fusions and integrations; and (8) consolidating gains and substituting nondissociative defenses to deal with life stress. Fusion and integration work is typically delayed until later in the course of therapy.

SIGNS THAT THE PATIENT IS READY FOR FUSIONS

Partial fusions will occur both in and out of the treatment setting. Some will be spontaneous, and some will be performed by the therapist. Before a therapist performs a partial or final fusion, he or she should try to determine whether the alters are ready for the fusion. Forced or coercive fusions, or fusions for which the patient has not been properly prepared, have a short half-life and almost universally come apart. Signs suggesting that two or more alters are ready for fusion usually indicate that the dissociative barriers maintaining separateness have eroded to a point where fusion is possible. The alters may report coconsciousness or other forms of simultaneously shared awareness. A nondysphoric, persistent sense of simultaneous copresence is a strong indicator that two or more alters are ready to attempt fusion. The alters may report an "identity crisis," in that they do not feel the way they used to and have a blurred or overlapping sense of identity. The alters may also report themselves ready to fuse or request that the therapist help them fuse. In some instances, the alters request fusion because continued separateness is uncomfortable (Kluft, 1984a).

GETTING THE PATIENT READY FOR FUSION

In general, alters who are going to be fused should be close to the same age. Age differences are probably most acute in fusions involving two or more child alters and less important in fusions among adult alters. Where significant age differences exist, younger alters can be age-progressed using the hypnotherapy techniques described in Chapter Nine.

If the therapist and patient have been using and updating personality system maps (described in Chapter Eight), these should be consulted prior to attempting fusion. Generally, alters who are adjacent to each other on the map or share a common connection in the map's overall metaphor will fuse together more easily than alters who belong to different families or are in divergent domains on the map. In the latter case, fusions should probably be attempted among similar alters, and these resulting larger constellations should be fused across domains. If there are blank areas on the maps separating alters who seek fusion, these must be explored. Blank areas can indicate unrecognized alters whose presence will disrupt fusion.

The patient as a whole must be prepared for the fusion process. When extensive fusions are planned, or in cases where the alters participating in the fusion perform significant functions in the patient's daily life (e.g., work personalities), the patient should be advised to take some time off from work or other demanding activities. In fact, patients should be urged to accumulate some sick leave or vacation time in anticipation of fusion or extensive abreactive work. Fusion can temporarily suppress some abilities, making it difficult for a patient to perform tasks related for these capacities. If placed in a situation that demands these abilities, the patient may have to redissociate to gain access to the temporarily suppressed skills.

Principles of Fusion Techniques

Most fusions occur between two alters, although fusion among several alters is not uncommon (Kluft, 1982). Successful fusions can only occur after the dissociative defensive barriers that serve to separate the alters have been significantly eroded by psychotherapy, usually augmented by hypnotherapeutic techniques. The alters begin to accept each other and to develop a sense of mutual self-identification. Each will also acknowledge memories possessed by the other alter, and other issues for which the alter in question was previously amnesic or denied knowledge. At this point, the alters will often indicate that they are uncomfortable with their separateness and report experiences of coconsciousness and feelings of being redundant (Kluft, 1982). The therapist then spends some time searching for residual areas of conflict between the alters. Each alter should be offered the opportunity to talk about any latent issues and probe for hidden conflicts. If any problems remain, these must be worked through until no further issues divide the alters to be fused.

The next step usually involves a ceremony or ritual, frequently augmented by hypnosis, though spontaneous fusion may also occur if the alters have worked through their differences completely (Braun, 1984c). Most ceremonies described in the literature, as well as those that I have witnessed or performed, involve the use of visual imagery and metaphors and are generally performed while the alters are in trance. The image or metaphor employed should be discussed ahead of time with the alters and the patient as a whole. Some apparently innocuous images may have highly charged meanings for the alters or patient and may thus be detrimental to the fusion process.

Kluft (1982) reports using images of embrace, dance, and other shared activities. He notes that his patients seem to prefer images of the blending together of light or the flowing together of water. He calls forth the two alters to be fused to "stand" side by side, and then incorporates them into the hypnotically enhanced imagery. The alters may then be told that they are surrounded by a glowing ball of light, and that as their light blends together, they also blend together to become a single glowing ball of light. He stresses that images of blending in which all elements are preserved and represented in the larger whole are preferable to images or metaphors that suggest death, elimination, subtraction, or banishment. Braun (1984c) uses a similar set of metaphors and images. He reports using images of mixing different colors of paint or ink to get a "solution" colored by each alter.

Likewise, I typically employ images of blending together of light or fluid as part of the fusion ceremony. Patients seem to need and demand these ceremonies, although the fusion process usually appears to be taking place on its own with the development of coconsciousness, the erosion of dissociative barriers, and the alters' increasing discomfort with separateness. I do not know what fusion is or is about. At times I find myself quite skeptical of the process and wonder whether we have bought into a magical expectation about treatment outcome. Everything we know about developmental psychopathological processes would suggest that the early trauma suffered by these patients has irreparably damaged them, so that a unified sense of self would be impossible to achieve in later adult life (Putnam, 1988a). Yet I have seen some patients undergo a transformation over the course of treatment, so that the alter personalities lose their separateness and appear to be absorbed into a more integrated sense of self. Francie Howland taught me long ago that integration should not be the treatment goal with multiples, but it can be a gratifying outcome in some cases.

Final Fusions

Final fusions—that is, fusions in which all of the alters are blended into a single entity—are simply extensions of the techniques described above. Usually final fusions are preceded by a series of partial fusions that consolidate the alters into two or more composite personalities, which then undergo the final fusion. Braun (1983b) provides a good account of a sequence of fusions/integrations occurring over a several-year period prior to the final fusions of two patients. Final fusions may be accompanied by changes in sensory perception by the patient (Braun, 1983b, 1984c). I have heard several patients spontaneously report that sounds were clearer ("less muffled"), colors brighter, and vision sharper following a final integration.

Failure of Fusions

The Need to Assess the Stability of a Fusion

It becomes obvious to anyone who works with or has followed several MPD patients over time that many so-called "final" fusions are not final at all. Braun often says in MPD workshops, "The first final fusion isn't!" Kluft (1985e) calmly states, "I learned to anticipate relapses" (p. 66). It is absolutely expectable for the patient either to come apart or not to fuse at all, and merely to *appear* to fuse during the initial "final" fusion. Relapses of fusions and failure to fuse are common events in the course of therapy and should be anticipated with the patient. If both therapist and patient learn to approach fusions with skeptical caution, and not to invest too much hope and expectation in them, relapses can be absorbed into the course of treatment without undue disappointment or disruption.

In some instances, the failure of the fusion is overtly demonstrated by the emergence of an alter thought to have been fused. In many cases, the fusion appears to be successful, and the therapist and often the patient believe that the patient is now "whole." A number of dynamics will perpetuate this illusion for a while. The patient may be unaware of the existence of unfused alters, because they are not overtly emerging and causing amnesia and time loss; however, they may still affect the patient's behavior through passive-influence phenomena. In other instances, the patient is aware of the existence of these alters and conceals this from the therapist.

A multiple has many reasons to deceive the therapist about the success of a fusion. Not infrequently, the multiple is pretending to be fused in order to please the therapist. The patient may sense strong needs on the part of the therapist to have the fusion be a success, and may fear that if the failure is revealed, the therapist will reject him or her. Deception is also a defense against having to face further painful uncovering and abreactive work. In some patients, there may be significant secondary gain associated with feigning fusion (e.g., discharge from a hospital or preservation of a relationship or job that requires the patient to be "cured"). Deception is part of the patient's lifestyle and is to be expected in the treatment as well as in many other areas of the patient's life. Kluft (1985e) has wisely observed that one should understand the practice of deception by MPD patients "as a reenactment in the transference of a desperate coping style rather than proof of 'poor character'" (p. 66).

Signs of Failure of Fusions

Assessing the patient for failure of a final fusion is similar to evaluating a patient for possible MPD. The advantage is that the therapist is now familiar with the personality system and the patient's dynamics. Most of the signs, symptoms, and strategies used in the diagnostic process are applicable to this assessment. As in the diagnostic process, it is important always to have a high index of suspicion for the existence of alters.

Evidence of amnesia is the single best sign of the failure of a final fusion. This may be manifested by unexplained behaviors and incidents for which the patient has little explanation or obviously confabulates details. The therapist must be alert for evidence of amnesia both in and out of the therapy setting. Amnesia in the treatment setting is manifested by intrasession microamnesias, in which the patient appears to forget something that has just happened or asks the same question several times, and by intersession amnesias, in which the patient appears to forget important details of previous sessions or becomes confused about changes in session scheduling. Amnesias outside of the treatment setting are manifested in all of the direct and indirect ways that one finds during diagnostic evaluation.

The therapist should always be alert to signs of possible switching during sessions. Sudden changes in voice, speech, facial appearance, body language, mannerisms, and affects suggest the possibility of covert switching. The therapist should follow up a possible switch with questions designed to test for amnesia for the material or events prior to the possible switch. Stress usually precipitates switching, and close attention should be paid to this possibility when the therapeutic process becomes intense. The therapist should also be alert for evidence of passive-influence phenomena within or outside of the treatment setting.

The persistence of self-destructive or suicidal behavior is a sign of continued dividedness. In my experience, this is one of the most common manifestations of a failure to fuse. The therapist should work through the chronology of any self-destructive act, looking for evidence of amnesia or passive-influence phenomena. Even if evidence of amnesia is not found, the therapist should strongly suspect that the self-destructive behavior is associated with an undiscovered alter.

Intense and inappropriate affects can be signs of unsuspected alters. Depression, while ubiquitous throughout the course of treatment with most MPD patients, may be a sign of hidden alters when it comes suddenly without clear causality. Inappropriate social behaviors (e.g., swearing in public in a previously demure female patient) should also suggest the covert presence of alters. Social withdrawal may be another sign that the patient is attempting to conceal the existence of alters. The appearance of new psychosomatic symptoms, the reappearance of old somatic phenomena, or the failure of an obviously psychosomatic symptom to remit with fusion should all be taken to indicate the possible presence of hidden alters.

The existence of covert alters may be detected in the dynamics of the therapeutic process. The patient may attempt to terminate therapy after a "successful" final fusion, claiming that no further treatment is necessary and everything is fine. Unfortunately, too many therapists, for reasons of their own, are willing to collude with such patients' denial. Kluft (1985e) has found that "the most frequent causes for stalemated or unsuccessful treatment were the existence of other unsuspected personalities, the persistence of personalities believed to be fused, and/or the clinician's fears of exploring lest other alters be found or an apparent fusion upset" (p. 66). If the therapy comes to a standstill, or if there is unending chaos that prevents productive work, the therapist should look for covert alters.

Transference and countertransference phenomena can indicate the presence of covert alters. If the patient continues to manifest a "multiple" transference reaction to the therapist (e.g., continues to place the therapist in situations that recapitulate earlier abusive experiences or maintains highly compartmentalized views of the therapist), then one should infer the existence of unsuspected alters. The therapist should also carefully observe his or her own responses and reactions for the possibility that he or she is overlooking evidence of alters or is in fact unconsciously responding to covert alters. A truly successful final fusion should have a marked effect on the patient's transference reaction, and the continuation of multiple-like dynamics in the therapy is a strong indication of the existence of covert alters.

Probes to Assess Fusion Stability

Given the high rate of relapse and/or failure to fuse in the first place, it is advisable to test the patient actively for evidence of fusion/integration stability. Kluft (1985e) has developed a formal interview protocol for assessing the stability of fusions in his patients. He begins by inquiring about signs and symptoms of MPD in general, and then focusing on signs and symptoms that were specific to the patient during the course of treatment. The patient is asked to provide a chronology of his or her interim history, and is also asked about the observations and opinions of others with regard to the fusion. Kluft then attempts, nonhypnotically, to elicit every one of the patient's alters whom he has met during the course of therapy or of whom he has heard. He uses whatever nonhypnotic techniques or cues have worked best in the past for the patient. If these measures fail to demonstrate multiplicity, he then initiates hypnotic inquiry. Kluft (1985e) states that this is the most fruitful item of the protocol. He has found that, pragmatically, it is best to attempt to contact suspected alters through the use of ideomotor signaling or inner vocalization, rather than trying to get them to emerge overtly. This tactic reduces the patient's anxieties about loss of control and decreases the time necessary to survey the list of past alters. Although this procedure may be upsetting for some patients, Kluft notes that "major disruptive events" are rare.

There are other ways to probe the patient to determine the stability of an integration. A final fusion should result in the recovery of relatively complete memory for traumatic events. In patients claiming to be fused, one can attempt to take a complete history of the events associated with the early creation of alters. Nonfused patients usually have great difficulty in providing a coherent history of these events. One can also provide the patient with sequential tasks, such as those described for diagnosis in Chapter Four.

A set of intriguing preliminary observations on the differential responses of fused versus nonfused multiples to hypnotic age regression suggests that this technique may provide a useful probe into the stability of a fusion/integration (Kluft, 1986c). Kluft observed that subjective experiences and recall of historical events during hypnotically induced age regression differed in fused and nonfused patients. In unfused multiples, memories of historical events recalled during the age regression procedure were accompanied by intense affects in those alters claiming to be reliving the events. Alters who did not experience the events directly might report "witnessing" them or might be amnesic for the historical material.

In patients whom Kluft regarded as integrated (i.e., they passed his above-described protocol), no formerly separate alters could be elicited, and events previously experienced with great affective intensity were now recalled with "less force and immediacy" (Kluft, 1986c, p. 151). The "ownership" of the events also underwent transformation, with half of the patients reporting the events as personal experiences and half qualifying their recall with such statements as this: "That happened to X, but now it is as if it were something that happened to me" (p. 151). Kluft speculates "that as integration begins, a process of cognitive restructuring is set in motion that changes recall, the affective sense of past events, and the sense of self and point-of-view from which past events are experienced" (1986c, p. 153). He extends this formulation to include the possibility that this restructuring process may extend to nontreatment settings in which there is an erosion of dissociative barriers, such as forensic or diagnostic evaluations.

Types of Fusion Failures and Fusion Relapse Events

Most "fusions" probably never occurred in the first place, so that the discovery of unfused and separate alters is not actually a relapse. In other cases, there seems to be a temporary merging of alter personalities that fails to hold, and the alters reappear as separate entities. Fusions that fail to "take" or relapse within a short time are usually due to incomplete working through of traumatic material contained in one or more of the involved alters (Kluft, 1986b). In some cases, patients may deliberately undo their fusions shortly afterwards in order to use dissociative defenses in coping with current life stresses. During the period immediately following a final fusion, many patients have little in the way of nondissociative defenses to protect them from the stress and strains of life as "singles." Not surprisingly, some elect to return to the more familiar condition of being multiples.

Other causes of relapse include the reactivation of fused alters by issues raised in or outside of treatment, particularly those dealing with traumatic material. The death of an abuser is a particularly potent activator of fused alters and may lead to the re-emergence of MPD in a previously stably integrated individual years after the final fusion. Some patients may be able to suppress alters or to feign fusion for prolonged periods. The longest-running case whom I have followed experienced the overt re-emergence of alters over 3 years after he appeared to be integrated. He had, however, made significant gains during this period of relative quiescence, and these were maintained in spite of the reappearance of overt alters.

Therapeutic Interventions for Fusion Failures

As with most areas of the therapeutic process, the response of patients to a failed final fusion is complex and multifaceted. Certain personalities (e.g., the host) often evince profound disappointment, which quickly turns into despair and hopelessness that anything will ever change. Crises and suicidal behavior can be precipitated by renewed or new evidence of dividedness. Multiples may become concerned about the possibility that the therapist will reject them or will lose interest in them because they have failed to "perform" or because they have concealed evidence of separateness. Other alters may be triumphant and gloating, viewing the failure of the fusion as a sign of their power and a victory in their struggle for control of the patient and the therapy.

Multiples often view fusion and the failure thereof as a tremendous test. Unfortunately, clinicians may reinforce this attitude by an overemphasis on fusion at the exclusion of other aspects of therapeutic progress. Varieties of this test include the following: Can the therapist detect the covert dividedness and thereby reaffirm his or her sensitivity to the internal world of the patient? Can the therapist accept being misled or lied to about the fusion? Will the therapist accept the multiple when the fusion is revealed to be a fraud? What will happen to the therapist's sense of competence/grandiosity when the fusion is found to be a sham? Will the therapist become punitive when he or she discovers the deception? These and many other questions and themes may be part of the testing experienced by a multiple when a final fusion is not achieved or sustained.

Not surprisingly, given the blurring of treatment boundaries that multiples often elicit, therapists' responses often mirror those of their patients. I have repeatedly observed competent therapists plunged into feelings of despair, helplessness, and hopelessness over the failure of fusions that they were certain had "cured" patients. Anger over deception, and humiliation over "gullibility," occasionally become transformed into resentment and rejection of a patient. If this is extreme, the therapist may attempt to initiate a transfer of the multiple to another therapist because he or she feels unable to "help" the patient.

The discovery of new alters and other layering phenomena may temporarily overwhelm a therapist. Therapists must remain aware of their countertransference wishes and needs for their patients to be "cured" or to be "successes." Most therapists will probably experience the wish to be rid of MPD patients from time to time during the course of therapy, and the most expedient means would be to fuse and thus "cure" the patients. Multiples, with their extreme interpersonal sensitivity, will pick up on this message and may feign fusion to please a therapist and/or set the therapist up for a fall at a later time.

When a therapist finds that a final fusion has failed to occur or hold, it is important to share this information clearly with the patient. In a case where the multiple is deliberately feigning fusion, there will be resistance or an argument about the "facts." The therapist should share with the patient the observations supporting the therapist's assessment that the patient remains divided. Arguments with the patient should be avoided, as should responding to the patient's demands for "proof" that he or she is still multiple. This is just a variation on the old theme of difficulty in accepting the diagnosis, so prominent during the early phase of treatment.

The next steps in working with a failed fusion are really the same as before. Newly discovered alters should be individually met, and information should be gathered on their life history, function, and place in the personality system as a therapeutic alliance is nurtured. Previously known alters who came unfused or feigned fusion must be directly addressed, and any unresolved traumas must be worked through completely. Residual traumatic memories and affects that have not been adequately explored are the major causes of fusion failures. The failure of a fusion does not indicate a major setback; it just underscores the fact that the therapy must continue to uncover and work through the massive amount of trauma suffered by the patient.

Work with patients who suffer relapses after long periods of apparent fusion suggests that most of these relatively late-occurring events fall short of full-scale multiplicity and often respond rapidly to treatment

(Kluft, 1986b). Holdout alters, who remained hidden when other alters fused, are often willing to fuse after some work. In many instances, these holdouts have been waiting to see what happened to the alters who fused and have had their concerns allayed by what they have witnessed. Latent alters, who were reactivated by the fusion of others and emerged to fill the vacuum created by the fusion, are usually less energized and less invested in separateness than the alters that they replaced; consequently, they are more willing to give up their autonomy and fuse. Those alters who fused and became unfused because of unresolved issues are often eager to re-fuse. Repeatedly, I have heard alters who re-emerged after a failed fusion use the metaphor of a jigsaw puzzle to describe this experience. They describe a feeling of "fitting together" that is natural and pleasant. The process of repeated final fusions is likened to rounding off the burrs along the edges until the parts fit tightly.

Postfusion Treatment

Importance of Postfusion Treatment

There is general agreement among experienced MPD therapists that final fusion of all of the alters, although an important milestone, does not mark the end of treatment. Braun (1984c) estimates that final fusion represents the 70% mark in the course of treatment. Kluft (1984a) observes that this unification is only "one aspect" of the treatment and may even be incidental in some patients. A patient should continue in active treatment until a new sense of identity is firmly rooted and the issues and reactions evoked by fusion/integration have been worked through.

The postfusion period is critical for the consolidation of internal unity and the development of a new and more integrated sense of personal identity. It is also during this period that the patient must actively develop and utilize nondissociative coping mechanisms for handling stress and crises. During the period immediately following fusion, which usually lasts for several months or longer, the patient will generally experience a number of predictable reactions to his or her new way of being. These often dysphoric responses need to be worked through if the patient is to remain fused and functional. During the postfusion period, the therapist must remain alert for evidence of covert multiplicity and would do well to regularly perform a systematic re-evaluation of the patient, using Kluft's protocol and/or other probes for hidden alters.

Stresses during the Postfusion Period

READJUSTMENTS IN IMPORTANT RELATIONSHIPS

The patient's new status as a fused multiple requires a readjustment in his or her sense of self. Virtually nothing is known about this process beyond the observations of therapists who have worked with such patients. The ease and comfort with which the patient adjusts to his or her new mode of being is probably influenced by a number of factors. In my limited experience with fused patients, it appears to me that those patients who have undergone a number of final fusions and relapses before stabilizing in a fused state are more comfortable with their new identity as "singles" than are patients who have not had as many chances to experience this new sense of self. Although Kluft (1986b) does not believe that an adult patient's age has any effect on the patient's prognosis, I believe that age at fusion does have an effect on the patient's ability to adjust to life as a single and to substitute nondissociative defenses for coping with stress. Older patients, who have spent 20 or more years of their adult lives as multiples, appear to have a more difficult time restructuring their self-image than patients who fuse in their 20s to mid-30s.

The issues raised by a new sense of identity are usually most apparent and problematic when the patient is faced with a readjustment in important relationships. It often becomes obvious to the patient at this point, if not sooner, that many of the significant others in the patient's life would prefer him or her to remain fragmented. Patients will often face strong overt or covert pressures to "be their old selves." One of the adaptive advantages that being a multiple formerly provided for a patient was the ability to be whomever or whatever was required to please and placate significant others. Families of origin often react strongly to fusion, and attempt to disrupt and undo the treatment and return patients to their former state. Unfortunately, spouses, friends, and children may also seek to undo treatment gains in an effort to preserve the gratification that they have received from patients' multiplicity. Multiples, with their strong tendency to recapitulate old trauma in current relationships, often are involved in pathological or at least problematic relationships that exacerbate this process of readjustment.

Therapists can help patients to critically examine the overt and covert demands to be multiple made upon them by significant others. In their new and fragile state of unification, most patients continue to see themselves as completely at fault for problems in their relationships and often feel that it is they who must change to please the other persons. Therapists should help patients work through the necessary readjustments in relationships and help them to recognize when inappropriate and pathological demands are being made by others. Patients need a great deal of support and reassurance during this period, as well as another perspective from which to view the pressures and demands placed upon them.

FACING PROBLEMS PREVIOUSLY EVADED THROUGH DISSOCIATION

One of the most difficult aspects of the fusion/integration process is a patient's having to come face to face with many painful issues that previously were avoided by dissociating. As the dissociative fog lifts following fusion, and the patient views his or her past and present life as a continuous whole for the first time, it is usually readily apparent that this life is a mess. The initial euphoria that accompanies the achievement of unity rapidly gives way to a profound depression as the patient is forced to face and cope with many problems that he or she had previously been unaware of or had avoided by dissociative behaviors. Each patient has his or her individual burden to bear, but most must face a combination of accepting the reality of the past trauma/abuse and responsibility for the pain and suffering that they may have caused.

Although a multiple may have been abreacting and working through past traumas during a major portion of the therapy, the patient will still have to come to a new understanding and acceptance of this same trauma following fusion/integration. The retrospective viewing of these experiences as a continuous whole, rather than as flashes and fragments of memory, changes the patient's perspective. The effect of this new perspective can be temporarily devastating to the patient as he or she more fully comprehends the horror of just what and how much was done to him or her. While still a multiple, the patient is usually able to maintain sets of contradictory feelings toward the abuser(s) side by side. This is not as easily done in the fused state, which forces the patient to face and resolve these very different perceptions. The therapist must help the patient assimilate his or her past history as a continuous experience and memory, while integrating the new continuous sense of self that now runs through the course of events. Not uncommonly, additional traumas will be uncovered and abreacted, though these residual traumas will not be personified by alters.

The patient must also face the consequences of his or her actions. Typically, while a multiple, the patient assumed responsibility for much of the trauma that was inflicted upon him or her, over which the patient actually had little control. Paradoxically, while still a multiple, the patient often ignored responsibility for his or her own hurtful or harmful actions toward others. Following fusion, these discrepancies must be reversed. Accepting responsiblity for his or her actions is often extremely painful for the patient to face, particularly when it involves the patient's spouse and/or children. While assuming this responsibility, the patient must be consoled and supported by the therapist and helped to understand that he or she was ill and often reflexively inflicted upon others what had originally been done to him or her.

GRIEF WORK

The newly fused/integrated multiple also has much grief work to do. Patients must grieve for the past, for the loss of an idealized view of their parents/abusers, and for the loss of what they could have been and done if they had not been dissociatively fragmented. The patient must also grieve for the loss of the alters. Kluft (1983) has referred to this last process as the "loneliness after fusion." In patients who were socially withdrawn and isolated prior to fusion, alters frequently functioned to keep the patients company. As one patient put it, "I could be all by myself, but I was never alone. Now I feel alone." A therapist must facilitate mourning for the divided state. One should remember that as painful and disruptive as being a multiple may have been for the patient, it was also a life-saving solution and refuge during moments of sheer horror. The internal worlds of many multiples contain elements of fairy-tale beauty, perfection, and peace that must be surrendered with fusion. These losses should be identified and mourned also.

In my experience, another area of grief work that should be addressed is the patient's disappointment at the experience of being fused/integrated. Even in cases where the importance of fusion/integration has been actively downplayed, the patient will still have great expectations about the joys of being a unified personality. Many multiples express frustration at the inability of "singles" to empathize with their worlds, but I find that multiples have equal difficulty in understanding what it means to be a unified personality. Many multiples have very unrealistic expectations about how good it feels to be unified. Usually a patient becomes rapidly disillusioned and should be helped to experience and express that disappointment. These are realistic feelings; they are part of the letting go of dividedness and accepting the imperfections and pain of the world as "singles" know it.

Therapeutic Considerations during the Postfusion Period

As is the case with fusion/integration, the clinical literature only briefly touches on therapy during the postfusion phase. All authors agree that treatment must continue beyond a final fusion and that the patient must understand this expectation from the very beginning. Kluft (1983) mentions using reassurance and calming and/or ego-building hypnotic techniques to help the patient weather postfusion difficulties. Braun (1984c) cites a variety of hypnotic techniques as useful for postfusion work. He suggests that if patients have not already been taught autohypnotic techniques, they should develop a repertoire at this time. He believes that these are useful in relaxation, assertiveness training, and rehearsal in fantasy. Deep trance techniques, described in Chapter Nine, are widely held to be useful both before and after integration (Braun, 1984c). Brassfield (1983) stresses the need to continue work in recognizing and coping with trauma and grieving over losses as necessary to prevent relapse into a dissociative coping style.

One area in which newly fused/integrated patients seem to need a great deal of help is the recognition and identification of feelings. In the past, strong affects were important factors in the genesis of new alters, and consequently were sequestered behind dissociative barriers. Newly unified patients typically have difficulty even in simply identifying their feelings and are frightened by the intensity of some affects. A therapist should be alert to this problem and help a patient to label feelings and make connections between feelings and life events. The patient must learn how to appropriately express and respond to feelings, particularly strong affects. The ability to experience, identify, express, and appropriately respond to strong feelings in a nondissociative way is one of the most important tasks facing the patient during the postfusion period.

Mixed feeling states are hard for a newly fused patient to cope with. As a multiple, the patient handled mixed feeling states and ambivalence by switching between or among a number of alters, each of whom relatively purely personified one particular feeling or point of view. The patient usually did not have to tolerate the simultaneous experience of intense contradictory feelings. Now, as a fused multiple, the patient must experience the anxiety and inner turmoil that come with mixed feelings and ambivalence. The intensity and distress that mixed feeling states generate may at times be mistaken by patient and/or therapist for new dissociative splitting.

The socialization of a newly fused/integrated multiple is a complex and all-encompassing task that the therapist should not undertake alone. This is a good time to get the patient involved in groups that seek to address specific problems, such as assertiveness training, socialization, and parenting. The patient should also be encouraged to actively expand social networks and to renew contact with old or estranged friends. In the long run, most integrated patients that I know report that they are more functional and happier than they were as multiples.

SUMMARY

This final chapter has covered two of the most complicated areas in the treatment of MPD: crisis intervention and therapeutic resolution. Crises are all too frequent and expectable events during treatment. They occur when some event or pressure disturbs the fragile balance of the personality system or overwhelms its ability to cope. Multiples are extremely vulnerable to crises and typically have few external resources or supports to sustain them during difficult moments.

Anticipation and prevention are the strongest crisis intervention steps one can take. Plumbing the personality system for its strengths and weaknesses, forecasting the existence of hidden alters and failures of fusion, and establishing plans to deal with potential traumas all help to prevent or reduce crises. A number of crises can be anticipated in advance, including the discovery of new alters, failed fusions, and intrusions by past abusers. In addition, the therapist must be able to tolerate a high level of "background noise" and must react cautiously to the patient's provocations, threats, and struggles for control.

When crises occur, every effort should be made to identify and negotiate with the alters involved. Suicide attempts and self-destructive behaviors are the most common crises. Hospitalization may be necessary, but a range of other interventions should be considered first, including contracting, helping angry alters to ventilate, symptom substitution, strengthening of protectors, and a host of hypnotic techniques. Dissociative crises (e.g., fugues and rapid switching) are usually driven by personality system conflicts or the intrusion of overwhelming traumatic memories. System conflicts respond well to working directly with the alters involved, whereas intrusive traumas can be handled by abreaction. Crises involving acute somatic symptoms can be handled in a similar fashion. Medical and external interventions may be required, but introduce a new level of complexity and often derail treatment.

Although the current clinical impression is optimistic about treatment outcome, little is really known about the nature of therapeutic resolution in MPD. A good prognosis appears to be associated with commitment to therapy and change, a willingness to use nondissociative coping strategies, and a lack of investment in the condition and the uniqueness of the alters. Less complicated patients with fewer alters, fewer traumas, and the absence of concurrent Axis II pathology do better. Even with appropriate treatment, many MPD patients probably will not achieve an integrated sense of self, though substantial functional improvement generally occurs. When fusion occurs, it is preceded by an extensive recovery and working through of dissociated affects and memories, and heralded by a discomfort with remaining divided. Fusion ceremonies have proven useful in concretizing this psychological restructuring.

Relapses of fusions and the discovery of hidden layers of alters are to be expected. The stability of apparent fusions can be assessed by periodic systematic inquiry. Even when a final fusion is achieved, much work remains to be done. New defenses to life's stresses have to be erected, readjustments in important relationships have to be negotiated, and pathological demands to return to the divided state have to be addressed. The loss of the alters may require mourning and grief work, and newly experienced feelings of ambivalence must be identified. Despite its complexities and difficulties, the treatment of MPD can be a professionally gratifying experience that opens one's eyes as a therapist.

References

Abeles M, Schilder P (1935). Psychogenic loss of personal identity. *Archives of Neurology and Psychiatry, 34*:587–604.

Akhtar S, Brenner I (1979). Differential diagnosis of fugue-like states. *Journal of Clinical Psychiatry, 40*:381–385.

Alexander V K (1956). A case study of a multiple personality. *Journal of Abnormal and Social Psychology, 52*:272–276.

Allison R B (1974a). A new treatment approach for multiple personalities. *American Journal of Clinical Hypnosis, 17*:15–32.

Allison R B (1974b). A guide to parents: How to raise your daughter to have multiple personalities. *Family Therapy, 1*:83–88.

Allison R B (1978a). A rational psychotherapy plan for multiplicity. *Svensk Tidskrift für Hypnos, 3–4*:9–16.

Allison R B (1978b). Psychotherapy of multiple personality. Paper presented at the annual meeting of the American Psychiatric Association, Atlanta, May.

Allison, R B (1978c). On discovering multiplicity. *Svensk Tidskrift für Hypnos, 2*:4–8.

Allison R B, Schwartz T (1980). *Minds in Many Pieces*. New York, Rawson, Wade.

Ambrose G (1961). *Hypnotherapy with Children*. London, Staples Press.

American Psychiatric Association (1980a). *Diagnostic and Statistical Manual of Mental Disorders, Third Edition*. Washington, DC, APA.

American Psychiatric Association (1980b). *A Psychiatric Glossary, Fifth Edition*. Washington, DC, APA.

American Psychiatric Association (1987). *Diagnostic and Statistical Manual of Mental Disorders, Third Edition Revised*. Washington, DC, APA.

Andorfer J C (1985). Multiple personality in the human information-processor: A case history and theoretical formulation. *Journal of Clinical Psychology, 41*:309–324.

Archibald H C, Tuddenham R D (1965). Persistent stress reaction after combat: A 20 year follow-up. *Archives of General Psychiatry, 12*:475–481.

Azam E E (1887). *Hypnotisme, Double Conscience et Altération de la Personnalité* (Préface de J M Charcot). Paris, J. B. Ballière.

Barkin R, Braun B G, Kluft R P (1986). The dilemma of drug treatment for multiple personality disorder patients. In Braun B G (Ed.) *The Treatment of Multiple Personality Disorder*. Washington, DC, American Psychiatric Press.

Baum E A (1978). Imaginary companions of two children. *Journal of the American Academy of Child Psychiatry, 49*:324–330.

Beahrs J O (1982). *Unity and Multiplicity*. New York, Brunner/Mazel.

Beahrs J O (1983). Co-consciousness: A common denominator in hypnosis, multiple personality, and normalcy. *American Journal of Clinical Hypnosis, 26*:100–113.

Beal E W (1978). Use of the extended family in the treatment of multiple personality. *American Journal of Psychiatry, 135*:539–542.

Benson D F, Miller B L, Signer S F (1986). Dual personality associated with epilepsy. *Archives of Neurology, 43*:471–474.

Benson R M, Pryor D B (1973). "When friends fall out": Developmental interference with the function of some imaginary companions. *Journal of the American Psychoanalytic Association, 21*:457–473.

Berman E (1974). Multiple personality: Theoretical approaches. *Journal of the Bronx State Hospital, 2*:99–107.

Bernheim K F, Levine, R R J (1979). *Schizophrenia: Symptoms, Causes, Treatments.* New York, Norton.

Bernstein E, Putnam F W (1986). Development, reliability and validity of a dissociation scale. *Journal of Nervous and Mental Disease, 174*:727–735.

Berrington W P, Liddell D W, Foulds G A (1956). A re-evaluation of the fugue. *Journal of Mental Science, 102*:280–286.

Bettelheim B (1979). *Surviving and Other Essays.* New York, Harcourt Brace Jovanovich.

Blank A S (1985). The unconscious flashback to the war in Viet Nam veterans: Clinical mystery, legal defense, and community problem. In Sonnenberg S M, Blank A S, and Talbot J A (Eds.) *The Trauma of War.* Washington, DC, American Psychiatric Press.

Bliss E L (1980). Multiple personalities: A report of 14 cases with implications for schizophrenia and hysteria. *Archives of General Psychiatry, 37*:1388–1397.

Bliss E L (1983). Multiple personalities, related disorders, and hypnosis. *American Journal of Clinical Hypnosis, 26*:114–123.

Bliss E L (1984a). Spontaneous self-hypnosis in multiple personality disorder. *Psychiatric Clinics of North America, 7*:135–148.

Bliss E L (1984b). A symptom profile of patients with multiple personalities, including MMPI results. *Journal of Nervous and Mental Disease, 172*:197–202.

Bliss E L (1986). *Multiple Personality, Allied Disorders and Hypnosis.* New York, Oxford University Press.

Bliss E L, Bliss J (1985). *Prism: Andrea's World.* New York, Stein & Day.

Bliss E L, Jeppsen E A (1985). Prevalence of multiple personality among inpatients and outpatients. *American Journal of Psychiatry, 142*:250–251.

Bliss E L, Larson E M (1985). Sexual criminality and hypnotizability. *Journal of Nervous and Mental Disease, 173*:522–526.

Bliss E L, Larson E M, Nakashima S R (1983). Auditory hallucinations and schizophrenia. *Journal of Nervous and Mental Disease, 171*:30–33.

Bluhm H (1949). How did they survive? *American Journal of Psychotherapy, 2*:3–32.

Boor M (1982). The multiple personality epidemic: Additional cases and inferences regarding diagnosis, etiology, dynamics and treatment. *Journal of Nervous and Mental Disease, 170*:302–304.

Boor M, Coons P M (1983). A comprehensive bibliography of literature pertaining to multiple personality. *Psychological Reports, 53*:295–310.

Bowers M K, Brecher-Marer S, Newton B W, Piotrowski Z, Spyer T C, Taylor W S, Watkins J G (1971). Therapy of multiple personality. *International Journal of Clinical and Experimental Hypnosis, 19*:57–65.

Brandsma J M, Ludwig A M (1974). A case of multiple personality: Diagnosis and therapy. *International Journal of Clinical and Experimental Hypnosis, 22*:216–233.

Brassfield P A (1980). *A discriminative study of a multiple personality*. Ann Arbor, MI, University Microfilms International.

Brassfield P A (1983). Unfolding patterns of the multiple personality through hypnosis. *American Journal of Clinical Hypnosis, 26*:146–152.

Braun B G (1980). Hypnosis for multiple personalities. In Wain H (Ed.) *Clinical Hypnosis in Medicine*. Chicago, Year Book Medical.

Braun B G (1983a). Psychophysiologic phenomena in multiple personality and hypnosis. *American Journal of Clinical Hypnosis, 26*:124–137.

Braun B G (1983b). Neurophysiological changes in multiple personality due to integration: A preliminary report. *American Journal of Clinical Hypnosis 26*:84–92.

Braun B G (1984a). Foreword to symposium on multiple personality. *Psychiatric Clinics of North America, 7*:1–2.

Braun B G (1984b). Hypnosis creates multiple personality: Myth or reality? *International Journal of Clinical and Experimental Hypnosis, 32*:191–197.

Braun B G (1984c). Uses of hypnosis with multiple personalities. *Psychiatric Annals, 14*:34–40.

Braun B G (1984d). Towards a theory of multiple personality and other dissociative phenomena. *Psychiatric Clinics of North America, 7*:171–193.

Braun B G (1985). The transgenerational incidence of dissociation and multiple personality disorder: A preliminary report. In Kluft R P (Ed.) *The Childhood Antecedents of Multiple Personality*. Washington, DC, American Psychiatric Press.

Braun B G (1986). Issues in the psychotherapy of multiple personality. In Braun B G (Ed.) *The Treatment of Multiple Personality Disorder*. Washington, DC, American Psychiatric Press.

Braun B G, Braun R (1979). Clinical aspects of multiple personality. Paper presented at the annual meeting of the American Psychiatric Association, Chicago, May.

Braun B G, Sachs R G (1985). The development of multiple personality disorder: Predisposing, precipitating, and perpetuating factors. In Kluft R P (Ed.) *The Childhood Antecedents of Multiple Personality*. Washington, DC, American Psychiatric Press.

Brende J O (1984). The psychophysiologic manifestations of dissociation. *Psychiatric Clinics of North America, 7*:41–50.

Brende J O, Benedict B D (1980). The Vietnam combat delayed stress response syndrome: Hypnotherapy of "dissociative symptoms." *American Journal of Clinical Hypnosis, 23*:34–40.

Brende J O, Rinsley D B (1981). A case of multiple personality with psychological automatisms. *Journal of the American Academy of Psychoanalysis, 2*:129–151.

Brenman M, Gill M M, Knight R (1952). Spontaneous fluctuations in depth of hypnosis and their implications for ego function. *International Journal of Psycho-Analysis, 33*:22–23.

Breuer J, Freud S (1895). *Studies on hysteria*. New York, Basic Books, 1957.

Brown G W (1983). Multiple personality disorder, a perpetrator of child abuse. *Child Abuse and Neglect, 7*:123–126.

Browne A, Finkelhor D (1986). Impact of child sexual abuse: A review of the research. *Psychological Bulletin, 99*:66–77.

Burks B S (1942). A case of primary and secondary personalities showing co-operation toward mutual goals. *Psychological Bulletin, 39*:462.

Carlson E T (1981). The history of multiple personality in the United States: I. The beginnings. *American Journal of Psychiatry, 138*:666–668.

Carlson E T (1982). Jane C. Rider and her somnambulistic vision. *Histoire des Sciences Medicales, 17*:110–114.

Carlson E T (1984). The history of multiple personality in the United States: Mary Reynolds and her subsequent reputation. *Bulletin of the History of Medicine, 58*:72–82.

Carlson E B, Putnam F W (1988). Unpublished data.

Caul D (1978a). Treatment philosophies in the management of multiple personality. Paper presented at the annual meeting of the American Psychiatric Association, Atlanta, May.

Caul D (1978b). Hypnotherapy in the treatment of multiple personality. Paper presented at the annual meeting of the American Psychiatric Association, Atlanta, May.

Caul D (1983). On relating to multiple personalities. Paper presented at the annual meeting of the American Psychiatric Association, New York.

Caul D (1984). Group and videotape techniques for multiple personality disorder. *Psychiatric Annals, 14*:43–50.

Caul D (1985a). Caveat curator: Let the caretaker beware. Paper presented at the annual meeting of the American Psychiatric Association, Dallas, May.

Caul D (1985b). Group therapy and the treatment of MPD. Paper presented at the annual meeting of the American Psychiatric Association, Dallas, May.

Caul D (1985c). Inpatient management of multiple personality disorder. Paper presented at the annual meeting of the American Psychiatric Association, Dallas, May.

Caul D (1985d). Determining the prognosis in the treatment of multiple personality disorder. Paper presented at the annual meeting of the American Psychiatric Association, Dallas, May.

Cocores J, Santa W, Patel M (1984). The Ganser syndrome: Evidence suggesting its classification as a dissociative disorder. *International Journal of Psychiatry in Medicine, 14*:47–56.

Confer W N, Ables B S (1983). *Multiple Personality: Etiology, Diagnosis, and Treatment.* New York, Human Sciences Press.

Congdon M H, Hain J, Stevenson I (1961). A case of multiple personality illustrating the transition from role-playing. *Journal of Nervous and Mental Disease, 132*:497–504.

Coons P M (1980). Multiple personality: Diagnostic considerations. *Journal of Clinical Psychiatry, 41*:330–336.

Coons P M (1984). The differential diagnosis of multiple personality: A comprehensive review. *Psychiatric Clinics of North America, 7*:51–65.

Coons P M (1985). Children of parents with multiple personality disorder. In Kluft R P (Ed.) *The Childhood Antecedents of Multiple Personality.* Washington, DC, American Psychiatric Press.

Coons P M (1986). Treatment progress in 20 patients with multiple personality disorder. *Journal of Nervous and Mental Disease, 174*:715–721.

Coons P M, Bradley K (1985). Group psychotherapy with multiple personality patients. *Journal of Nervous and Mental Disease, 173*:515–521.

Coons P M, Milstein V (1984). Rape and post-traumatic stress in multiple personality. *Psychological Reports, 55*:839–845.

Coons P M, Milstein V (1986). Psychosexual disturbances in multiple personality: Characteristics, etiology and treatment. *Journal of Clinical Psychiatry, 47*:106–110.

Coons P M, Sterne A L (1986). Initial and follow-up psychological testing on a group of patients with multiple personality disorder. *Psychological Reports, 58*:43–49.

Cory C E (1919). A divided self. *Journal of Abnormal Psychology, 14*:281–291.

Crabtree A (1986). Dissociation: Explanatory concepts in the first half of the twentieth century. In Quen J M (Ed.) *Split Minds/Split Brains.* New York, New York University Press.

Culpin M (1931). *Recent Advances in the Study of the Psychoneuroses.* London, J & A Churchill.

Cutler B, Reed J (1975). Multiple personality: A single case study with a 15 year follow-up. *Psychological Medicine, 5*:18–26.

Damgaard J, Benschoten S V, Fagan J (1985). An updated bibliography of literature pertaining to multiple personality. *Psychological Reports, 57*:131–137.

Dancsino A, Daniels J, McLaughlin T J (1979). Jo-Jo, Josephine, and Jonanne: A study of multiple personality by means of the Rorschach test. *Journal of Personality Assessment, 43*:300–313.

Davidson K (1964). Episodic depersonalization: Observations on 7 patients. *British Journal of Psychiatry, 110*:505–513.

Davis P H, Osherson A (1977). The concurrent treatment of a multiple-personality woman and her son. *American Journal of Psychotherapy, 31*:504–515.

Devinsky O, Putnam F W, Grafman J, Bromfield E, Theodore W H (1988). Dissociative states and epilepsy. Unpublished manuscript.

Dickes R (1965). The defensive function of an altered state of consciousness: A hypnoid state. *Journal of the American Psychoanalytic Association, 13*:356–403.

Dixon J C (1963). Depersonalization phenomena in a sample population of college students. *British Journal of Psychiatry, 109*:371–375.

Dor-Shav K N (1978). On the long-range effects of concentration camp internment on Nazi victims: 35 years later. *Journal of Consulting and Clinical Psychology, 46*:1–11.

Ellenberger H F (1970). *The Discovery of the Unconscious: The History and Evolution of Dynamic Psychiatry.* New York, Basic Books.

Elliott D (1982). State intervention and childhood multiple personality disorder. *Journal of Psychiatry and the Law, 10*:441–456.

Emde R N, Gaensbauer T J, Harmon R J (1976). *Emotional Expression in Infancy: A Biobehavioral Study (Psychological Issues,* Monograph 37, Vol. 10). New York, International Universities Press.

Enoch M D, Trethowan W H (1979). *Uncommon Psychiatric Syndromes.* Bristol, Wright.

Erickson M H, Erickson E M (1941). Concerning the nature and character of post-hypnotic behavior. *Journal of General Psychology, 24*:95–133.

Erickson M H, Kubie L S (1939). The permanent relief of an obsessional phobia by means of communications with an unsuspected dual personality. *Psychoanalytic Quarterly, 8*:471–509.

Ewalt J R, Crawford D (1981). Posttraumatic stress syndrome. *Current Psychiatric Therapy, 20*:145–153.

Fagan J, McMahon P (1984). Incipient multiple personality in children: Four cases. *Journal of Nervous and Mental Disease, 172*:26–36.

Fenichel O (1945). *The Psychoanalytic Theory of Neurosis.* New York, Norton.

Ferenczi S (1934). Gedanken über das trauma. *International Zeitschrift für Psychoanalyse, 20*:5–12.

Fischer K W, Pipp S L (1984). Development of the structures of unconscious thought. In Bowers K, Meichenbaum D (Eds.) *The Unconscious Reconsidered.* New York, Wiley.

Fisher C (1945). Amnesic states in war neuroses: The psychogenesis of fugues. *Psychoanalytic Quarterly, 14*:437–468.

Fisher C (1947). The psychogenesis of fugue states. *American Journal of Psychotherapy, 1*:211–220.

Fisher S (1973). *Body Consciousness.* London, Calder & Boyars.

Fliess R (1953). The hypnotic evasion: A clinical observation. *Psychoanalytic Quarterly*, 22:497–511.

Frankel F H (1976). *Hypnosis: Trance as a Coping Mechanism.* New York, Plenum.

Frankel F H (1979). Scales measuring hypnotic responsivity: A clinical perspective. *American Journal of Clinical Hypnosis*, 21:208–218.

Frankel F H, Orne M T (1976). Hypnotizability and phobic behavior. *Archives of General Psychiatry*, 37:1036–1040.

Frankenthal K (1969). Autohypnosis and other aids for survival in situations of extreme stress. *International Journal of Clinical and Experimental Hypnosis*, 17:153–159.

Frankl V E (1962). *Man's Search for Meaning: An Introduction to Logotherapy.* Boston, Beacon.

Freud S (1941). A disturbance of memory on the Acropolis. *International Journal of Psycho-Analysis*, 22:93–101.

Freud S, Breuer J (1893). On the psychical mechanism of hysterical phenomena. In *Collected Papers, Vol. 1.* London, International Psychoanalytic Press, 1924.

Fullerton D T, Harvy R F, Klein M H, Howell T (1981). Psychiatric disorders in patients with spinal cord injuries. *Archives of General Psychiatry*, 38:1369–1371.

Gardner G G (1974). Hypnosis with children and adolescents. *International Journal of Clinical and Experimental Hypnosis*, 22:20–38.

Gardner G G (1977). Hypnosis with infants and preschool children. *American Journal of Clinical Hypnosis*, 19:158–162.

Gardner G G, Olness K (1981). *Hypnosis and Hypnotherapy with Children.* New York, Grune & Stratton.

Geleerd E R (1956). Clinical contribution to the problem of the early mother–child relationship. *Psychoanalytic Study of the Child*, 11:336–351.

Geleerd E R, Hacker F J, Rapaport D (1945). Contribution to the study of amnesia and allied conditions. *Psychoanalytic Quarterly*, 14:199–220.

Goddard H H (1926). A case of dual personality. *Journal of Abnormal and Social Psychology*, 21:170–191.

Greaves G B (1980). Multiple personality: 165 years after Mary Reynolds. *Journal of Nervous and Mental Disease*, 168:577–596.

Green C (1968). *Out-of-the-Body Experiences.* London, Hamish Hamilton.

Green R, Money J (1969). *Transsexualism and Sex Reassignment.* Baltimore, Johns Hopkins University Press.

Greyson B (1985). A typology of near-death experiences. *American Journal of Psychiatry*, 142:967–969.

Grinker R R, Spiegel J P (1943). *War Neuroses in North Africa.* New York, Josiah Macy, Jr., Foundation.

Gruenewald D (1977). Multiple personality and splitting phenomena: A reconceptualization. *Journal of Nervous and Mental Disease*, 164:385–393.

Hale E (1983). Inside the divided mind. *New York Times Magazine*, April 17, pp. 100–106.

Halifax J (1982). *Shaman: The Wounded Healer.* New York, Crossroad.

Hall R C, LeCann A F, Schoolar J C (1978). Amobarbital treatment of multiple personality. *Journal of Nervous and Mental Disease*, 166:666–670.

Harner M (1982). *The Way of the Shaman.* New York, Bantam.

Harper M (1969). Deja vu and depersonalization in normal subjects. *Australian and New Zealand Journal of Psychiatry*, 3:67–74.

Harriman P L (1937). Some imaginary companions of older subjects. *American Journal of Orthopsychiatry*, 7:368–370.

Harriman P L (1942a). The experimental production of some phenomena related to the multiple personality. *Journal of Abnormal and Social Psychology, 37*:244–255.

Harriman P L (1942b). The experimental induction of a multiple personality. *Psychiatry, 5*:179–186.

Harriman P L (1943). A new approach to multiple personalities. *American Journal of Orthopsychiatry, 13*:638–643.

Hart B (1926). The concept of dissociation. *British Journal of Medical Psychology, 10*:241–263.

Hart H (1954). ESP projection: Spontaneous cases and the experimental method. *Journal of the American Society for Psychical Research, 48*:121–141.

Hart W L, Ebaugh F, Morgan D C (1945). The amytal interview. *American Journal of Medical Sciences, 210*:125–131.

Henderson J L, Moore M (1944). The psychoneuroses of war. *New England Journal of Medicine, 230*:273–279.

Herman J (1986). Recovery and verification of memories of childhood sexual trauma. Paper presented at the annual meeting of the American Psychiatric Association, Washington, DC, May.

Herold C M (1941). Critical analysis of the elements of psychic functions: Part I. *Psychoanalytic Quarterly, 10*:513–544.

Herzog A (1984). On multiple personality: Comments on diagnosis and therapy. *International Journal of Clinical and Experimental Hypnosis, 22*:216–233.

Hilgard E R (1965). *Hypnotic Susceptibility*. New York, Harcourt Brace Jovanovich.

Hilgard E R (1973). A neodissociation interpretation of pain reduction in hypnosis. *Psychological Review, 80*:396–411.

Hilgard E R (1977). *Divided Consciousness: Multiple Controls in Human Thought and Action*. New York, Wiley.

Hilgard E R (1984). The hidden observer and multiple personality. *International Journal of Clinical and Experimental Hypnosis, 32*:248–253.

Horevitz R P (1983). Hypnosis for multiple personality disorder: A framework for beginning. *American Journal of Clinical Hypnosis, 26*:138–145.

Horevitz R P, Braun B G (1984). Are multiple personalities borderline? *Psychiatric Clinics of North America, 7*:69–88.

Horowitz M J (1985). Disasters and psychological responses to stress. *Psychiatric Annals, 15*:161–167.

Horsley J S (1943). *Narcoanalysis*. New York, Oxford Medical Publications.

Horton P, Miller D (1972). The etiology of multiple personality. *Comprehensive Psychiatry, 13*:151–159.

Hurlock E B, Burstein W (1932). The imaginary playmate. *Journal of General Psychology, 41*:380–392.

Irwin H J (1980). Out of the body down under: Some cognitive characteristics of Australian students reporting OOBEs. *Journal of the Society for Psychical Research, 50*:448–459.

Jacobson E (1977). Depersonalization. *Journal of the American Psychoanalytic Association, 7*:581–609.

Jahoda G (1969). *The Psychology of Superstition*. London, Hogarth Press.

Janet P (1889). *L'Automatisme Psychologique*. Paris, Alcan.

Janet P (1890). *The Major Symptoms of Hysteria*. New York, Macmillan.

Jeans R F (1976). The three faces of Evelyn: A case report. I. An independently validated case of multiple personalities. *Journal of Abnormal Psychology, 85*:249–255.

John R, Hollander B, Perry C (1983). Hypnotizability and phobic behavior: Further supporting data. *Journal of Abnormal Psychology*, 92:390–392.

Kales A, Kales J D (1974). Sleep disorders: Recent findings in the diagnosis and treatment of disturbed sleep. *New England Journal of Medicine*, 290:487–499.

Kales A, Paulson M, Jacobson A, Kales J D (1966a). Somnambulism: Psychophysiological correlates. II. Psychiatric interviews, psychological testing, and discussion. *Archives of General Psychiatry*, 14:595–604.

Kales A, Paulson M, Jacobson A, Kales J D, Walter R D (1966b). Somnambulism: Psychophysiological correlates. I. All-night EEG studies. *Archives of General Psychiatry*, 14:586–594.

Kales A, Soldatos C R, Caldwell A B, Kales J D, Humphery F J, Charney D S, Schweitzer P K (1980). Somnambulism. *Archives of General Psychiatry*, 37:1406–1410.

Kampman R (1974). Hypnotically induced multiple personality: An experimental study. *Psychiatria Fennica*, 10:201–209.

Kampman R (1975). The dynamic relation of the secondary personality induced by hypnosis to the present personality. *Psychiatria Fennica*, 11:169–172.

Kampman R (1976). Hypnotically induced multiple personality: An experimental study. *International Journal of Clinical and Experimental Hypnosis*, 24:215–227.

Kanzer M (1939). Amnesia: A statistical study. *American Journal of Psychiatry*, 96:711–716.

Kempe C H, Silverman F N, Steele B F, Droegemueller W, Silver H K (1962). The battered-child syndrome. *Journal of the American Medical Association*, 181:17–24.

Kempf E F (1915). Some studies in the psychopathology of acute dissociation of the personality. *Psychoanalytic Review*, 2:361–389.

Kennedy A, Neville J (1957). Sudden loss of memory. *British Medical Journal*, vii:428–433.

Kenny M G (1981). Multiple personality and spirit possession. *Psychiatry*, 44:337–358.

Kenny M G (1984). "Miss Beauchamp's" true identity. *American Journal of Psychiatry*, 141:920

Kirshner L A (1973). Dissociative reactions: An historical review and clinical study. *Acta Psychiatrica Scandinavica*, 49:698–711.

Kiraly S J (1975). Folie a deux. *Canadian Psychiatric Association Journal*, 20:223–227.

Kline M V (1976). Emotional flooding: A technique in sensory hypnoanalysis. In Olsen P (Ed.) *Emotional Flooding.* New York, Human Sciences Press.

Kline N, Angst J (1979). *Psychiatric Syndromes and Drug Treatment.* New York, Jason Aronson.

Kluft R P (1982). Varieties of hypnotic interventions in the treatment of multiple personality. *American Journal of Clinical Hypnosis*, 24:230–240.

Kluft R P (1983). Hypnotherapeutic crisis intervention in multiple personality. *American Journal of Clinical Hypnosis*, 26:73–83.

Kluft R P (1984a). Treatment of multiple personality disorder: A study of 33 cases. *Psychiatric Clinics of North America*, 7:9–29.

Kluft R P (1984b). Multiple personality disorder in childhood. *Psychiatric Clinics of North America*, 7:135–148.

Kluft R P (1984c). An introduction to multiple personality disorder. *Psychiatric Annals*, 14:19–24.

Kluft R P (1984d). Aspects of the treatment of multiple personality disorder. *Psychiatric Annals*, 14:51–55.

Kluft R P (1985a). The natural history of multiple personality disorder. In Kluft R P (Ed.) *The Childhood Antecedents of Multiple Personality.* Washington, DC, American Psychiatric Press.

Kluft R P (1985b). Childhood multiple personality disorder: Predictors, clinical findings, and treatment results. In Kluft R P (Ed.), *The Childhood Antecedents of Multiple Personality*. Washington, DC, American Psychiatric Press.

Kluft R P (1985c). On malingering and MPD: Myths and realities. Paper presented at Multiple Personality Disorder and the Legal System, a workshop given at the annual meeting of the American Psychiatric Association, Dallas, May.

Kluft R P (1985d). The treatment of multiple personality disorder (MPD): Current concepts. In Flach F F (Ed.) *Directions in Psychiatry*. New York, Hatherleigh.

Kluft R P (1985e). Using hypnotic inquiry protocols to monitor treatment progress and stability in multiple personality disorder. *American Journal of Clinical Hypnosis, 28*:63–75.

Kluft R P (1986a). The simulation and dissimulation of multiple personality disorder by defendants. Paper presented at the annual scientific meeting of the American Society of Clinical Hypnosis, Seattle, March 20.

Kluft R P (1986b). Personality unification in multiple personality disorder (MPD). In Braun B G (Ed.) *The Treatment of Multiple Personality Disorder*. Washington, DC, American Psychiatric Press.

Kluft R P (1986c). Preliminary observations on age regression in multiple personality disorder patients before and after integration. *American Journal of Clinical Hypnosis, 28*.147–156.

Kluft R P (1987). First-rank symptoms as a diagnostic clue to multiple personality disorder. *American Journal of Psychiatry, 144*:293–298.

Kluft R P, Braun B G, Sachs R (1984). Multiple personality, intrafamilial abuse and family psychiatry. *International Journal of Family Psychiatry, 5*:283–301.

Kolb L C (1985). The place of narcosynthesis in the treatment of chronic and delayed stress reactions of war. In Sonnenberg S M, Blank A S, Talbott J A (Eds.) *The Trauma of War*. Washington, DC, American Psychiatric Press.

Krystal H (1969). *Massive Psychic Trauma*. New York, International Universities Press.

Langs R J (1974a). *The Technique of Psychoanalytic Psychotherapy, Vol. 1*. New York, Jason Aronson.

Langs R J (1974b). *The Technique of Psychoanalytic Psychotherapy, Vol. 2*. New York, Jason Aronson.

Larmore K, Ludwig A M, Cain R L (1977). Multiple personality—An objective case study. *British Journal of Psychiatry, 131*:35–40.

Leavitt H C (1947). A case of hypnotically produced secondary and tertiary personalities. *Psychoanalytic Review, 34*:274–295.

Levenson J, Berry S L (1983). Family intervention in a case of multiple personality. *Journal of Marital and Family Therapy, 9*:73–80.

Levitan H (1980). The dream in traumatic states. In Natterson J M (Ed.) *The Dream in Clinical Practice*. New York, Jason Aronson.

Lief H I, Dingman J F, Bishop M P (1962). Psychoendocrinologic studies in a male with cyclic changes in sexuality. *Psychosomatic Medicine, 24*:357–368.

Lindy J B (1985). The trauma membrane and other clinical concepts derived from psychotherapeutic work with survivors of natural disasters. *Psychiatric Annals, 15*:153–160.

Lipton S D (1943). Dissociated personality: A case report. *Psychiatric Quarterly, 17*:33–56.

Lister E D (1982). Forced silence: A neglected dimension of trauma. *American Journal of Psychiatry, 139*:872–876.

Loewald H W (1955). Hypnoid state, repression, abreaction and recollection. *Journal of the American Psychoanalytic Association, 3*:201–210.

Loewenstein R J, Hamilton J, Alagna S, Reid N, Devries M (1987). Experiential sampling in the study of multiple personality disorder. *American Journal of Psychiatry*, *144*:19–21.

Loewenstein R J, Putnam F W, Duffy C, Escobar J, Gerner R (1986). Males with multiple personality disorder. Paper presented at the 3rd annual meeting of the International Society for the Study of Multiple Personality and Dissociative States, Chicago, September.

London P (1965). Developmental experiments in hypnosis. *Journal of Projective Techniques and Personality Assessment*, *29*:189–199.

London P, Cooper L M (1969). Norms of hypnotic susceptibility in children. *Developmental Psychology*, *1*:113–124.

Lovinger S L (1983). Multiple personality: A theoretical view. *Psychotherapy: Theory, Research, and Practice*, *20*:425–434.

Lovitt R, Lefkof G (1985). Understanding multiple personality with the comprehensive Rorschach system. *Journal of Personality Assessment*, *49*:289–294.

Ludlow C, Putnam F W (1988). Unpublished data.

Ludwig A M (1966). Altered states of consciousness. *Archives of General Psychiatry*, *15*:225–234.

Ludwig A M (1983). The psychobiological functions of dissociation. *American Journal of Clinical Hypnosis*, *26*:93–99.

Ludwig A M, Brandsma J M, Wilbur C B, Bendfeldt F, Jameson H (1972). The objective study of a multiple personality. *Archives of General Psychiatry*, *26*:298–310.

Luparello T J (1970). Features of fugue: A unified hypothesis of regression. *Journal of the American Psychoanalytic Association*, *18*:379–398.

Maoz B, Pincus C (1979). The therapeutic dialogue in narco-analytic treatments. *Psychotherapy: Theory, Research, and Practice*, *16*:91–97.

Marcos L R, Trujillo M (1978). The sodium amytal interview as a therapeutic modality. *Current Psychiatric Therapies*, *18*:129–136.

Marmer S S (1980a). The dream in dissociative states. In Natterson J M (Ed.) *The Dream in Clinical Practice*. New York, Jason Aronson.

Marmer S S (1980b). Psychoanalysis of multiple personality. *International Journal of Psycho-Analysis*, *61*:439–459.

Mason R O (1893). Duplex personality. *Journal of Nervous and Mental Disease*, *18*:593–598.

Mason R O (1895). Duplex personality: Its relation to hypnotism and to lucidity. *Journal of Nervous and Mental Disease*, *22*:420–423.

Mayeux R, Alexander M, Benson F, Brandt J, Rosen J (1979). Poriomania. *Neurology*, *29*:1616–1619.

Mayo T (1845). Case of double consciousness. *Medical Gazette* (London, New Series), *1*:1202–1203.

McKellar P (1977). Autonomy, imagery, and dissociation. *Journal of Mental Imagery*, *1*:93–108.

Messerschmidt R (1927–1928). A quantitative investigation of the alleged independent operation of conscious and subconscious processes. *Journal of Abnormal and Social Psychology*, *22*:325–340.

Mesulam M M (1981). Dissociative states with abnormal temporal lobe EEG: Multiple personality and the illusion of possession. *Archives of Neurology*, *38*:178–181.

Miller R D (1984). The possible use of auto-hypnosis as a resistance during hypnotherapy. *International Journal of Clinical and Experimental Hypnosis*, *32*:236–247.

Mischel W, Mischel F (1958). Psychological aspects of spirit possession. *American Anthropologist*, *60*:249–260.

Mitchell, S W (1888). Mary Reynolds: A case of double consciousness. *Transactions of the College of Physicians of Philadelphia, 10*:366–389.

Money J (1974). Two names, two wardrobes, two personalities. *Journal of Homosexuality, 1*:65–78.

Money J, Primrose C (1968). Sexual dimorphism and dissociation in the psychology of male transsexuals. *Journal of Nervous and Mental Disease, 147*:472–486.

Morselli G E (1930). Sulla dissoziazione mentale. *Rivista Sperimentale di Freniatria, 54*:209 322.

Morton J H, Thoma E (1964). A case of multiple personality. *American Journal of Clinical Hypnosis, 6*:216–225.

Murphy G (1947). *Personality: A Biosocial Approach to Origins and Structure.* New York, Harper & Row.

Myers D, Grant G (1970). A study of depersonalization in students. *British Journal of Psychiatry, 121*:59–65.

Myers F W H (1886). Multiplex personality. *Proceedings of the Society for Psychical Research, 4*:496–514.

Myers W A (1976). Imaginary companions, fantasy twins, mirror dreams and depersonalization. *Psychoanalytic Quarterly, 45*:503–524.

Nagera H (1969). The imaginary companion: Its significance for ego development and conflict solution. *Psychoanalytic Study of the Child, 24*:165–196.

Nemiah J C (1981). Dissociative disorders. In Freeman A M, Kaplan H I (Eds.) *Comprehensive Textbook of Psychiatry, Third Edition.* Baltimore, Williams & Wilkins.

Nissen M J, Ross J L, Willingham D B, MacKenzie T B, Schacter D L (1988). Memory and awareness in a patient with multiple personality disorder. *Brain and Cognition, 8*: 117–134.

Noyes R, Hoenk P R, Kupperman B A (1977). Depersonalization in accident victims and psychiatric patients. *Journal of Nervous and Mental Disease, 164*:401–407.

Noyes R, Kletti R (1977). Depersonalization in response to life-threatening danger. *Psychiatry, 18*:375–384.

Noyes R, Slymen D J (1978–1979). The subjective response to life-threatening danger. *Omega, 9*:313–321.

O'Brien P (1985). The diagnosis of multiple personality syndromes: Overt, covert, and latent. *Comprehensive Therapy, 11*:59–66.

Oesterreich T K (1966). *Possession: Demoniacal and Other among Primitive Races in Antiquity, the Middle Ages, and Modern Times.* New York, New York University Press.

Orne M T (1977). The construct of hypnosis: Implications of the definition for research and practice. *Annals of the New York Academy of Sciences, 296*:14–33.

Palmer J, Dennis M (1975). *A Community Mail Survey of Psychic Experiences in Research in Parapsychology.* Metuchen, NJ, Scarecrow Press.

Palmer J, Lieberman R (1975). The influence of psychological set on ESP and out-of-body experiences. *Journal of the American Society for Psychical Research, 69*:193–213.

Palmer J, Vassar C (1974). ESP and out-of-body experiences: An exploratory study. *Journal of the American Society for Psychical Research, 68*:257–280.

Pattison E M, Wintrob R M (1981). Possession and exorcism in contemporary America. *Journal of Operational Psychiatry, 12*:13–20.

Peck M W (1922). A case of multiple personality: Hysteria or dementia praecox. *Journal of Abnormal and Social Psychology, 17*:274–291.

Perry J C, Jacobs D (1982). Overview: Clinical applications of the amytal interview in psychiatric emergency settings. *American Journal of Psychiatry, 139*:552–559.

Pettinati H M, Horne R L, Staats J M (1985). Hypnotizability in patients with anorexia nervosa and bulimia. *Archives of General Psychiatry*, *42*:1014–1016.

Piotrowski Z A (1977). The movement responses. In Rickers-Ovsiankina M (Ed.) *Rorschach Psychology*. Huntington, NY, Robert E. Krieger.

Place M (1984). Hypnosis and the child. *Journal of Child Psychology and Psychiatry*, *25*:339–347.

Prechtl H F R, O'Brien M J (1982). Behavioral states of the full term newborn: Emergence of a concept. In Stratton P (Ed.) *Psychobiology of the Human Newborn*. New York, Wiley.

Prechtl H F R, Theorell K, Blair A W (1973). Behavioral state cycles in abnormal infants. *Developmental Medicine and Child Neurology*, *15*:606–615.

Prince M (1890). Some of the revelations of hypnotism. In Hale N G (Ed.) *Morton Prince: Psychotherapy and Multiple Personality, Selected Essays*. Cambridge, MA, Harvard University Press, 1975.

Prince M (1906). *Dissociation of a Personality*. New York, Longman, Green.

Prince M (1909a). Experiments to determine co-conscious (subconscious) ideation. *Journal of Abnormal Psychology*, *3*:33–42.

Prince M (1909b). The psychological principles and field of psychotherapy. In Hale N G (Ed.) *Morton Prince: Psychotherapy and Multiple Personality, Selected Essays*. Cambridge, MA, Harvard University Press, 1975.

Prince M (1929). *Clinical and Experimental Studies in Personality*. Cambridge, MA, Sci-Art.

Prince M, Peterson F (1908). Experiments in psycho-galvanic reactions from co-conscious (subconscious) ideas in a case of multiple personality. *Journal of Abnormal Psychology*, *3*:114–131.

Prince W F (1917). The Doris case of quintuple personality. *Journal of Abnormal Psychology*, *11*:73–122.

Putnam F W (1984a). The psychophysiological investigation of multiple personality disorder: A review. *Psychiatric Clinics of North America*, *7*:31–41.

Putnam F W (1984b). The study of multiple personality disorder: General strategies and practical considerations. *Psychiatric Annals*, *14*:58–62.

Putnam F W (1985a). Dissociation as a response to extreme trauma. In Kluft R P (Ed.) *The Childhood Antecedents of Multiple Personality*. Washington, DC, American Psychiatric Press.

Putnam F W (1985b). Multiple personality. *Medical Aspects of Human Sexuality*, *19*:59–74.

Putnam F W (1985c). Pieces of the mind: Recognizing the psychological effects of abuse. *Justice for Children*, *1*:6–7.

Putnam F W (1986a). The scientific investigation of multiple personality disorder. In Quen J M (Ed.) *Split Minds/Split Brains*. New York, New York University Press.

Putnam F W (1986b). The treatment of multiple personality: State of the art. In Braun B G (Ed.) *The Treatment of Multiple Personality Disorder*. Washington, DC, American Psychiatric Press.

Putnam F W (1988a). The disturbance of "self" in victims of childhood sexual abuse. In Kluft R P (Ed.) *Incest-Related Syndromes of Adult Psychopathology*. Washington, DC, American Psychiatric Press.

Putnam F W (1988b). Unpublished data.

Putnam F W (1988c). The switch process in multiple personality disorder and other state-change disorders. *Dissociation*, *1*:24–32

Putnam F W, Guroff J J, Silberman E K, Barban L, Post R M (1986). The clinical phenomenology of multiple personality disorder: A review of 100 recent cases. *Journal of Clinical Psychiatry*, *47*:285–293.

Putnam F W, Loewenstein R J, Silberman E K, Post R M (1984). Multiple personality in a hospital setting. *Journal of Clinical Psychiatry, 45*:172 175.

Putnam F W, Post R M (1988). Multiple personality disorder: An analysis and review of the syndrome. Unpublished manuscript.

Quimby L C, Andrei A, Putnam F W (1986). De-institutionalization of chronic MPD patients. Paper presented at the 3rd annual meeting of the International Society for the Study of Multiple Personality and Dissociative States, Chicago, September.

Rapaport D (1942). *Emotions and Memory* (Menninger Clinic Monograph Series No. 2). Baltimore, Williams & Wilkins.

Rapaport D (1971). *Emotions and Memory.* New York, International Universities Press.

Ravenscroft K (1965). Voodoo possession: A natural experiment in hypnosis. *International Journal of Clinical and Experimental Hypnosis, 13*:157–182.

Redlich F C, Ravitz L J, Dession G H (1951). Narcoanalysis and truth. *American Journal of Psychiatry, 107*:586–593.

Rendon M (1977). The dissociation of dissociation. *International Journal of Social Psychiatry, 23*:240–243.

Ribot T (1910). *The Diseases of Personality.* Chicago, Kegan Paul, Trench, Trubner.

Riggall R M (1931). A case of multiple personality. *Lancet, ii*:846–848.

Roberts W (1960). Normal and abnormal depersonalization. *Journal of Mental Science, 106*:478–493.

Rosen H, Myers H J (1947). Abreaction in the military setting. *Archives of Neurology and Psychiatry, 57*:161–172.

Rosenbaum M (1980). The role of the term schizophrenia in the decline of multiple personality. *Archives of General Psychiatry, 37*:1383–1385.

Rosenbaum M, Weaver G M (1980). Dissociated state: Status of a case after 38 years. *Journal of Nervous and Mental Disease, 168*:597–603.

Ross, C A (1984). Diagnosis of a multiple personality during hypnosis: A case report. *International Journal of Clinical and Experimental Hypnosis, 32*:222–235.

Rubenstein R, Newman R (1954). The living out of "future experiences" under hypnosis. *Science, 119*:472–473.

Russell D (1986). The incest legacy. *The Sciences, 26*:28–32.

Sabom M B (1982). *Recollections of Death: A Medical Investigation.* New York, Harper & Row.

Sachs R G, Braun B G (1985). The evolution of an outpatient multiple personality disorder group: A seven year study. Paper presented at the 2nd annual meeting of the International Society for the Study of Multiple Personality and Dissociative States, Chicago, October.

Sachs R G, Braun B G (1986). The role of social support systems in the treatment of multiple personality disorder. In Braun B G (Ed.) *The Treatment of Multiple Personality Disorder.* Washington, DC, American Psychiatric Press.

Salley R D (1988). Subpersonalities with dreaming functions in a patient with multiple personalities. *Journal of Nervous and Mental Disease, 176*:112–115.

Saltman V, Solomon R (1982). Incest and multiple personality. *Psychological Reports, 50*:1127–1141.

Sargant W, Slater E (1941). Amnesic syndromes in war. *Proceedings of the Royal Society of Medicine, 34*:757–764.

Schapiro S A (1975–1976). A classification for out-of-body phenomena. *Journal of Altered States of Consciousness, 2*:259–265.

Schenk L, Bear D (1981). Multiple personality and related dissociative phenomena in patients with temporal lobe epilepsy. *American Journal of Psychiatry, 138*:1311–1315.

Schreiber F R (1974). *Sybil.* New York, Warner Paperbacks.

Sedman G (1966). Depersonalization in a group of normal subjects. *British Journal of Psychiatry, 112*:907–912.

Seeman M V (1980). Name and identity. *Canadian Journal of Psychiatry, 25*:129–137.

Shelley W B (1981). Dermatitis artefacta induced in a patient by one of her multiple personalities. *British Journal of Dermatology, 105*:587–589.

Shiels D (1978). A cross cultural study of beliefs in out of the body experiences. *Journal of the American Society for Psychical Research, 49*:697–741.

Shorvon H J (1946). The depersonalization syndrome. *Proceedings of the Royal Society of Medicine, 39*:779–792.

Shorvon H J, Sargant W (1947). Excitatory abreaction: With special reference to its mechanism and the use of ether. *Journal of Mental Science, 43*:709–732.

Silber A (1979). Childhood seduction, parental pathology and hysterical symptomatology: The genesis of an altered state of consciousness. *International Journal of Psycho-Analysis, 60*:109–116.

Silberman E K, Putnam F W, Weingartner H, Braun B G, Post R M (1985). Dissociative states in multiple personality disorder: A quantitative study. *Psychiatry Research, 15*:253–260.

Simpson M M, Carlson E T (1968). The strange sleep of Rachel Baker. *Academy Bookman, 21*:3–13.

Slater E, Roth M (1974). *Clinical Psychiatry, Third Edition.* Baltimore, Williams & Wilkins.

Smith J R (1985). Rap groups and group therapy for Viet Nam veterans. In Sonnenberg S M, Blank A S, Talbott J A (Eds.) *The Trauma of War.* Washington, DC, American Psychiatric Press.

Solomon R (1983). The use of the MMPI with multiple personality patients. *Psychological Reports, 53*:1004–1006.

Solomon R, Solomon V (1982). Differential diagnosis of multiple personality. *Psychological Reports 51*:1187–1194.

Solomon R, Solomon V (1984). Unusual case: The sexuality of a multiple personality. *Human Sexuality, 18*:235.

Sonnenberg S M, Blank A S, Talbott J A (Eds.) (1985). *The Trauma of War.* Washington, DC, American Psychiatric Press.

Spanos N P, Ansari F, Henderikus J S (1979). Hypnotic age regression and eidetic imagery: A failure to replicate. *Journal of Abnormal Psychology, 88*:88–91.

Spanos N P, Weekes J R, Bertrand L D (1985). Multiple personality: A social psychological perspective. *Journal of Abnormal Psychology, 94*:362–376.

Spiegel D (1984). Multiple personality as a post-traumatic stress disorder. *Psychiatric Clinics of North America, 7*:101–110.

Spiegel H (1963). The dissociation–association continuum. *Journal of Nervous and Mental Disease, 136*:374–378.

Spiegel H (1981). Hypnosis: Myth and reality. *Psychiatric Annals, 11*:16–23.

Spiegel H, Spiegel D (1978). *Trance and Treatment.* New York, Basic Books.

Stamm J L (1969). The problems of depersonalization in Freud's "Disturbance of memory on the Acropolis." *American Imago, 26*:356–372.

Stengel E (1941). On the aetiology of fugue states. *Journal of Mental Science, 87*:572–599.

Stengel E (1943). Further studies on pathological wandering (fugues with the impulse to wander). *Journal of Mental Science, 89*:224–241.

Stern C R (1984). The etiology of multiple personalities. *Psychiatric Clinics of North America, 7*:149–160.

Stevenson I, Pasricha S (1979). A case of secondary personality with xenoglossy. *American Journal of Psychiatry, 136*:1591–1592.

Stone C W (1916). Dual personality. *The Ohio State Medical Journal, 12*:672–673.

Sutcliffe J P, Jones J (1962). Personal identity, multiple personality, and hypnosis. *International Journal of Clinical and Experimental Hypnosis, 10*:231–269.

Taylor E (1982). *William James on Exceptional Mental States: The 1896 Lowell Lectures.* New York, Scribner's.

Taylor W S, Martin M F (1944). Multiple personality. *Journal of Abnormal and Social Psychology, 39*:281–300.

Thames L (1984). Limit setting and behavioral contracting with the client with multiple personality disorder. Paper presented at the 1st International Meeting on Multiple Personality and Dissociative Disorders, Chicago, September.

Thigpen C H, Cleckley H (1954). A case of multiple personality. *Journal of Abnormal and Social Psychology, 49*:135–151.

Thigpen C H, Cleckley H (1957). *The Three Faces of Eve.* New York, McGraw-Hill.

Torrie A (1944). Psychosomatic casualties in the Middle East. *Lancet, 29*:139–143.

Tuchman B W (1978). *A Distant Mirror: The Calamitous 14th Century.* New York, Knopf.

Twemlow S W, Gabbard G O, Jones F C (1985). The out-of-body experience: A phenomenological typology based on questionnaire responses. *American Journal of Psychiatry, 139*:450–455.

Varma V K, Bouri M, Wig N N (1981). Multiple personality in India: Comparisons with hysterical possession state. *American Journal of Psychotherapy, 35*:113–120.

Victor G (1975). Grand hysteria or folie a deux? *American Journal of Psychiatry, 132*:202.

Vonnegut K (1970). *Slaughterhouse Five.* London, Panther Books.

Wagner E E (1978). A theoretical explanation of the dissociative reaction and a confirmatory case presentation. *Journal of Personality Assessment, 42*:312–316.

Wagner E E, Allison R B, Wagner C F (1983). Diagnosing multiple personalities with the Rorschach: A confirmation. *Journal of Personality Assessment, 47*:143–149.

Wagner E E, Heise M (1974). A comparison of Rorschach records of three multiple personalities. *Journal of Personality Assessment, 38*:308–331.

Walker J I (1982). Chemotherapy of traumatic war stress. *Military Medicine, 147*:1029–1033.

Watkins J G (1971). The affect bridge: A hypnoanalytic technique. *International Journal of Clinical and Experimental Hypnosis, 19*:21–27.

Weitzenhoffer A M (1980). Hypnotic susceptibility revisited. *American Journal of Clinical Hypnosis, 22*:130–146.

Weitzman E L, Shamoain C A, Golosow N (1970). Identity diffusion and the transsexual resolution. *Journal of Nervous and Mental Disease, 151*:295–302.

West L J (1967). Dissociative reaction. In Freeman A M, Kaplan H I (Eds.) *Comprehensive Textbook of Psychiatry.* Baltimore, Williams & Wilkins.

White R W, Shevach B J (1942). Hypnosis and the concept of dissociation. *Journal of Abnormal and Social Psychology, 37*:309–328.

Wholey C C (1926). Moving picture demonstration of transition states in a case of multiple personality. *Psychoanalytic Review, 13*:344–345.

Wilbur C B (1982). Psychodynamic approaches to multiple personality. Paper presented at Multiple Personality: Diagnosis and Treatment, a workshop given at the annual meeting of the American Psychiatric Association, Toronto, May.

Wilbur C B (1984a). Multiple personality and child abuse. *Psychiatric Clinics of North America, 7*:3–7.

Wilbur C B (1984b). Treatment of multiple personality. *Psychiatric Annals, 14*:27–31.

Wilbur C B (1985). The effect of child abuse on the psyche. In Kluft R P (Ed.) *The Childhood Antecedents of Multiple Personality*. Washington, DC, American Psychiatric Press.

Williams D T (1981). Hypnosis as a psychotherapeutic adjunct with children and adolescents. *Psychiatric Annals, 11*:47–54.

Wilson S C, Barber T X (1982). The fantasy-prone personality: Implications for understanding imagery, hypnosis and parapsychology. In Sheikh A A (Ed.) *Imagery: Current Theory, Research and Application*. New York, Wiley.

Wise T N, Reading A J (1975). A woman with dermatitis and dissociative periods. *International Journal of Psychiatry in Medicine, 6*:551–559.

Wittkower E D (1970). Transcultural psychiatry in the Caribbean: Past, present and future. *American Journal of Psychiatry, 127*:162–166.

Wolff P H (1987). *The Development of Behavioral States and the Expression of Emotions in Early Infancy*. Chicago, University of Chicago Press.

Yap PM (1960). The possession syndrome: A comparison of Hong Kong and French findings. *Journal of Mental Science, 106*:114–137.

Young W C (1986). Restraints in the treatment of a patient with multiple personality. *American Journal of Psychotherapy, 50*:601–606.

Zamansky H S, Bartis S P (1984). Hypnosis as dissociation: Methodological considerations and preliminary findings. *American Journal of Clinical Hypnosis, 26*:246–251.

Zolik E S (1958). An experimental investigation of psychodynamic implications of the hypnotic "previous existence" fantasy. *Journal of Clinical Psychology, 14*:179–183.

Index